Computer Synthesized Speech Technologies: Tools for Aiding Impairment

John Mullennix
University of Pittsburgh at Johnstown, USA

Steven Stern
University of Pittsburgh at Johnstown, USA

Medical Information Science REFERENCE

MEDICAL INFORMATION SCIENCE REFERENCE
Hershey · New York

Director of Editorial Content:	Kristin Klinger
Director of Book Publications:	Julia Mosemann
Acquisitions Editor:	Lindsay Johnston
Development Editor:	Christine Bufton
Publishing Assistant:	Kurt Smith
Typesetter:	Jamie Snavely, Sean Woznicki
Production Editor:	Jamie Snavely
Cover Design:	Lisa Tosheff
Printed at:	Yurchak Printing Inc.

Published in the United States of America by
Medical Information Science Reference (an imprint of IGI Global)
701 E. Chocolate Avenue
Hershey PA 17033
Tel: 717-533-8845
Fax: 717-533-8661
E-mail: cust@igi-global.com
Web site: http://www.igi-global.com/reference

Library of Congress Cataloging-in-Publication Data

Computer synthesized speech technologies : tools for aiding impairment / John Mullennix and Steven Stern, editors.
p. ; cm.
Includes bibliographical references and index.
Summary: "This book provides practitioners and researchers with information that will allow them to better assist the speech disabled who wish to utilize computer synthesized speech (CSS) technology"--Provided by publisher.
ISBN 978-1-61520-725-1 (h/c)
1. Voice output communication aids. I. Mullennix, John W. II. Stern, Steven, 1966-
[DNLM: 1. Speech Disorders--rehabilitation. 2. Communication Aids for Disabled. 3. Self-Help Devices. WL 340.2 C7385 2010]
HV1569.5.C676 2010
681'.761--dc22

2009035180

British Cataloguing in Publication Data
A Cataloguing in Publication record for this book is available from the British Library.

Table of Contents

Detailed Table of Contents

The authors present a brief overview of the current research topics and future directions of research in the area encompassing CSS as used in augmentative and alternative communication for people with speech impairments. Issues that are especially important for practitioners who work with people with speech impairments are also discussed. This overview presents an integrated vision of research where practitioners need to be appraised of the latest research and technological developments and where researchers need to solicit feedback from practitioners in order to pursue fruitful future directions for research.

The development of computer synthesized speech technology over time is delineated. Beginning with early synthesis machines from the 18th century, the progression of individual and industrial advancements over time is briefly discussed. The chapter proceeds to examine modern (and more recent) developments from the business and industry sector involved in creating assistive and educational technologies using CSS. The chapter concludes with a discussion on CSS developments related to the fields of neuroprosthetics, robotics, composition and the arts, as well as how CSS has become a part of popular culture as captured through the medium of film.

The focus of this chapter is on developing personalized CSS voices for speech impaired persons suffering from dysarthria, an articulatory disorder affecting movement of speech articulators and control of respiration. The chapter discusses various reasons for development of natural sounding synthesized voices, especially the facilitation of social interaction with others. A brief review of current voice personalization techniques is followed by a detailed description of a Hidden Markov Modeling (HMM) based synthesis system designed to create an acceptable synthesized voice for a dysarthric individual. A study evaluating the system is described and the results summarized in terms of the efficacy of the authors' system.

An innovative approach to using artificially generated speech via hypothetical visual humanoid displays is described. The concept revolves around using signals originating at some point in the speech production system of the speech impaired individual. A brief overview of the speech production process and the recording of speech signals are provided. Methods of mapping of input signals to speech representations are discussed, with the emphasis on a priori knowledge to facilitate the process. Specific applications including communication enhancement, aids for the speech impaired and language training are discussed.

The research literature on use of CSS with children is reviewed. The factors that influence the intelligibility of CSS for children are examined, including context, speech rate, age, the listener's native language, experience with CSS and background noise. Comprehension of CSS by children is also discussed. The chapter concludes with an overview of children's preferences and attitudes toward CSS and the special considerations that should be factored in to providing a means of spoken output for children who possess communicative disabilities.

Section 5
Case Studies

Preface

As social scientists often define it, technology refers to devices and processes that extend our natural capabilities. Microscopes make it possible to see smaller things and telescopes enable us to see things that are further away. Cars extend the amount of space that we are able to travel far beyond where our feet can take us during a given period of time.

To us, this definition is most applicable and particularly pragmatic when we consider people whose natural capabilities are limited by a disability. There is nothing particularly new about using technologies to make up for individual shortcomings. Eyeglasses have been around since the thirteenth century. Carved earlike extensions that served as early hearing aids have been around since at least the sixteenth century.

With the advent of electronics and computers, as well as advancements in engineering, medicine and related fields, there has been tremendous, if not miraculous progress in the application of technology toward assisting people with disabilities. This book focuses on just one technology as applied toward one specific disability; that is, the use of computer synthesized speech (CSS) to help speech impaired people communicate using voice.

CSS is used commonly for a variety of applications, such as talking computer terminals, training devices, warning and alarm systems and information databases. Most importantly, CSS is a valuable assistive technology for people with speech impairment and visual impairments. Other technologies such as the internet are made more accessible to people with disabilities through the use of CSS.

When a person loses their voice, or is speech impaired, they are encumbered by a tremendously inconvenient disability coupled with a powerful stigma. The inability to speak is often accompanied by decreased feelings of self-worth and increased incidence of depression, feelings of isolation, and social withdrawal. The use of CSS or other assistive technologies is only one of many adaptations that a person with a serious speech impairment can make, particularly if the underlying cause (e.g., stroke, thoracic cancer) creates other difficulties for the person outside of speech problems.

OVERALL MISSION/OBJECTIVE OF THE BOOK

Our mission is to provide practitioners and future practitioners with information that will allow them to better assist the speech disabled who wish to utilize CSS technology.

In this book, an international panel of experts across numerous disciplines cover a variety of areas pertinent to understanding the many concerns in the implementation of CSS for practitioners working with speech disabled populations. This book serves to ground this work in current theory and research while at the same time existing as an approachable book used in the classroom or used as a reference book from one's bookshelf. Each chapter is geared toward providing information that practitioners should know, or even better, *can use*.

Throughout the book, there are a number of terms referring to various speech technologies, many of which are overlapping. Although we favor the acronym CSS to refer to computer synthesized speech, our contributors may use terms such as Speech Generating Device (SGDs), Voice Output Communication Aids (VOCAs), or may refer to more general Augmentative and Alternative Communication (AAC) aids. There are several ways in which CSS can be generated. One technique is synthesis by rule, which refers to synthetic speech that is generated via linguistic rules that are represented in a computer program. Another technique involves what is called concatenated speech, which is synthetic speech comprised of pre-recorded human phonemes (bits of speech) strung together. Both techniques can be embedded into what are called Text-to-Speech (TTS) systems, where the user inputs text through a keyboard and then an output device creates the audible speech. CSS systems should be distinguished from digitized human speech samples, where prerecorded messages are used in such applications as voice banking and telephone voice menus. In terms of assistive speaking aids, CSS is the "gold standard" because of its flexibility and its ability to be tailored to many different situations.

In preparing this book, we had five objectives. In overview:

- To provide an overview of CSS technology and its history.
- To present recent developments in CSS and novel applications of this evolving technology.
- To examine how CSS is used as a speaking aid for people with various speech impairments and how CSS is used in these cases as a speaking prosthesis.
- To better understand how social perceptions of CSS users are affected by attitudes toward CSS users, including prejudice and stereotyping.
- To provide case study examples of the issues that practitioners and users face when adopting CSS technology as a speaking aid.

Section 1: CSS Technology and History

CSS systems have evolved much over time. The history of these developments is covered in the book along with an explanation of the various types of techniques used in generating CSS in typical systems used today.

Section 2: Emerging Technologies

The successful implementation of a CSS system is affected by the quality of the synthetic voices used. Some CSS systems are more intelligible, natural sounding, and comprehensible than others. In addition, there is evidence that listening to synthetic speech puts a greater strain on the listener in terms of their paying attention to the speech. We devoted a portion of this book to an examination of cutting-edge approaches to CSS systems that will result in improved, more user-friendly CSS. Higher-quality CSS output will help to minimize the cognitive requirements incurred by attending to synthetic speech and will facilitate comprehension of CSS output.

Section 3: Specific Applications

There are numerous concerns regarding the use of CSS technology for people with speech disabilities. Many concerns are rooted in the physical realities of the presenting disorder. Disorders that progress slowly permit the patient more time to learn the technology than disorders that have a sudden onset. Some disorders also leave the patient more able to use their hands than others. Several chapters are written by experts on the application of CSS with children, people with intellectual disabilities and people with articulatory disorders for which CSS may offer new avenues of treatment.

Section 4: Social Factors

Those who work with CSS users can benefit from an understanding of how the combination of disability and technology affects social interactions between CSS users and other people. Two chapters discuss how attitudes toward CSS users (including stereotyping, prejudice, and discrimination) can affect how people react to CSS speech output from users with speech impairments.

Section 5: Case Studies

Finally, we felt that the practical value of this book would be enhanced by including case studies of people with speech impairments who are adopting CSS technology as a speaking aid. Two chapters were contributed by practitioners working directly with clients with significant speech impairments who were learning how to use CSS as an assistive speaking aid. In these chapters, the day to day issues and obstacles encountered by both the clients and the practitioners are highlighted.

OVERVIEW OF INDIVIDUAL CHAPTERS

To introduce the major themes of the book, John W. Mullennix and Steven E. Stern, in *Overview: Important Issues for Researchers and Practitioners Using Computer Synthesized Speech as an Assistive Aid*, present a brief overview of the current research topics and future directions of research in the area encompassing CSS as used in augmentative and alternative communication for people with speech impairments. Issues that are especially important for practitioners who work with people with speech impairments are also discussed. This overview presents an integrated vision of research where practitioners need to be appraised of the latest research and technological developments and where researchers need to solicit feedback from practitioners in order to pursue fruitful future directions for research.

The first section of this book is comprised of two chapters that provide the reader with an overview of the past and present of the technology behind computer synthesized speech. In Debbie Rowe's chapter, *From Wood to Bits to Silicon Chips: A History of Developments in Computer Synthesized Speech*, the development of computer synthesized speech technology over time is delineated. Beginning with early synthesis machines from the 18th century, the progression of individual and industrial advancements over time is briefly discussed. The chapter proceeds to examine modern (and more recent) developments from the business and industry sector involved in creating assistive and educational technologies using CSS. The chapter concludes with a discussion on CSS developments related to the fields of neuroprosthetics, robotics, composition and the arts, as well as how CSS has become a part of popular culture as captured through the medium of film.

In H.S. Venkatagiri's chapter, *Digital Speech Technology: An Overview*, the current status of digital speech technology is reviewed. Digital speech is divided into the categories of digitized human speech and synthesized speech. A detailed review of the technological details of how speech is digitized speech is presented. Then, a detailed look at manner in which speech is synthesized is covered, with various implementations in terms of algorithms discussed. The chapter concludes with an extended discussion of the considerations that must be taken into account when deciding whether digitized speech or synthesized speech is the best choice for a person in need of an augmented expressive communication capability.

The second section moves past the current state of CSS and examines emerging technologies. Four chapters examine some of the most recent advancements in the technology and application of CSS.

In D. Jeffery Higginbotham's chapter, he provides a look at where CSS has been and where it is going, with a description of how CSS is currently used in Signal Generating Devices (SGDs) and how speech intelligibility, sentence and discourse comprehension, social interaction, and emotion and identity factors into the use of SGDs by people with speech impairments. Of importance is the use of SGDs in social interaction, with recent developments oriented towards facilitating social interaction discussed. As well, the importance of having personalized and emotive voices is considered as part of what the future holds in order to development more functional SDGs for users who make use of these devices.

In H. Timothy Bunnell and Chris Pennington's chapter, *Advances in Computer Speech Synthesis and Implications for Assistive Technology*, a cutting-edge concatenation-based speech synthesis system, the ModelTalker TSS system, is described. The pros and cons of rule-based speech synthesis versus concatenation-based speech synthesis are briefly discussed followed by a description of a new approach to building personalized voices for users of SGDs. Issues of intelligibility and naturalness are considered as well as the technical constraints and numerous user issues that must be considered with such a system. The ultimate goal of this work is to allow users of this technology the ability to use fully natural sounding and expressive speech to communicate with others. The work the researchers discuss in this chapter represent a significant step forward in terms of developing user-friendly computer-based speech for people with speech impairments.

Sarah Creer, Phil Green, Stuart Cunningham, and Junichi Yamagishi's chapter, *Building Personalized Synthetic Voices for Individuals with Dysarthria Using the HTS Toolkit* focuses on developing personalized CSS voices for people suffering from dysarthria, an articulatory disorder affecting movement of speech articulators and control of respiration. The chapter discusses various reasons for development of natural sounding synthesized voices, especially the facilitation of social interaction with others. A brief review of current voice pesonalization techniques is followed by a detailed description of a Hidden Markov Modeling (HMM) based synthesis system designed to create an acceptable synthesized voice for a dysarthric individual. A study evaluating the system is described and the results summarized in terms of the efficacy of the authors' system.

Gérard Bailly, Pierre Badin, Denis Beautemps, and Frédéric Elisei's *Speech Technologies for Augmented Communication* describes an innovative approach to using artificially generated speech via hypothetical visual humanoid displays. The concept revolves around using signals originating at some point in the speech production system of the speech impaired individual. A brief overview of the speech production process and the recording of speech signals are provided. Methods of mapping of input signals to speech representations are discussed, with the emphasis on a priori knowledge to facilitate the process. Specific applications including communication enhancement, aids for the speech impaired and language training are discussed.

The third section of this book describes specific applications of CSS on different populations with specific disabilities. In particular, five chapters examine the use of CSS with children, individuals with

Broca's and global aphasias, adults with intellectual disabilities and the perception of CSS when used by people with intellectual and communicative disabilities.

Kathryn D.R. Drager and Joe Reichle, in *CSS and Children: Research Results and Future Directions*, review the research literature on use of CSS with children. The factors that influence the intelligibility of CSS for children are examined, including context, speech rate, age, the listener's native language, experience with CSS and background noise. Comprehension of CSS by children is also discussed. The chapter concludes with an overview of children's preferences and attitudes toward CSS and the special considerations that should be factored in to providing a means of spoken output for children who possess communicative disabilities.

Rajinder Koul, Diana Petroi, and Ralf Schlosser, in *Systematic Review of Speech Generating Devices for Aphasia* describe the results of a large meta-analysis of studies from 1980 to 2007 evaluating the effects of augmentative and alternative communication (AAC) intervention using speech generating devices (SGDs) on several quantitative outcome measures in individuals with severe Broca's and global aphasia. The data extracted from the studies included participant characteristics, treatment characteristics, treatment integrity design, and outcomes. Each study was assessed for methodological quality. The results are valuable for interpreting the efficacy of SGDs on aphasic populations and are important in terms of future applications with aphasic individuals.

Dean Sutherland, Jeff Sigafoos, Ralf W. Schlosser, Mark F. O'Reilly, and Giulio E. Lancioni, in *Are Speech-Generating Devices Viable AAC Options for Adults with Intellectual Disabilities?* describe the use of speech generating devices (SGDs) with the intellectually disabled. The chapter begins with a full description and definition of intellectual disability. Various issues resulting in a reluctance to use SGDs as interventions with the intellectually disabled are considered. A large scale systematic empirical review of intervention studies that involve teaching the use of SGDs to the intellectually disabled is described. The results of the review provide valuable evidence-based information to guide clinicians who work with this particular population in terms of the suitability for using SGDs as an intervention.

Rajinder Koul and James Dembowski in *Synthetic Speech Perception in Individuals with Intellectual and Communicative Disabilities* review the research on perception of CSS by individuals with intellectual, language and hearing impairments. Perception by the intellectually impaired (ranging from mild to severe) is examined in terms of perception of single words, sentences, discourse and how practice with CSS affects listening performance. Perception of CSS by those with hearing impairment and specific language impairment is also covered. The chapter concludes with a discussion on the role of CSS in the acquisition and learning of graphic symbols by individuals with little to no functional speech capability.

Oscar Saz, Eduardo Lleida, Victoria Rodriguez, W.-Ricardo Rodriguez, and Carlos Vaquero, in *The Use of Synthetic Speech in Language Teaching Tools: Review and a Case Study,* discuss the use of CSS in the development of speech therapy tools for the improvement of communication abilities in handicapped individuals is discussed. CSS is required for providing alternative communication to users with different impairments and for reinforcing the correct oral pronunciation of words and sentences. Different techniques can be used, such as pre-recorded audio, embedded Text-to-Speech (TTS) devices, talking faces, etc. These possibilities are reviewed and the implications of their use with handicapped individuals are discussed, including the experience of the authors in the development of tools for Spanish speech therapy. Finally, a preliminary experience in the use of computer-based tools for the teaching of Spanish to young children shows how removing the synthetic speech feature in the language teaching tool produces increased difficulty for the students.

The fourth section of this book contains two chapters that focus on social psychological approaches to understanding how users of CSS are evaluated by others.

John W. Mullennix and Steven E. Stern, in *Attitudes toward Computer Synthesized Speech* examine attitudes toward users of CSS technology as an assistive aid are examined. The research literature on attitudes toward the speech disabled and users of augmented and alternative communication are briefly reviewed and then discussed within the larger context of people's reactions to speaking computers. Research on attitudes towards CSS and persuasion of CSS is examined as a function of people's prejudicial attitudes toward the disabled. The chapter concludes with a discussion about the social factors that affect listeners' perception of CSS speech that go beyond simple intelligibility of CSS.

Steven E. Stern, John W. Mullennix's, Ashley Davis Fortier and Elizabeth Steinhauser*'s Stereotypes Of People With Physical Disabilities and Speech Impairments as Detected by Partially Structured Attitude Measures* focuses on stereotypes that people hold toward people with speech impairment and physical disabilities. The literature on stereotypes of people with physical disabilities is examined. Two empirical studies are described that examine six specific stereotypes. Their research provides evidence that people with physical disabilities and speech impairments are stereotyped as being asexual, unappealing, dependent, entitled, isolated, and unemployable.

The book concludes with two chapters on specific case studies that focus on practical issues encountered in the process of implementing CSS.

In Martine Smith, Janice Murray, Stephen von Tetzchner, and Pearl Langan's chapter, *A Tale of Transitions: The Challenges of Integrating Speech Synthesis in Aided Communication*, aided language development in persons with communicative disability is addressed. Aided language development refers to the fact that persons using technology aids to communicate must adapt to many changes in the technology over time. The focus of this chapter is on the issues that occur when a switch is made from a manual communication board to an electronic device. The chapter begins with a brief review of simple and complex aided communication and aided communication competence. Then, the complexity of the issues encountered during transition from one technology to another are aptly illustrated through two detailed case studies of aided communicators. Overall, the chapter provides excellent insight into the practical problems that occur in this situation and the factors that affect the adoption of high tech devices using voice output.

In Jeff Chaffee's *Tossed in the Deep End... Now What?! ...*, the author provides some useful strategies for the practitioner in order to help minimize the shock and stigma of adding device users to a caseload in a school, medical, or rehabilitation setting. To this end, the author provides a number of strategic rules for adapting the device to the therapy setting and a number of strategic rules for improving carryover into activities of daily living, the classroom, and other settings with caregivers and loved ones. To illustrate each of these strategies, a detailed and in-depth case of Corey, an adult AAC device user, is presented. His case illustrates many of the difficulties that are encountered during the adoption of an SGD for a client and highlights the need for clinicians and support staff to work together towards the common goal of improving communication through the use of CSS.

WHO WILL THIS BOOK BENEFIT?

This book is oriented towards educators, students, and practitioners in the areas of Psychology, Communication Disorders, Speech Pathology, Computer Science, Rehabilitation Sciences, Social Work,

Gerontology, Nursing, Special Education, and any other discipline where the use of CSS is applicable. The book's primary emphasis is on providing information based on scholarly and clinical work that will assist both clinical practitioners and future practitioners in making informed decisions about applications of synthetic speech with the speech disabled. Additionally, as the book is based on scholarly research with an applied perspective, researchers across multiple disciplines will find inspiration for future research ideas. Although the book is focused on CSS and speech disorders, scholars and practitioners in the more encompassing areas of human factors, human-computer interaction, disability legislation, and product development may find that the issues addressed are applicable to other forms of computer mediated communication as well.

We also hope that this book will be adopted as a primary or supplemental text for courses at the graduate and undergraduate level. These courses potentially span a number of different disciplines including but not limited to Communication Disorders and Sciences, Rehabilitation Sciences, Health-Related Fields, and Social and Behavioral Sciences. We also expect that the book will be useful to individual faculty, researchers and scholars as a reference and research source.

CONCLUSION

When a person with a speech impairment has an opportunity to use CSS as an assistive technology, they are gaining a measure of control that would have been unheard of half a century ago. In today's day and age, practitioners must be familiar with the latest advances in speech technology in order to properly serve their clients. However, just as important is the practitioner's understanding of how specific client needs affect the use of CSS, how cognitive factors related to comprehension of CSS affect its use, and how social factors related to perceptions of the CSS user affect interactions with other people. Armed with this information, we can hope for improved outcomes in the future for people using CSS as a speaking aid.

Acknowledgment

This volume is the result of a scholarly collaboration that has borne much fruit, beginning in the Fall of 1996. Both of us had been hired by the University of Pittsburgh's Johnstown Campus during the previous spring. One of us, John Mullennix, was a cognitive psychologist who specialized in psycholinguistics. The other, Steven Stern, was a social psychologist who had been examining how technological change led to changes in social interaction. Although we had much in common in many ways, neither of us guessed that we had any common ground for research endeavors.

Midway through our first semester, however, during a lunch, we discussed some of the research we had conducted earlier in our careers. John had been involved in research on perception and comprehension of synthetic speech with Dr. David Pisoni during a postdoctoral fellowship position at Indiana University. This work was purely cognitive, if not perceptual, in nature. As a student of the impacts of technological change, Steve wondered, out loud, if there had been any work on social psychological reactions to computerized voice. To our surprise, very little research in this area had been performed. Soon enough, we were conducting a series of studies of persuasiveness of computer synthesized speech, eventually examining how perceptions of disability played a role in how people felt about users of synthetic speech.

Over the years, our interest in the use of computer synthesized speech intensified and expanded. The work first focused on simple differences in attitudes toward natural and synthetic speech. Eventually, we found that the listener's knowledge about the disability status of a synthetic speech user was important, as well as the purpose that a spoken passage was being used for. This work has led us to incorporate scholarly findings in the area of prejudice and stereotyping into our research program. As we look at our research today, we realize that one never knows which direction research findings will take you.

Both of us would like to acknowledge the following people who were instrumental in our research over the years. A multitude of undergraduate researchers have worked with us on issues related to computer synthesized speech. These include Stephen Wilson, Corrie-Lynn Dyson, Benjamin Grounds, Robert Kalas, Ashley Davis Fortier, Elizabeth Steinhauser, Donald Horvath, Lynn Winters and Ilya Yaroslavsky. Without their enthusiastic assistance, diligent efforts, and their insights and intellectual curiosity, we would not have been able to be as productive in our research program.

We are also grateful for the constant support from both our campus in Johnstown and the University of Pittsburgh. We have received numerous research grants from the University of Pittsburgh Central Research and Development Fund and the University of Pittsburgh at Johnstown Faculty Scholarship Program to support our work. We were also both awarded sabbaticals by the University of Pittsburgh during the last decade which enhanced our ability to focus on research. We are also grateful for the collegial support that we have received over the years from our colleagues in the Psychology Department.

We would also like to extend our thanks to the Hiram G. Andrews Center in Johnstown, PA. Meeting with us on several occasions, the professionals at this center for vocational rehabilitation helped us to better understand disability in a real-life context and provided access to equipment and materials that we otherwise may not have been able to obtain.

John would like to thank all his colleagues who have provided support and advice over the years of his career, with special thanks to Dr. Richard Moreland, Dr. James Sawusch and Dr. David Pisoni for allowing me to grow and progress as a young "grasshopper" in the field. Steven would like to extend special thanks to his colleagues at the Catholic University of Louvain in Louvain la Neuve, Belgium, Particularly Olivier Corneille, Jacques-Philippe Leyens, Muriel Dumont, and Vincent Yzerbyt. And with all his heart, Steven is thankful to his wife Bea, and his daughters, Abby and Helen, for being the most supportive family anyone could ever ask for.

John Mullennix
Steven Stern
Editors

Chapter 1
Overview:
Important Issues for Researchers and Practitioners Using Computer Synthesized Speech as an Assistive Aid

John W. Mullennix
University of Pittsburgh at Johnstown, USA

Steven E. Stern
University of Pittsburgh at Johnstown, USA

ABSTRACT

A brief overview of the current research topics and future directions of research in the area encompassing CSS as used in augmentative and alternative communication for people with speech impairments. Issues that are especially important for practitioners who work with people with speech impairments are mentioned. This overview presents an integrated vision of research where practitioners need to be apprised of the latest research and technological developments and where researchers need to solicit feedback from practitioners in order to pursue fruitful future directions for research.

INTRODUCTION

Stephen Hawking is the most famous theoretical physicist of our generation. He is best known for books such as *A Brief History of Time*, *The Universe in a Nutshell*, and *On the Shoulders of Giants*, as well as hundreds of publications on topics related to theoretical cosmology, quantum gravity, and black holes. It is common knowledge that Dr. Hawking has suffered for over 40 years from amyotrophic lateral sclerosis (ALS), a disease of the nerve cells in the brain and spinal cord that control voluntary muscle movement. As a result of this disorder, Dr. Hawking lost the ability to speak many years ago. As he describes it:

The tracheotomy operation removed my ability to speak altogether. For a time, the only way I could communicate was to spell out words letter by letter, by raising my eyebrows when someone pointed to the right letter on a spelling card. It is pretty difficult to carry on a conversation like that, let alone write a scientific paper. (Hawking, 2009)

Eventually, Dr. Hawking was put into contact with developers working on early versions of speech

DOI: 10.4018/978-1-61520-725-1.ch001

synthesizers for use by people with speech impairments. Dr. Hawking describes the apparatus he adopted for use:

... David Mason, of Cambridge Adaptive Communication, fitted a small portable computer and a speech synthesizer to my wheel chair. This system allowed me to communicate much better than I could before. I can manage up to 15 words a minute. I can either speak what I have written, or save it to disk. I can then print it out, or call it back and speak it sentence by sentence. Using this system, I have written a book, and dozens of scientific papers. I have also given many scientific and popular talks. They have all been well received. I think that is in a large part due to the quality of the speech synthesizer... (Hawking, 2009)

Dr. Hawking started out using a system controlled with a hand switch that allowed him to choose words by moving a cursor through menus on a computer. Later modifications involved infrared beam switches that respond to head and eye movements. For many years, Dr. Hawking was satisfied with the "voice" provided by his Speech Plus™ synthesizer. However, a few years ago Dr. Hawking had a change of heart and decided to upgrade his speech synthesizer to one marketed by Neospeech™ that outputs a more realistic and natural sounding voice (www.neospeech.com/NewsDetail.aspx?id=50).

The story of Stephen Hawking is a heartwarming and uplifting story for many reasons, one of which, of course, is the triumph of human will and spirit over difficult circumstances. For those of us who research and develop speaking aids or who work with clients using speaking aids, however, his story offers great encouragement because it illustrates how a severe speech impairment can be dealt with through computer technology. Dr. Hawking has faced the same obstacles and issues that numerous persons with speech impairments have encountered when they have decided to adopt a computer-based speaking aid. Dr. Hawking has firsthand knowledge of some of the limitations of this technology and he has participated in the same decision processes that many people with speech impairments go through when they decide whether to update their speaking device or not. So in many respects, his story stands as a good example illustrating some of the major issues surrounding the use of computer-based speaking aids.

Stephen Hawking is not alone. There are many people around the world who suffer from disorders that result in various degrees of speech impairment. Some disorders are present from birth, such as cerebral palsy or disorders tied to intellectual disability, such as fetal alcohol syndrome or Down's syndrome. There are neurological disorders that do not show themselves until later in adulthood that have a severe impact on speech, such as ALS or Parkinson's disease. There are articulatory disorders like dysarthria where speech is impeded by poor or absent control of speech articulation. And there are other situations where speech loss is acquired through a sudden and unexpected event such as stroke or accidents involving traumatic brain injury (TBI). When considering the circumstances surrounding a speech impairment, each of these situations comes with its own special set of circumstances and its own set of unique challenges that must be dealt with. Researchers such as those in the present volume who work on computer synthesized speech (CSS) systems or those who investigate the use of CSS in alternative and augmentative communication (AAC) systems realize only too well that "one size does not fit all." This is one of the major themes addressed in the present volume by researchers who are concerned with how CSS is used in different populations with different speaking needs.

THE TECHNOLOGY

There exists a cornucopia of acronyms related to technologies designed to help people communicate and speak. The most general term is AAC, which is defined by the American Speech and Hearing

Association as "All forms of communication (other than oral speech) that are used to express thoughts, needs, wants, and ideas." (ASHA, 2009). In the research and clinical literature on speaking aids, experts refer to SGDs (speech generating devices), VOCAs (voice output communication aids), CSS (computer synthesized speech) and TTS (text to speech). SGDs and VOCAs refer to the actual user device, while CSS refers to speech synthesized on computer (usually software driven). TTS is a particular type of system where typed text is converted by the system to spoken voice output. In the present volume, the focus is on CSS. The development of speaking devices over time, including CSS systems, has been reviewed by others (e.g., Rowe, present volume), hence we will not discuss that history here. However, we wish to emphasize that changes in CSS technology are occurring rapidly and as a result are influencing the manner in which we think about using CSS as a speaking aid.

THE ISSUES

The common thread running through the research discussed in this volume is how CSS is useful when embedded into AAC devices for people with speech impairment. For researchers and clinical practitioners who work with clients, it is important to keep abreast of the latest developments in CSS technology and the research on use of CSS. Researchers need to know what new developments are in the works in order to make informed decisions about the appropriate research avenues to follow. Clinicians need to know what technology is currently available and what is on the horizon in order to ensure the appropriate choice of device for the user, in terms of current and future use. There is no question that there is a symbiotic relationship between research and practice. Without feedback (e.g., research data) from users of CSS technology and the practitioners who implement the technology, researchers would have a difficult time assessing what works and what does not work in terms of practical applications of CSS. And without knowing the latest research literature on CSS systems and their use, clinicians are lacking important information that they need to decide how to provide their clients with the best possible advice and care.

Intelligibility and Naturalness

Over the years, the intelligibility of CSS and the degree to which the CSS voices sound "natural" have proved to be stumbling blocks in terms of CSS usability. Good intelligibility is a basic aspect of a good CSS system. If listeners cannot understand the sounds produced by a CSS device, then all other aspects of the system are rendered moot. Over the years, much research has examined the intelligibility of synthesized speech produced by different systems (Greene, Logan, & Pisoni, 1986; Logan & Pisoni, 1989; Mirenda & Beukelman, 1987, 1990; Venkatagiri, 2003, 2004). Comprehension of synthesized utterances and the cognitive load involved in listening to CSS have been studied also (Duffy & Pisoni, 1992; Luce, Feustel, & Pisoni, 1983; Ralston, Pisoni, & Mullennix, 1995). Generally speaking, the higher the quality of CSS, the more intelligible it is and the easier it is for the listener's cognitive system to process it.

In recent work on CSS systems, newer speech synthesis techniques such as concatenation and Hidden Markov Modeling (HMM) (see Bunnell & Pennington, Creer et al., Venkatagiri, this volume) have allowed significant strides to be made in improving both intelligibility and naturalness. This bodes well in terms of making CSS users and the people around them more comfortable with speech output from these devices. Moreover, recent developments in personalization of CSS, including greater choices of voices and the ability to develop a tailor-made voice for a user, hold great promise for encouraging people with speech impairments to adopt this technology. The personalization of voice is an issue that is frequently overlooked, yet may be as important to the CSS user as intelligibility is. As an example, the famous movie critic and Chicago Sun-Times columnist Roger Ebert discusses his attempts to find a suitable synthesized voice after losing his own voice through surgery related to a bout with cancer:

One day I was fooling around with the built-in Speech program on my Mac, and started playing with some of the voices. One of the beauties of Speech for Mac is that it will speak anything on the screen--e-mail, file names, web pages, anything. That was a godsend. Most of the voices, however, left a lot to be desired. Their voice named Fred sounded too much like someone doing a bad Paul Lynde imitation. (Ebert, 2009)

Ebert goes on to talk about trying out a couple different CSS voices he found on the internet, with each voice being an improvement, yet he reports still not being completely satisfied:

But on those occasions I've appeared in public or on TV with a computer voice, I nevertheless sound like Robby the Robot. Eloquence and intonation are impossible. I dream of hearing a voice something like my own. (Ebert, 2009)

Recently, Ebert finds a new company on the web and cites their advertisement:

CereProc offers a range of voices in many accents. We can create amazing new voices quickly due to our innovative voice creation system. Many of our voices are built exclusively for specific customers and applications. (Ebert, 2009)

Finally, Ebert concludes, "That's me!" (Ebert, 2009). Ebert's trials and tribulations illustrate how important it can be to find the appropriate CSS voice, especially when the CSS user may work in an environment where speaking is especially critical to their vocation. This issue is addressed in the present volume by a number of authors (Bunnell & Pennington; Creer et al.; Higginbotham), indicating the relative importance now placed on tailoring CSS voices to the user.

Different Needs for Different People

As mentioned above, there are many different disorders and conditions which give rise to the need for speaking aids based on CSS for persons with speech impairments. The disorders vary greatly in terms of origin (congenital or acquired), the severity of speech impairment incurred, whether the speech impairment is correlated with intellectual disability, and whether the impairment is accompanied by other physical impairments. Because of the variety of different conditions involved, again the phrase "one size does not fit all" applies. CSS systems need to be flexible and adaptable to different situations and different users. For example, perhaps one finds that a visually oriented interface is more appropriate for a child or an adult with intellectual disability. For stroke victims or people with cerebral palsy or multiple sclerosis, there are questions about the physical interface for the device. Should a hand switch be used? Is an infrared beam eye tracker necessary? Can the person type text on a keyboard and have a text to speech convertor output the speech? The special needs of different populations represent a strong theme in the present volume (see Drager & Reichle; Koul & Dembowski; Koul et al.; Sutherland et al.). This research has important implications for practitioners who may have to deal with different clients with different problems. In two chapters in the present volume, Chaffee and Smith et al. describe detailed case studies that illustrate very clearly the practical difficulties that emerge when training a client to use a CSS system and when training a client to transition from one system to another. It is apparent that the strategies practitioners use when working with clients using CSS need to be flexible as well. As mentioned above, developments in AAC and CSS technology are occurring rapidly. Practitioners must make informed decisions about the worthiness of changing the system a client is using. They must gauge the potential benefit of shifting to a system that may have improved intelligibility, naturalness or ease of use against the potential disruption to the client's life and the difficulty of re-training them. This situation was illustrated by the case of Stephen Hawking, who persisted in using an older CSS system despite improvements in the technology over the course of many years. But, as mentioned above eventually he decided it was worth the disruption to transition to a newer and more sophisticated system.

Social Aspects

To some extent, all of us sound different from one another. Our individual voice, to an extent, is an important part of our individual identity. Loss of voice is also terrifically inconveniencing considering the extent to which people communicate by speaking.

It is no surprise that loss of voice will have massive ramification on how one sees themselves as well as how they interact with others. To go back to the case of Roger Ebert, Ebert first attempted to communicate with others using handwritten notes. He noted:

Business meetings were a torture. I am a quick and I daresay witty speaker. Now I came across as the village idiot. I sensed confusion, impatience and condescension. I ended up having conversations with myself, just sitting there. (Ebert, 2009)

The difficulties Ebert experienced with written notes also apply to people communicating via CSS. We believe that the manner in which CSS users interact with people in their social environment has been neglected somewhat in the research literature. Depending on the situation, a conversation with a CSS user can result in frustration and impatience on the part of the listener. For example, in 2005 a reporter from The Guardian, a UK newspaper, interviewed Stephen Hawking. She reported:

Stupidly, given that I have read all about it, I fail to realise just how arduous and time-consuming the process of live communication is. If I did, I wouldn't squander the time on asking a joke, warm-up question. I tell him I have heard he has six different voices on his synthesizer and that one is a woman's. Hawking lowers his eyes and starts responding. After five minutes of silence the nurse sitting beside me closes her eyes and appears to go to sleep. I look around. On the windowsill are framed photos stretching back through Hawking's life. There are photos of one of his daughters with her baby. I notice Hawking's hands are thin and tapering. He is wearing black suede Kickers. Another five minutes pass. There are pictures of Marilyn Monroe on the wall, one of which has been digitally manipulated to feature Hawking in the foreground. I see a card printed with the slogan: 'Yes, I am the centre of the universe.' I write it down and turn the page in my notebook. It makes a tearing sound and the nurse's eyes snap open. She goes over to Hawking and, putting her hand on his head, says, 'Now then, Stephen,' and gently wipes saliva from the side of his mouth. Another five minutes pass. Then another. Hawking's assistant, who sits behind him to see what is going on on his screen, nods slightly. Here it comes: 'That was true of one speech synthesizer I had. But the one I use normally has only one voice. It is 20 years old, but I stick to it because I haven't found better and because I'm known by it worldwide.' That's it? The fruit of 20 minutes' effort? This man is a Hercules. (The Guardian, 2005)

As Higginbotham (present volume) points out, the temporal dynamics and collaborative nature of conversation between speaker and listener can be disrupted when the speaker is a CSS user. The pattern of conversational give and take is an important aspect of CSS usability and one that needs addressed. Higginbotham notes that most AAC systems are not designed to properly facilitate real time social interaction between user and listener. However, he describes some possible ways that CSS systems can be adjusted to preserve the normal conversational rhythm that is so important for fluid social interaction.

There is also evidence that people with speech impairments are stigmatized (Anderson & Antonak, 1992; Weitzel, 2000) and that listeners' reactions to their CSS speech is affected as a result (Stern, Mullennix, & Wilson, 2002). Stern et al. (present volume) indicate that people with impairments are viewed as asexual, unappealing, dependent, entitled, isolated, and unemployable. We have also demonstrated in a series of studies that people don't like to listen to CSS. However, when listeners know that the user has a speech impairment, they may experience a "positive prejudice" toward the speaker, which then disappears if the user is perceived as using CSS for a "negative purpose" such as a telephone campaign (Mullennix, present volume, Stern, Dumont, Mullennix, & Winters, 2007). The attitudes that people have towards those with speech impairments who use CSS may prove to be the most intractable problem of all. Not only do strangers have attitudes toward people with speech impairments that may affect their perception of a CSS user's speech, but even people close to the user, such as family, friends, caretakers, co-workers, etc., may possess these attitudes. It's reasonable to assume that one day CSS technology will progress to the point where CSS is perfectly intelligible, natural sounding, and easy to use. But how do you change a person's attitude toward a CSS user? It is clear that a significant amount of future social psychological research needs to address this problem and hopefully arrive at possible ways to change the culture from which the average person views the speech impaired using this technology to speak.

THE FUTURE

So what does the future hold for CSS, especially as utilized in AAC devices? There are many indications that research currently in progress will soon result in speaking aids that are much more sophisticated than what are available today. For example, Bailly et al. (present volume) on augmented speech communication (ASC) discuss systems that convert non audible murmur and silent cued speech into audiovisual speech. There is work emerging on Brain Computer Interfaces (BCI's) where users may be able to train a CSS system to output speech based on specific brain wave patterns (e.g., Guenther & Brumberg, 2009). There is also research that is beginning to explore the use of what are called "talking heads" or animated visual avatars that would provide a person with a speech impairment a visual depiction of their speech synchronized with auditory output (Massaro, 1998; 2004). Hence, in terms of the technology, we are on the cusp of many exciting developments that hold promise for the future. But advancements in technology represent only one portion of progress. No matter how good the technology is, we still have to come up with ways to tailor the technology to different populations of users. We still need to address the social dynamics that underlie the conversational event between CSS user and listener. We also need to develop better training techniques and better ways to change the culture surrounding persons with speech impairments, which is part of the large picture of how people with impairments are viewed by society. It is our hope that the present volume represents a significant step in accomplishing these goals.

REFERENCES

American Speech and Hearing Association (ASHA). Retrieved September 14, 2009, http://www.asha.org/public/speech/disorders/AAC.htm

Anderson, R. J., & Antonak, R. F. (1992). The influence of attitudes and contact on reactions to persons with physical and speech disabilities. *Rehabilitation Counseling Bulletin*, *35*, 240–247.

Duffy, S. A., & Pisoni, D. B. (1992). Comprehension of synthetic speech produced by rule: A review and theoretical interpretation. *Language and Speech*, *35*, 351–389.

Ebert. (2009). *Finding my own voice.* Retrieved September 14, 2009 from http://blogs.suntimes.com/ebert/2009/08/finding_my_own_voice.html

Greene, B. G., Logan, J. S., & Pisoni, D. B. (1986). Perception of synthetic speech produced automatically by rule: Intelligibility of eight text-to-speech systems. *Behavior Research Methods, Instruments, & Computers*, *18*, 100–107.

Guenther, F., & Brumberg, J. (2009, May). *Real-time speech synthesis for neural prosthesis*. Paper presented at the 157th Meeting of the Acoustical Society of America, Portland, OR.

Hawking, S. (2009). *Prof. Stephen Hawking's disability advice*. Retrieved September 14, 2009, from http://www.hawking.org.uk/index.php/disability/disabilityadvice

Logan, J. S., Greene, B. G., & Pisoni, D. B. (1989). Segmental intelligibility of synthetic speech produced by rule. *The Journal of the Acoustical Society of America*, *86*, 566–581. doi:10.1121/1.398236

Luce, P. A., Feustel, T. C., & Pisoni, D. B. (1983). Capacity demands in short-term memory for natural and synthetic speech. *Human Factors*, *25*, 17–32.

Massaro, D. W. (1998). *Perceiving talking faces: From speech perception to a behavioral principle.* Cambridge, MA: MIT Press.

Massaro, D. W. (2004). From multisensory integration to talking heads and language learning. In G. Calvert, C. Spence, & B.E. Stein (Eds.), *Handbook of multisensory processes* (pp. 153-176). Cambridge, MA: MIT Press.

Mirenda, P., & Beukelman, D. R. (1987). A comparison of speech synthesis intelligibility with listeners from three age groups. *Augmentative and Alternative Communication*, *3*, 120–128. doi:10.1080/07434618712331274399

Mirenda, P., & Beukelman, D. R. (1990). A comparison of intelligibility among natural speech and seven speech synthesizers with listeners from three age groups. *Augmentative and Alternative Communication*, *6*, 61–68. doi:10.1080/07434619012331275324

Ralston, J. V., Pisoni, D. B., & Mullennix, J. W. (1995). Perception and comprehension of speech. In A. Syrdal, R. Bennet, & S. Greenspan (Eds.), *Applied speech technology* (pp. 233-288). Boca Raton, FL: CRC Press.

Stern, S. E., Dumont, M., Mullennix, J. W., & Winters, M. L. (2007). Positive prejudice towards disabled persons using synthesized speech: Does the effect persist across contexts? *Journal of Language and Social Psychology*, *26*, 363–380. doi:10.1177/0261927X07307008

Stern, S. E., Mullennix, J. W., & Wilson, S. J. (2002). Effects of perceived disability on persuasiveness of computer synthesized speech. *The Journal of Applied Psychology*, *87*, 411–417. doi:10.1037/0021-9010.87.2.411

The Guardian. (2005). *Return of the time lord.* Retrieved September 14, 2009, from http://www.guardian.co.uk/science/2005/sep/27/scienceandnature.highereducationprofile

Venkatagiri, H. S. (2003). Segmental intelligibility of four currently used text-to-speech synthesis methods. *The Journal of the Acoustical Society of America*, *113*, 2094–2104. doi:10.1121/1.1558356

Venkatagiri, H. S. (2004). Segmental intelligibility of three text-to-speech synthesis methods in reverberant environments. *Augmentative and Alternative Communication*, *20*, 150–163. doi:10.1080/07434610410001699726

Weitzel, A. (2000). Overcoming loss of voice. In D.O. Braithwaite & T.L. Thompson (Eds.), *Handbook of communication and people with disabilities: Research and application* (pp. 451-466). Mahwah, NJ: Erlbaum.

Section 1
Overview of Computer Synthesized Speech

Chapter 2
From Wood to Bits to Silicon Chips:
A History of Developments in Computer Synthesized Speech

Debbie A. Rowe
Rensselaer Polytechnic Institute, USA

ABSTRACT

This chapter lists some of the key inventions and applications in the history of computer synthesized speech (CSS). Starting with a brief look at the early synthesis machines—precursors to the computerized renditions of the 20th century—the chapter proceeds to look at the strides made by corporations, such as Bell Labs, IBM, Apple Inc., and Microsoft, in creating assistive technologies that tap into the benefits of CSS. There is also a discussion on developments in the fields of Neuroscience, Robotics, and the non-scientific fields of Composition and the Arts. Finally, the chapter explores how CSS has permeated the popular culture mediums of film and television, sometimes in parallel and sometimes as antecedents to current day inventions.

INTRODUCTION

Attempts to simulate human speech with inanimate objects have been in force well before the dawn of computers in the 20th Century. Some scholars have indicated that initial attempts go as far back as the ancient world of the Romans and the Greeks, where high priests would project their voices through statues of idols as if they were puppets (Cater, 1983; Coker et al, 1963). However, many would agree that the first legitimate attempt to have inanimate objects replicate the sounds of a human voice came in 18th Century Europe, where mechanical devices were engineered to produce certain vowel and consonant sounds. It would take approximately another 150 years for man to progress from machine-generated synthetic speech to electronically-generated versions, and then several decades more to streamline a computer-generated form. During that time, speech synthesis would go from a way to study human speech patterns, to a component of telecommunications, to an assistive technology tool, and beyond. This chapter will look at these developments.

DOI: 10.4018/978-1-61520-725-1.ch002

INDIVIDUAL INNOVATION

As is the case with many modern technologies produced en masse today, we have the inventive spirit of individuals to thank for laying the groundwork to today's computer synthesized speech. Researchers point to 18th century Europe as the birth place of mechanical speech synthesizers. **Wolfgang Ritter von Kempelen**, a Hungarian nobleman, engineer, and government official, invented one of the first synthesizer machines (Coker et al., 1963; Schroeder, 2004). According to Manfred Schroeder's research (2004), von Kempelen began development of his earliest "speaking machine" in 1769, designing it from wood and leather to replicate the functions of human lungs, vocal cords, and vocal tracts. The mechanism was manually operated, with air blown through the various parts to produce sounds (Cater, 1983). The first rendition of the machine created vowel sounds. A later version had a "tongue" and "lips" that enabled it to produce consonants with plosive sounds, "such as the *b* (as in *bin*) and *d* (as in *din*)" (Schroeder, 2004, p.26). It is unclear why von Kempelen decided to make the device. During the period of his inventions, there was a growing interest in "spring-operated automatons" that replicated human actions (Coker et al., 1963, p. 3). This could have influenced his decision to make the speaking machine, and to subsequently publish his 1791 book documenting his work. What is noted, however, is that von Kempelen's "early forays into synthetic speech stimulated much research into the physiology of speech production and experimental phonetics" (Schroeder, 2004, p. 26).

Paralleling von Kempelen's work was **Christian Gottlieb Kratzenstein**'s 1779 entry into the Imperial Russian Academy of St. Petersburg's annual competition. Kratzenstein, a physiologist, won the competition by providing the best explanation of the physiological differences between five vowel sounds, along with his construction of a model made of resonators that could produce those sounds (Cater, 1983; Coker et al., 1963; Schroeder, 2004). Like von Kempelen's device, Kratzenstein's invention was modeled after the human vocal tract, and produced sounds by manipulating airflow over vibrating structures or reeds. It too was not automated, requiring someone to operate it.

By the nineteenth century, Sir **Charles Wheatstone** built upon ideas from von Kempelen's machine and the theories purported by Kratzenstein and one **W. Willis** of Britain. Kratzenstein and Willis independently theorized that machine-generated vowels could come from "different shapes having identical resonances" (Schroeder, 2004, p. 27). Using this knowledge in combination with his musical expertise, Wheatstone made his own speaking machine—a more sophisticated rendition of the von Kempelen device (Cater, 1983).

By the middle of the nineteenth century, **Joseph Faber** of Vienna built a talking machine that was said to be able to "hold a conversation in normal speech, it could whisper, and it could even sing" (Coker et al., 1963, p. 4-5). According to researchers Coker, Denes, and Pinson, Faber's machine also spoke with the use of bellows pushing air over vibrating reeds. The machine was fairly large, and required an operator who would manipulate it like an organ or piano.

According to the research of John P. Cater (1983), a young **Alexander Graham Bell** also entered the realm of speech synthesizer designs during this period. Bell happened to witness Wheatstone's speaking machine in action in the mid-1800s. What Bell saw inspired him to make his own speaking machine, with the assistance of his brother and his father—an elocutionist. Bell's machine was in the shape of a human skull "complete with rubber lips and a wooden tongue" (Schroeder, 2004, p. 28). As fate would have it, his work on his speaking machine helped to lay the groundwork for his invention of the telephone, for which he received a patent in 1876.

INDUSTRIAL INNOVATION: THE ROAD TO COMPUTER SYNTHESIZED SPEECH

The twentieth century marked the shift from individual innovation to more corporate-sponsored, industrial innovation of speech synthesizers. At the forefront of such enterprise were Bell Laboratories and Haskins Laboratories.

Bell Telephone Laboratories

Under the auspices of Bell Labs (then called "Bell Telephone Laboratories"), **Homer W. Dudley** proffered a theory on electronic speech coding, in 1928, as a means of transmitting speech signals across the Atlantic for telecommunication purposes (Schroeder, 2004). Based on this idea, he designed a voice coder, or "vocoder" (alternately referred to as a "voder")—the first electronic speech synthesizer—in 1937 (Alcatel-Lucent, 2009; Bell Telephone Laboratories, Inc., 1981; Coker et al., 1963; Schroeder, 2004). Though electronic, Dudley's vocoder required someone to operate it; someone with "about the same amount of training as a concert pianist" (Rodman, 1999, p. 178). Like some of its predecessors, the vocoder speech synthesizer worked through the manipulation of keys and a foot pedal (Coker et al., 1963; Rodman, 1999) not unlike Faber's device from the 1800s. Bell Labs demonstrated Dudley's device to the general public at the 1939 New York World's Fair. (To hear what Dudley's vocoder sounded like, visit Dennis Klatt's webpage of historic voice synthesizer recordings at http://cslu.cse.ogi.edu/tts/research/history/ (Klatt, 1986).)

The vocoder was capable of speech analysis/recognition as well as synthesis. These features led to its transatlantic use for signaling secret information between Roosevelt and Churchill during World War II (Bell Telephone Laboratories, Inc., 1981). Schroeder calls the vocoder the "grandfather of modern speech and audio compression" that makes live voice communication possible across the Internet (p. 3). Subsequent versions of the vocoder are still used today for encrypted communication within the secret service and military communities (Bell Telephone Laboratories, Inc., 1981), and even for use in movie sound effects (see the section on "Film" below).

Just as electronic synthesized speech was born at Bell Labs, so too was *computer* synthesized speech. In 1962, more than two decades after the vocoder was first launched, **John L. Kelly** and **Carol Lochbaum** used an IBM 704 computer to make another vocoder at Bell Labs—one that could sing "Bicycle Built for Two" (Alcatel-Lucent, 2009; Schroeder, 2004). With that creation, computer synthesized speech (CSS) was born.

However, generating an acceptable singing voice from a computer is easier than generating an acceptable speaking voice. According to Schroeder (2004), "a singing computer, although perhaps unintelligible, is much more impressive to lay audiences than a speaking computer with its electronic accent" (p. 29). Bell Labs' **Cecil H. Coker** and **Joe Olive** took the lead in working on "articulatory synthesis" in the 1960s and "concatenative synthesis" in the 1970s, elements that dictate how natural computer synthesized speech sounds (Alcatel-Lucent, 2009).

Haskins Laboratories

The original mission behind Haskins research on synthesized speech was to assist blind war veterans. Building upon Bell Telephone Laboratories' work with sound spectrographs, the researchers at Haskins developed, in the 1940s, photographic spectrograms that represented sound (Smithsonian, 2002). With their Pattern Playback Synthesizer created in the 1950s by **Franklin Cooper**, they developed a type of reading machine that "convert[ed] pictures of the acoustic patterns of speech back into sound" (Haskins, 2008b). According to the Smithsonian Institution, "The Pattern Playback produce[d] a monotone output and was used extensively to identify the acoustic cues of speech until it was displaced by a computer-driven synthesizer built in the mid 1960s" (Smithsonian, 2002). News of Haskins Labs research with the Pattern Playback Machine reached the general public in 1954, when Cooper, Alvin Liberman and Pierre Delattre demonstrated it on the CBS show "Adventure" (Haskins, 2008a). Creating a speech synthesizer to work for the needs of the blind may have been born out of their work on the war effort for the National Academy of Sciences (Haskins, 1953, p. 25), but this invention and its demonstration to the world on television marks another important milestone. Speech synthesizers would go on from there to find their most lucrative market to date within the arena of assistive technology.

ASSISTIVE AND EDUCATIONAL TECHNOLOGY

Though Bell Labs and Haskins Labs scientists were the initial innovators in designing and applying computer synthesized speech, the baton was taken up by other companies in getting the technology to the masses. Two companies, **Industrial Business Machines Corporation** (IBM) and **Kurzweil Computer Products** (KCP) have played key parts in finding a successful, long term market for computer synthesized speech—accessibility for people with sensory and learning disabilities. Other companies have worked on applying the technologies to the education market, while others still have applied it to telephony and everyday computing uses.

IBM

IBM began work on making devices capable of audio responses as early as 1969 (IBM, 2009c), in conjunction with their work on speech recognition. (In fact, a lot of IBM's discussions on their synthesized speech developments are done as an offshoot of the discussions on speech recognition.) By 1971, they had launched their "first operational application of speech recognition [that enabled] customer engineers servicing equipment to "talk" to and receive "spoken" answers from a computer that [could] recognize about 5000 words" (IBM, 2009a). Continuing the work of helping their equipment users, IBM designed a computer with audio capabilities as a service to those who had vision problems. By 1988, just seven years after they put their first personal computer on the market (IBM, 2009b), IBM would put their mark on the assistive technology field with the launch of their **IBM Independence Series** of products for computer users with special needs. The **Personal System/2 Screen Reader** was the first product to be released. It gave blind and low vision users the chance to hear what was on their computer screens. To date, there have been only two other CSS-related developments from IBM, both of which were for the assistive technology market. There was the release of the **Screen Reader/2** in 1992, and the **Home Page Reader for Windows,** which was designed in 1997 and released in 1998. Home Page Reader was "a talking Web browser that opens the World Wide Web with spoken Internet access to blind and visually impaired users."

Kurzweil

Like a lot of clever computer software, [the OCR program] was a solution in search of a problem. —Ray Kurzweil (Kurzweil, 1999, p.174).

Ray Kurzweil is probably the designer and company founder with the longest standing reputation for creating assistive technologies that make use of CSS. In 1974, four years after getting his Bachelor's degree from Massachusetts Institute of Technology (MIT), he started his second company—Kurzweil Computer Products (KCP). He founded the company to engineer the first Optical Character Recognition (OCR) program that could read all fonts used in print. The market then was limited to OCR programs that could only decipher "one or two specialized type styles" (Kurzweil, 1999, p. 174). The next year, through a chance encounter with a fellow passenger on a plane, he realized that his OCR program could be put to use to resolve a yet unaddressed problem. The passenger, who happened to be blind, mentioned that his only real hurdle in life was reading "ordinary printed material" (Kurzweil, 1999, p. 174). Kurzweil's OCR program was not enough to address this problem, but it did become a part of the solution. KCP went about creating a computer hardware and software package that provided the visually disabled with print access through the development of a flat bed scanner and a text-to-speech (TTS) synthesizer that, bundled with the OCR program, could read any text (Kurzweil, 1999; Smithsonian, 2002b). The Kurzweil Reading Machine (KRM), the first "print-to-speech reading machine," was launched to such acclaim in January 1976 that Walter Cronkite demonstrated on air, using it 'to read aloud his signature sign-off: "And that's the way it was, January 13, 1976." '

The KRM device introduced Kurzweil the person to the world stage. It led to the development of several other pieces of equipment and several other companies, often with visually disabled users in mind. In 1980, he sold his OCR and scanning technology to Xerox. They in turn used that technology to develop the software, TextBridge (still in existence today, but marketed by the company Nuance). By 1982, Kurzweil started a new company—the Kurzweil Music Systems. The keyboards he would develop under the advisement of Stevie Wonder, led to the dominant synthesizer sound in western music in the 1980s. The keyboard allowed musicians to synthesize the sounds of several different instruments while only playing the keys of a keyboard, lessening the need to learn to play multiple instruments, or even forming an entire band. This was of use to all populations, including the visually disabled.

Concurrent with the launch of the Kurzweil Music Systems (KMS) in 1982 was the launch of another of his companies—the Kurzweil Artificial Intelligence (KAI). This company focused on the sometimes counterpart invention to speech synthesis—that of speech recognition. The programs that came out of that company include a dictation software specifically for doctors, called Kurzweil VoiceMed, and a dictation program for the general public, called Voice Xpress Plus. Fifteen years after it was founded, KAI was sold in 1997 to a European company called Lernout & Hauspie (L&H). L&H specialized in both speech synthesis and speech recognition. Kurzweil (1999) notes, "[KAI] arranged a strategic alliance between the dictation division of L&H...and Microsoft." This would lead to the subsequent inclusion of L&H computer voices, LH Michelle and LH Michael, in Microsoft products.

Lernout & Hauspie

Jo Lernout and **Pol Hauspie** founded L&H in 1987, in Belgium. As mentioned above, the company specialized in speech synthesis and recognition. By 1995, the business became very lucrative and began buying up several other speech companies, including Kurzweil Artificial Intelligence (KAI). Other companies of note that were acquired included Dragon Systems, the maker of the popular speech recognition software Dragon NaturallySpeaking. L&H developers also worked on synthesized voices, the most popular of which were LH Michelle and LH Michael, as noted above. Unfortunately, L&H was part of the bursting of the dot-com bubble at the turn of the 21st century, which saw the rapid rise and growth in wealth of technology companies that declined at an even more meteoric rate. The company went bankrupt after its founders were arrested for fraud in 2001 (Hesseldahl, 2001; Greenberg, 2001). Products from the company were sold off. Dragon NaturallySpeaking was purchased by ScanSoft, (called Nuance today), which has nurtured Dragon NaturallySpeaking into arguably the most popular speech recognition software, with playback capabilities in the voice of computer synthesized speech or the voice of the person who made the dictation recording.

Texas Instruments

When thinking of Texas Instruments (TI), developments in calculators often come to mind. Texas Instruments, however, was one of the first companies to produce a computerized speech synthesis mechanism not specifically marketed to people with disabilities. Their "Speak and Spell" device, released in 1978, was an educational toy that could teach children how to pronounce and spell words. The toy gained extensive popularity when it was featured in the movie "E.T.: The Extra-Terrestrial" (1982), as E.T. used the Speak and Spell with other items to build his communicator to phone home.

Apple Inc.

In 2004, O'Reilly Media Inc's MacDevCenter writer F.J. de Kermadec noted:

The new audio capabilities of Mac OS X, along with the renewed commitment from Apple to this amazing technology have concurred to produce what is widely considered to be the most convenient and advanced speech technology available in this field (de Kermadec, 2004).

Though the very first Macintosh computer, launched in 1984, used the MacInTalk computer voice to declare its arrival to the world stating "Hello, I'm Macintosh," there was little more that that model could do by way of speech synthesis. Speech synthesis requires such extensive computing power to adapt to the on demand needs of end users, it took almost another 20 years, with Mac OS X, for the launch of a fully capable speech synthesizer, with both screen reading and text-to-speech capabilities. However, Apple has more than made up for the long wait with the quantity and quality of voice options bundled with its operating system today.

Within the Universal Access and Speech centers of the Leopard edition of OS X (version 10.5, released in 2005), there are several components that make use of computer synthesized speech. The VoiceOver Utility (Apple, 2009a) offers customizable features, including two dozen CSS voices from which to choose. There are talking dialog boxes, and even the option to get time announcements from the computer's clock.

Apple's strides in speech synthesis do not stop with its computers, but rather extends to telephony and the feature films. The VoiceOver technology applied to the computers are also applied to iPhones (Apple, 2009b), as part of the company's commitment to accessibility. Also, the MacInTalk computer voice made its feature film "acting" debut in 2008. In the movie *WALL-E*, we have what is probably the first instance of a CSS voice playing an actor's part; MacInTalk is given actual voice credit for the role of a non-Mac computer character on film, that of "Auto" the autopilot computer that controls the cruise ship "Axiom" (Stanton, 2008).

Microsoft Corporation

On Microsoft Corporation's commitment to accessibility, Bill Gates wrote on the corporation's website, "Our vision is to create innovative technology that is accessible to everyone and that adapts to each person's needs. Accessible technology eliminates barriers for people with disabilities and it enables individuals to take full advantage of their capabilities." (Microsoft, 2009b)

MS Windows Operating Systems

While Microsoft (MS) has had a legacy of working on accessibility issues from the days of DOS, most specifically AccessDOS, it has not always included computer synthesized speech as part of its solution. Accessibility tools were often based on customizable screen sizes, commands for the keyboards, simple sound alerts, and magnifiers. Putting the volume button on the taskbar to provide quick access was even one of their measures to improve accessibility. Computer synthesized speech, however, did not come to Microsoft Windows until the advent of Windows 2000, released in February of that year. In the operating system, the "Narrator" program was introduced and is still in use two Windows generations later with Windows Vista. Microsoft describes Narrator as "a text-to-speech utility that reads what is displayed on the screen—the contents of the active window, menu options, or text that has been typed" (Microsoft, 2009d). (It should be noted that Narrator acts more like a screen reader than a text-to-speech program. Screen readers are capable of announcing all text on a computer, including dialog boxes and menu choices like "File," "View," "Copy," "Paste." Text-to-speech programs on the other hand tend to read only the text generated *within* the boundaries of a document or webpage.)

Text-to-speech had even more capabilities when Microsoft Windows XP was released in 2001. In this incarnation, users had choices in CSS voices. Microsoft Sam, the voice for "Narrator" was still in use, but you could also select from Microsoft Mary, Microsoft Mike, as well as LH Michelle or LH Michael (as noted in the Lernout & Hauspie section above). You could also add other CSS voices purchased through third-party software manufacturers.

Surprisingly, Microsoft scaled down the number of voices bundled with the operating system for its next operating system—Windows Vista. Possibly because of the failing of Lernout & Hauspie (the company), LH Michelle and LH Michael voices were no longer bundled with the operating system. Users got access to a new Microsoft voice for the Narrator feature; Microsoft Anna replaced Microsoft Sam. New with Vista, however, was a more expansive list of accessibility options in the Ease of Access center which included audio descriptions of what was happening in videos displayed.

MS Office Products

Though computer synthesized speech (CSS) was not bundled within the standard office suite of products until Office 2003, Microsoft had made grounds in making its products compatible with third party CSS programs, such as screen readers, as far back as Office 2000. They made the decision to make Outlook 2000 more screen reader-friendly by giving users the option to change images and icons to text, and to customize columns and fields to display as much, or as little information as the user wanted to hear (Microsoft, 2009a).

Word 2003 had, arguably, taken the most advantage of CSS technology of all the MS Office programs to date. Microsoft introduced its "Language Bar" which offered speech recognition and text-to-speech read back capabilities. Users could dictate their documents then play them back to check for errors and the like, whether or not those users were visually disabled or not. This feature made the Language Bar more than an accessibility tool because its function was of value to all users of Word, including those who would not want the verbosity of Narrator that reads what sighted users would not need to hear.

MS Internet Explorer

Microsoft started taking into consideration some of the requirements of screen readers for web browsers with version 4.0 of Internet Explorer (IE). With that version, they introduced "The ability to disable smooth scrolling and other effects that can confuse screen reading utilities" (Microsoft, 2009c). IE version 6 came with the option to load pages without their built-in sound files turned on. This was useful, for example, for those sites that load with musical sounds playing, which would often prove to be a distraction to those listening to their screen readers. Though there have been many other features built into other versions of Internet Explorer, they do not impact the use of speech synthesis.

Third-Party Software Companies

Nuance Communications, Inc.

Many important but less widely known companies have made significant strides in developing and applying computer synthesized speech over the last two decades, sometimes by procuring other speech-specialization companies that have become defunct. Nuance Communications, Inc., which today has Dragon NaturallySpeaking as a star product, is one such company. As mentioned earlier, Dragon was once owned by Lernout & Hauspie. Upon that company's demise, the Dragon technology was acquired by ScanSoft (Lee, 2001), which merged with Nuance in 2005. According to CNET Blog Network's Steve Toback (2008), after acquiring or merging with 40+ different companies over time, Nuance Communications "is far and away the 800-pound gorilla of speech technology," compared to its competitors at IBM, Microsoft, and the like.

Dragon NaturallySpeaking version 9 was the first incarnation of the program released after Nuance merged with ScanSoft. This version allowed users to dictate their documents and choose to either listen to their documents read aloud by a CSS voice—the "Read That" feature—or listen to the recording of their own voice as the speech recognition technology picked it up—the "Play That Back" feature. This tapped into the writing styles of users who like to read aloud, or have someone read aloud to them, as they work to revise their documents.

Dragon in its many forms—Standard, Preferred, Medical, Legal—is not the only speech synthesis product that Nuance brings to the marketplace. Their voice technologies, such as "RealSpeak," are applied in telephony, automotive, and mobile technologies.

To list all the other software developers that work on CSS technologies today would be near impossible, and beyond the scope of this chapter. However, some important ones bear mentioning here:

- FreedomScientific: Manufacturers of **JAWS** for Windows screen reading software, which even *The New York Times* labels as ***the*** "most popular screen-reading software" (Tedeshi, 2006).
- Ai Squared: Manufacturers of **ZoomText** Magnifier/Reader, another leading assistive technology software that uses both a screen reader and text-to-speech technology.
- NeoSpeech: Makers of CSS voices **NeoSpeech Kate** and **NeoSpeech Paul**, two of the most popular United States-accented CSS voices in use today.
- Oddcast Inc.: Makers of **SitePal**, a "speaking avatar solution that enables small businesses to enhance their web presence and improve business results with virtual speaking characters." (Oddcast, 2008)

A NOTE ON NEUROPROSTHETICS AND SPEECH IMPAIRMENT APPLICATIONS

Most of the assistive technologies discussed thus far in this chapter have dealt with aids for visual impairment. Speech impairment—from mild forms such as stuttering or a lisp, to chronically severe forms such as those caused by a stroke or complete paralysis—is also served by computerized speech technology. Neuroprosthetics "is an area of neuroscience concerned with neural prostheses—using artificial devices to replace the function of impaired nervous systems or sensory organs" (Brain-computer, 2009). One of the most recognizable figures today who uses a neuroprosthetic device is British physicist **Stephen Hawking**. Stricken by a form of amyotrophic lateral sclerosis (ALS), Hawking is almost completely paralyzed, and uses a speech synthesizer which he activates through twitches of his cheek muscles (Hawking, 2009; Henderson & Naughton, 2009). A noted speaker, he often composes what he wants to say to an audience before meeting them, by starting and stopping a cursor on a computer screen that he controls through a switch in his hand. (To see a video of Dr. Hawking communicating via his computer, please see the TED video "Stephen Hawking asks big questions about the universe" at http://www.ted.com/talks/stephen_hawking_asks_big_questions_about_the_universe.html (TED, 2008).)

Dr. Hawking's neuroprosthetics are external to his body, but advances in this research area have led to developments of brain-computer interfaces (BCI), sometimes referred to as brain-machine interface (BMI). BCIs allow for direct connections between a computer and a user's brain, which can lead to action controlled by thoughts. (See reference on Tony Fitzpatrick's 2006 article about a teenager who could play a video game just by thinking about it.) In a segment entitled "Brain Power," CBS Television's "60 Minutes" news program aired a story on Scott Mackler and his use of a BCI to communicate with the world. Mackler, who at age 40 was also stricken with ALS, could only use his eyes to communicate, "saying" yes or no indicated by the direction of his stare. With his BCI, however, he could communicate with full sentences on a computer that used the NeoSpeech Paul voice (mentioned above). (The entire "60 Minutes" video segment can be viewed at: http://www.cbsnews.com/video/watch/?id=4564186n&tag=contentMain;contentBody (Cetta, 2008).)

ROBOTICS

ASIMO—the Advanced Step in Innovative MObility robot—is another familiar figure in the world today. Perhaps the most recognizable, non-fictional, robot at the turn of the 21st century, its creators at Honda tout it as "The World's Most Advanced Humanoid Robot." Not much is written on ASIMO regarding its CSS technology. Dean Creehan of PopularRobotics.com states that Honda is usually quite cautious about disclosing information on its robotics research (Creehan, 2003). However, it may really just be a case that CSS is not considered one of the innovative features of the robot. Creehan did find out at a 2003 conference that ASIMO speaks using an IBM ProTalker speech synthesis engine. But according to Gearlog.com, ASIMO "never speaks for itself—Asimo's voice is typically generated by an off-stage handler" (Ulanoff, 2009).

In 2009, ASIMO entered the world of neuroprosthetics by becoming a brain-machine interface controlled robot. "Without electrode array implants or special training of the user" a human being can control certain features of an ASIMO robot through thoughts alone, including its ability to speak (Honda, 2009).

While ASIMO makes a significant leap in robotics and speech synthesis, there are many other types of robots, designed for different duties that follow it in capabilities and features. ASIMO is a service droid made for assisting humans. There are also speaking "toybots" (Skillings, 2009) of which the now defunct robot dog, Sony's AIBO (Borland, 2006) was the most popular. While both ASIMO and AIBO looked like artificial objects, there are human-looking robots called "Actroids" (Actroid, 2009) who are able to depict human emotion in their facial features and other body parts. The Japanese teacher robot, Saya, is able to smile and say thank you to her students (Kageyama, 2009). Another actroid robot, CB2 (the Child-robot with Biomimetic Body), has the capacity to learn through observation and interaction, imitating breathing, walking, but not yet speaking (Suzuki, 2009).

COMPOSITION RESEARCH

There are instances where having an alternate reader, such as CSS technology, may or may not prove beneficial. In my own research, I am investigating the use of text-to-speech (TTS) technology applied in instances where people prefer to hear their writing read aloud as they work on revising it. There are multiple iterations of this reading aloud activity—1) those who prefer to read aloud to themselves, 2) those who prefer to read to someone else, and 3) those who like to have someone read their work to them. The Dragon NaturallySpeaking version discussed earlier in this chapter provides TTS technology that can address iterations 1) and 3). In one study conducted thus far, research subjects who typically read their writing aloud for themselves were asked to use a TTS program—NaturalSoft's NaturalReader program—to substitute for their own reading. The subjects, who had not worked with TTS technology prior to the study, had varying degrees of objection to how robotic-sounding the voice options were. While this particular reaction is common among new TTS users, there were other more important findings that can be applied to other CSS application research. In trying to replicate an established practice, such as the read-aloud habits of the writers in the study, it came to light that that practice entailed more than hearing and seeing the text at the same time—the previously perceived key components in reading aloud. Some writers realized upon their application of the technology that they had a physical need to feel themselves saying the words in their mouths as they read, as a means of detecting problems that needed correcting—the benefits of which are lost when the computer performs the reading task for them. They also lost the opportunity to "perform" their work, as though telling their story to an audience, to physically engage their entire bodies in enacting the words and emotions behind what they had written. These significant issues of embodiment were not clear to the participants until CSS was brought in to duplicate the basic components of their read-aloud practice. So what can be learned about other everyday social practices and habits of reading or speaking when we study the effects of CSS "replacing" those functions? There is far more research yet to be done in many fields that could address this question.

THE ARTS

The Arts is another field that makes use of CSS technology. A robot, named **"Kiru,"** was part of a 2001 art installation at the **Whitney Museum of American Art** in New York City. The installation was part of an exhibit entitled "Data Dynamics," of which Kiru was part of artist **Adrianne Wortzel**'s work entitled "Camouflage Town." Kiru lived in the museum for the duration of the spring exhibit, moving about the main floor, speaking to visitors in his CSS voice as they interacted with him. He could be directed to do or say a number of things, both through built-in commands, as well as remote instructions sent from visitors within the museum or those using the internet to view life through his "eyes." (To see a video of Kiru asking visitors to press the 4th floor button in the museum's elevator, see the artist's website at http://www.adriannewortzel.com/. For more of Kiru and the Camouflage Town experience, you may also go to http://www.adriannewortzel.com/robotic/camouflagetown/index.html.)

In December 2002, also at the Whitney Museum, the installation "**Listening Post**" was unveiled.

Listening Post is an art installation that culls text fragments in real time from thousands of unrestricted Internet chat rooms, bulletin boards and other public forums. The texts are read (or sung) by a voice synthesizer, and simultaneously displayed across a suspended grid of more than two hundred small electronic screens (EAR Studio, 2009).

Created with the collaboration of **Ben Rubin**, a sound designer and multimedia artist, and **Mark Hansen**, formerly of the Statistics and Data Mining Research Department at Bell Labs, Listening Post gave voice to anonymous statements and declarations gleaned from the internet—statements as benign as "I am 14," or "I'm from Argentina," to stronger statements about what was breaking in the news at the time. (To see a video sampling of this award winning work, please visit http://video.google.com/videoplay?docid=-121912060 8081240028 (EAR Studio, 2002).)

COMPUTER SYNTHESIZED SPEECH ON FILM

During the era of the space race—from the late 1950s to 1960s—it became increasingly common for U.S. popular culture to embrace what citizens were reading about in their newspapers, hearing on the radio, or seeing on their televisions, just as it is today. The imagination of authors, screenwriters, and filmmakers alike tapped into the heightened, collective consciousness of what life could be like beyond earth. Some of the more notable works of science fiction generated during that time borrowed facts from real world developments in science and technology, including developments in computer synthesized speech.

The most notable of these was the film, ***2001: A Space Odyssey***, released in 1968. The story revolves around mysterious monoliths that appear at different points in man's history—on earth, the moon, and eventually orbiting Jupiter during a manned space mission. During that mission to Jupiter, the ship's computer—the **Heuristically programmed ALgorithmic (HAL) 9000 Computer**—controls all ships functions, though under the supervision of two astronauts. HAL is quite interactive—he speaks and recognizes speech. As the ship nears Jupiter, HAL appears to malfunction and proceeds to not only disobey human commands but kills all but one of the astronauts on board, including three that were in hibernation.

The character of the HAL-9000 computer was voiced and played by a human actor (Douglas Rain), as is the case with almost all computer characters in film and on television. However, HAL was based, in part, on what writer **Arthur C. Clarke** had witnessed on a visit to Bell Labs in 1962. He happened to be visiting a friend at the labs when the first computerized vocoder demonstrated the singing of Harry Dacre's "Bicycle Built for Two." In a scene in the movie *2001*, the HAL-9000 sings the very same "Bicycle Built for Two" as he is being dismantled and taken offline by the sole surviving astronaut.

Though illustrating what a computer voice might be like in the 21st century setting of the movie, Douglas Rains spoke with great clarity and intelligibility, but with an extreme lack of emotion. In instances where humans may show alarm in their voice, for example the line "Just what do you think you're doing, Dave?" (Kubrick, 1968), HAL has the same tone and inflection as he does in every other situation. Despite or because he is a highly evolved computer, he continues to speak only of logical things in logical terms. For example, he terminates his conversation with someone he is leaving for death, by matter-of-factly stating that "the conversation can serve no purpose anymore" as the person tries to save someone's life. This is just one example of his logic on verbal display, while lacking any emotional intonation.

Though we are in the 21st century now, speech synthesis developments have not quite lived up to the predictions of the movie. In the 40 years since the movie's release, there have been many instances where computer synthesized speech has played a role, even if the role was <u>not</u> enacted by a computer. Below is a list of some of the instances where CSS technology has appeared on the small and big screens:

- ***Star Trek*** (Roddenberry & Butler, 1966): This television and movie franchise actually has the longest running CSS voice. The Enterprise and Starfleet computers have been played by actress Majel Barrett from the first season of the television series in 1966 (Roddenberry & Hart, 1966; IMDb, 2009b) to the 2009 release of the motion picture *Star Trek* (Abrams, 2009).
- ***Alien***: Viewers are introduced to a computer called "Mother." Like HAL and the Enterprise computer, she controls the ship

at the behest of humans. She does not, however, have speech recognition capabilities, and must have commands typed in for functionality. The movie is released in 1979.

- ***2010***: The SAL-9000 computer is introduced. It is a wholly interactive system like its male counterpart HAL, which makes a reappearance in this film. This computer also lacks emotion, though there are really no lines in the film that warrant a display of emotion. The movie is released in 1984.
- ***E.T.: The Extra-Terrestrial:*** As mentioned earlier in this chapter, the Texas Instruments educational toy—Speak and Spell—was featured in the film. E.T. picks up the English language by watching television and playing with the toy. He subsequently uses the toy as one part of his custom-made communicator which he uses to call home. The movie is released in 1982.
- ***Alien Resurrection***: The computer controlling the medical space lab featured in this film is called "Father." It is a male counterpart to "Mother" featured in the first installment of the Alien movie franchise. This computer has limited speech recognition capabilities, responding only to specific command structures. The movie is released in 1997.
- ***AI: Artificial Intelligence*** (2001), ***I, Robot*** (2004), ***Star Trek: The Next Generation*** (1987-2002), ***Star Wars*** series (1977-present), ***The Terminator*** *series (1984-2009)*: Each of these films feature robots, androids, and cyborgs with artificial intelligence capabilities. Where they differ from the movies listed above is that these machines are given emotions—emotions which can sometimes be deactivavted, as is the case with **Lt. Commander Data**'s emotion chip in ***Star Trek: Generations*** (Carson, 1994). The capacity for emotion, of course, has an impact in the alleged CSS voice quality of the synthetic life forms.

In 2008, two films were released that marked an important step in CSS on film: ***Eagle Eye*** (Caruso, 2008) and ***WALL-E*** (Stanton, 2008). Unlike all the movies listed above which are set in the future, *Eagle Eye* is set in present day America. The two main characters go through half the film before realizing that the voice they've been hearing all along on a telephone is that of a computer. While there is a certain degree of anthropomorphism or human naturalness built into several of today's CSS voices, it is highly unlikely that it would take several hours of interaction for a lay person to realize that there is a computer generating the voice. (But this can be debated by the researchers who specialize in CSS design.)

In the movie *WALL-E*, CSS technology is used in front of and behind the camera. As discussed previously, the actual MacInTalk CSS voice is used as a character's voice on the film. It is perhaps no surprise that the MacInTalk voice is used on a Pixar film, since Steve Jobs, the current CEO of Apple Inc. founded Pixar Studios in 1986.

Behind the scenes of *WALL-E*, a modern day vocoder software program is used to make a human actress—Elissa Knight–sound like a robot, the character "EVE." Legendary sound designer Ben Burtt, of *Invasion of the Body Snatchers* (1978), the *Star Wars* franchise, and the *Indiana Jones* franchise fame (IMDb, 2009a), demonstrates how he arrived at this and other sound effects for *WALL-E* in the bonus featurette *Animation Sound Design: Building Worlds From The Sound Up*, on DVD versions of *WALL-E*.

RESEARCH DIRECTIONS AND APPLICATIONS

We are approaching new frontiers in the research and application of CSS today. There is the rapid acceptance of speaking Global Positioning System (GPS) devices that lead some to wonder today how we drove and read maps at the same time. As we slowly start to move away from print publications to their electronic forms, e-Readers such as Amazon's "Kindle," come bundled with text-to-speech technology that can read the entire collection of an electronic library's worth of books. These developments look at non-traditional applications of speech synthesis that can benefit from having someone else or something else performing a reading task for the primary user.

To explore new questions, share knowledge, and discuss the roles that computer synthesized speech can have in the world in the near and distant future, many entities have come together to form various consortia on developing and applying CSS. Conferences such as INTERSPEECH, International Conference on Spoken Language Processing, and The Acoustical Society of America are but a handful of the important conferences discussing the advances in speech technology. Universities such as Massachusetts Institute of Technology (MIT) and Carnegie Mellon University (CMU) sponsor collaborative projects and even speech synthesizer contests, such as the annual Blizzard Challenge. As time progresses with advances in hardware and software capacities, the fields of Artificial Intelligence(AI) and Natural Language Processing (NLP) will go further in giving CSS voices…"a soul" as Ben Burtt of the movie *WALL-E* (Stanton, 2008) puts it, referring to what feels lacking in synthesized voices.

CONCLUSION

We as a species have been working on replicating ourselves, our functions, and our tasks, perhaps as soon as we came into being. We've been curious about how some of us are able to speak and others not, and that curiosity about our speech led to the first speaking machines of the 1700s. As our knowledge and technological capacities grew, we found better, more effective ways to artificially generate our speech, finding a way to enable some to read for themselves when otherwise they could not, or speak for themselves when their bodies proved silent. The same kind of enquiry that led us over 200 years ago to examine how we generate speech is now leading us to take a closer look at all the things we do or do not use speech for, and why. The primary purpose of computer synthesized speech has been that of making communication possible. But that is only where we are today. We have yet to see CSS at its fullest and varied potential when it becomes ubiquitous and fully integrated into our everyday lives.

REFERENCES

Abrams, J. J. (Director). (2009). *Star Trek* [Motion picture]. United States: Paramount Pictures.

Acoustical Society of America. (2009). *Meetings of the Acoustical Society of America*. Retrieved from http://asa.aip.org/meetings.html.

Actroid. (n.d.). Retrieved July 2, 2009, from Wikipedia: http://en.wikipedia.org/wiki/Actroid

Ai Squared. (2009). *Corporate homepage*. Retrieved from http://aisquared.com/

Alcatel-Lucent. (2009). *Bell Labs Historical Timeline*. Retrieved from http://www.alcatel-lucent.com/wps/portal/!ut/p/kcxml/Vc5LDoIwGATgs3CCvxKKuqxIJBIeCkhh00BaFW0LwQfh9sLCGHeTb5LJQAkFlLp6N5fq2bS6kkChtBlhlu3P1RxNF0PxZ4iRnwReq8TkxXICvPMhBYosltxQt08zHCQ8j7nbheO49k-pg8JtfdgMncYvKuWY52VUazs7Kynqux3xSjoPhwTmtWXEgCP4EM-fvuN5LzQXPXQqo8Ni5SliGB_8NTlf/delta/base64xml/L3dJdyEvd0ZNQUFzQUsvNElVRS82XzlfSVA!

Apple Inc. (2009a). *Accessibility-VoiceOver in Depth*. Retrieved from http://www.apple.com/accessibility/voiceover/

Apple Inc. (2009b). *iPhone-Accessibility.* Retrieved from http://www.apple.com/iphone/iphone-3gs/accessibility.html

Bell Telephone Laboratories, Inc. (1981). *Impact: A compilation of Bell System innovations in science and engineering that have led to the creation of new products and industries, while improving worldwide telecommunications* (2nd ed.), (L.K. Lustig, Ed.). Murray Hill, NJ: Bell Laboratories.

Borland, J. (2006, January 26). *Sony puts Aibo to sleep.* Retrieved from http://news.cnet.com/Sony-puts-Aibo-to-sleep/2100-1041_3-6031649.html?tag=mncol

Brain-computer interfaces. (n.d.) Retrieved July 1, 2009, from The Psychology Wiki http://psychology.wikia.com/wiki/Brain-computer_interfaces

Cameron, J. (Director). (1984). *The Terminator* [Motion picture]. United States: Helmdale Film.

Carnegie Mellon University. (2009). *Festvox—Blizzard Challenge.* Retrieved from http://festvox.org/blizzard/

Carson, C. (1994). *Star Trek: Generations* [Motion picture]. United States: Paramount Pictures.

Caruso, D. J. (Director). (2008). *Eagle Eye* [Motion picture]. United States: DreamWorks SKG.

Cater, J. (1983). *Electronically Speaking: Computer Speech Generation.* Indianapolis: Howard W. Sams & Co., Inc.

Cetta, D.S. (Producer). (2008, November 4). Brain Power [segment]. *60 Minutes* [Television series]. New York: CBS News.

Coker, C. H., Denes, P. B., & Pinson, E. N. (1963). *Speech Synthesis: An Experiment in Electronic Speech Production.* Baltimore: Waverly Press.

Creehan, D. (2003). *Artificial Intelligence for ASIMO.* Retrieved from http://popularrobotics.com/asimo_ai.htm de Kermadec, F.J. (2004). *Are You Talking to Me? Speech on Mac OS X.* Retrieved from http://www.macdevcenter.com/pub/a/mac/2004/03/17/speech.html

EAR Studio, Inc. (Producer). (2002, December). *Listening Post – Part 1.* Video posted to http://video.google.com/videoplay?docid=-1219120608081240028

EAR Studio, Inc. (n.d.). *Listening Post Homepage.* Retrieved July 1, 2009 from http://www.earstudio.com/projects/listeningpost.html.

Fitzpatrick, T. (2006) *Teenager moves video icons just by imagination.* Retrieved from http://news-info.wustl.edu/news/page/normal/7800.html

FreedomScientific. (2009). *Products page.* Retrieved from http://www.freedomscientific.com/product-portal.asp

Greenberg, H. (2001, June 25). Watch It! The Traps Are Set The best investing advice is the most basic: Beware of getting too clever. *Fortune.* Retrieved from http://money.cnn.com/magazines/fortune/fortune_archive/2001/06/25/305449/index.htm

Haskins Laboratories. (1953). *Haskins Laboratories.* Retrieved from http://www.haskins.yale.edu/history/haskins1953.pdf

Haskins Laboratories. (2008a). *The "Adventure" Film.* Retrieved from http://www.haskins.yale.edu/history/Adventure.html

Haskins Laboratories. (2008b). *Decades of Discovery–1950s.* Retrieved from http://www.haskins.yale.edu/decades/fifties.html

Hawking, S. (n.d.). *Prof. Stephen Hawking's Computer.* Retrieved June 30, 2009, from http://www.hawking.org.uk/index.php/disability/thecomputer

Henderson, M., & Naughton, P. (2009, April 21). Prof Stephen Hawking 'comfortable' in hospital after health scare. *TimesOnline*. Retrieved from http://www.timesonline.co.uk/tol/news/uk/science/article6139493.ece

Hesseldahl, A. (2001, January 19). Disaster Of The Day: Lernout & Hauspie. *Forbes*. Retrieved from http://www.forbes.com/2001/01/19/0119disaster.html

Honda Motor Company, Ltd. (2009, March 31). *Honda, ATR and Shimadzu Jointly Develop Brain-Machine Interface Technology Enabling Control of a Robot by Human Thought Alone*. Retrieved from http://world.honda.com/news/2009/c090331Brain-Machine-Interface-Technology/

Hyams, P. (Director). (1984). *2010* [Motion picture]. United States: Metro-Goldwyn-Mayer

IBM. (2009a). *1971*. Retrieved from http://www-03.ibm.com/ibm/history/history/year_1971.html

IBM. (2009b). *The First 10 Years*. Retrieved from http://www-03.ibm.com/ibm/history/exhibits/pc25/pc25_tenyears.html

IBM. (2009c). *History of IBM.* Retrieved from http://www-03.ibm.com/ibm/history/history/history_intro.html

IMDb. (2009). *Ben Burtt*. Retrieved from http://www.imdb.com/name/nm0123785/

IMDb. (2009). *Filmography by TV series for Majel Barrett*. Retrieved from http://www.imdb.com/name/nm0000854/filmoseries#tt0060028

International Speech Communication Association. (2009). *Interspeech 2009*. Retrieved from http://www.interspeech2009.org/

Jeunet, J. (Director). (1997). *Alien: Resurrection* [Motion picture]. United States: Twentieth Century Fox.

Kageyama, Y. (2009, March 11). *Human-like robot smiles, scolds in Japan classroom*. Retrieved from http://www.physorg.com/news155989459.html.

Klatt, D. H. (1986). *Audio recordings from the Appendix of D. Klatt, "Review of text-to-speech conversion for English."* Retrieved from http://cslu.cse.ogi.edu/tts/research/history/

Kubrick, S. (Director). (1968). *2001: A Space Odyssey* [Motion picture]. United Kingdom: Metro- Goldwyn-Mayer.

Kurzweil, R. (1999). *The Age of Spiritual Machines*. New York: Penguin.

Lee, J. (2001, November 29). Buyers of Units Of Lernout Are Disclosed. *New York Times*. Retrieved from http://www.nytimes.com/2001/11/29/business/buyers-of-units-of-lernout-are-disclosed.html?scp=1&sq=Buyers%20of%20Units%20Of%20Lernout%20Are%20Disclosed&st=cse

Lucas, G. (Director). (1977). *Star Wars* [Motion picture].United States: Twentieth Century Fox.

Massachusetts Institute of Technology. (2009). *University homepage*. Retrieved from http://mit.edu

Microsoft Corporation. (2009a). *Accessibility in Microsoft Products*. Retrieved from http://www.microsoft.com/enable/products/default.aspx

Microsoft Corporation. (2009b). *Microsoft's Commitment to Accessibility*. Retrieved from http://www.microsoft.com/enable/microsoft/default.aspx

Microsoft Corporation. (2009c). *Older Versions of Microsoft Internet Explorer.* Retrieved from http://www.microsoft.com/enable/products/IE.aspx

Microsoft Corporation. (2009d). *Windows 2000 Professional Accessibility Resources*. Retrieved from http://www.microsoft.com/enable/products/windows2000/default.aspx

NaturalSoft Limited. (2009). *NaturalReaders homepage*. Retrieved from http://naturalreaders.com/

NeoSpeech. (2009) Corporate homepage. Retrieved from http://neospeech.com/

Nuance Communications, Inc. (2009). *Nuance Corporate Website*. Retrieved from http://www.nuance.com/

Oddcast Inc. (2008). *SitePal homepage*. Retrieved from http://www.sitepal.com/

Proyas, A. (Director). (2004). *I, Robot* [Motion picture]. United States: Twentieth Century Fox.

Roddenberry, G. (Writer) & Butler, R. (Director). (1966). The Cage [Television series episode]. In G. Roddenberry (Producer), *Star Trek*. Culver City, CA: Desilu Studios.

Roddenberry, G. (Writer) & Hart, H. (Director). (1966). Mudd's Women [Television series episode]. In G. Roddenberry (Producer), *Star Trek*. Culver City, CA: Desilu Studios.

Roddenberry, G. (Writer) & Allen, C. (Director). (1987). Encounter at Farpoint [Television series episode]. In G. Roddenberry (Executive Producer). *Star Trek: The Next Generation*. Los Angeles: Paramount Television.

Rodman, R. D. (1999). *Computer Speech Technology*. Boston: Artech.

Schroeder, M. (2004).*Computer Speech: recognition, compression, synthesis*. Berlin: Springer.

Scott, R. (Director). (1979). *Alien* [Motion picture]. United States: Brandywine Productions.

Skillings, J. (2009, May 27). *Look out, Rover. Robots are man's new best friend*. Retrieved from http://news.cnet.com/Look-out%2C-Rover.-Robots-are-mans-new-best-friend/2009-11394_3-6249689.html?tag=mncol

Smithsonian Institution. (2002a). *Haskins Laboratories*. Retrieved from http://americanhistory.si.edu/archives/speechsynthesis/ss_hask.htm

Smithsonian Institution. (2002b). *Kurzweil Company Products, Inc*. Retrieved from http://americanhistory.si.edu/archives/speechsynthesis/ss_kurz.htm

Spielberg, S. (Director). (1982). *E.T.: The Extra-Terrestrial*. United States: Universal Pictures.

Spielberg, S. (Director). (2001). *AI: Artificial Intelligence* [Motion picture]. United States: Warner Brothers.

Stanton, A. (Director). (2008). *WALL-E* [Motion picture]. United States: Pixar Animation Studios.

Suzuki, M. (2009, April 5). *Japan child robot mimicks infant learning*. Retrieved from http://www.physorg.com/news158151870.html

TED Conferences, LLC. (Producer). (2008, April) Stephen Hawking asks big questions about the universe. *Talks*. Video posted to http://www.ted.com/talks/stephen_hawking_asks_big_questions_about_the_universe.html

Tedeshi, B. (2006, November 6). Do the Rights of the Disabled Extend to the Blind on the Web? *New York Times*. Retrieved from http://www.nytimes.com/2006/11/06/technology/06ecom.html?_r=1&scp=1&sq=Do%20the%20Rights%20of%20the%20Disabled%20Extend%20to%20the%20Blind%20on%20the%20Web?&st=cse

Toback, S. (2008). *Wonder why everything isn't speech controlled?* Retrieved from http://news.cnet.com/8301-13555_3-10023024-34.html?tag=mncol

Ulanoff, L. (2009, March 31). *Honda Asimo Responds to Thought Control--Horror Film Makers Rejoice*. Retrieved from http://www.gearlog.com/2009/03/honda_asimo_responds_to_though.php

Wortzel, A. (2001). *Camouflage Town homepage*. Retrieved from http://www.adriannewortzel.com/robotic/camouflagetown/index.html

Wortzel, A. (n.d.). *Homepage*. Retrieved July 1, 2009 from http://www.adriannewortzel.com/

ADDITIONAL READING

Bowman, L. M. (2003, April 25). *IBM, ScanSoft pair up for speech software*. http://news.cnet.com/IBM%2C-ScanSoft-pair-up-for-speech-software/2100-1012_3-998371.html

Dutoit, T. (2001). *An Introduction to Text-to-Speech Synthesis*. Dordrecht: Kluwer.

Holmes, J. N. (1993). *Speech synthesis and recognition*. London: Chapman & Hall.

Kell, E., Bailly, G., Monaghan, A., Terken, J., & Huckvale, M. (Eds.). (2002). *Improvements in Speech Synthesis*. West Sussex: John Wiley & Sons.

Microsoft Corporation. (2009e). *Accessibility*. Retrieved from http://www.microsoft.com/ENABLE/

Microsoft Corporation. (2009f). *Research About Accessibility*. Retrieved from http://www.microsoft.com/enable/research/default.aspx.

Pitt, I., & Edwards, A. (2003). *Design of Speech-based Devices: a practical guide*. London: Springer.

Sharma, D. C. (2004, November 17). *Microsoft, Scansoft pair up for speech software*. Retrieved from http://news.cnet.com/Microsoft%2C-ScanSoft-pair-up-for-speech-software/2100-1012_3-5456577.html

Smithsonian Institution. (2002). *Smithsonian Speech Synthesis History Project (SSSHP) 1986 - 2002*. Retrieved from http://americanhistory.si.edu/archives/speechsynthesis/ss_hask.htm.

Speech Synthesis. (n.d.). Retrieved July 2, 2009, from Wikipedia http://en.wikipedia.org/wiki/Speech_synthesis

Sproat, R. (Ed.). (1998). *Multilingual text-to-speech synthesis: the Bell Labs approach*. Dordrecht: Kluwer.

Stork, D. G. (Ed.). (1997). *HAL's Legacy: 2001's computer as dream and reality*. Cambridge, MA: MIT Press.

Sydik, J. (2007) *Design Accessible Websites: Thirty-six keys to Creating Content for All Audiences and Platforms*. Raleigh: Pragmatic Bookshelf.

Tatham, M., & Morton, K. (2005). *Developments in Speech Synthesis*. West Sussex: John Wiley & Sons.

Weinschenk, S., & Barker, D. T. (2000). *Designing effective speech interfaces*. New York: John Wiley & Sons.

Wenzel, E. (2007). Leopard looks great. But what if you can't see? Retrieved from http://news.cnet.com/8301-10784_3-9808510-7.html

APPENDIX

Computer Speech Synthesis Timeline (Table 1)

Who	*When*	*What Happened*
Wolfgang Ritter von Kempelen	1769	Designed the first mechanical speaking machine
Christian Gottlieb Kratzenstein, physiologist	1779	Won prize for his theory on the physiology of certain vowel sounds and for his mechanical speaking machine
Wolfgang Ritter von Kempelen	1791	Published his book on speech synthesis
Charles Wheatstone	early 1800s	Made his own rendition of von Kempelen's device
W. Willis	1800s	Theorized that machine-generated vowels could come from "different shapes having identical resonances
Joseph Faber	mid-1800s	Built his piano-sized talking machine
Alexander Graham Bell	mid-1800s	Made his own synthesizer after having seen Wheatstone's device
Bell Labs/Homer Dudley	1928-39	Theory on and development of first electronic synthesizer—voder/vocoder
Haskins Labs/Franklin Cooper	1950s	Pattern Playback Synthesizer for the blind developed.
Bell Labs/John L. Kelly and Carol Lochbaum	1962	A computerized vocoder—the first computerized speech synthesizer
Bell Labs/Cecil H. Coker	1960s	Worked on articulatory synthesis
Desilu Productions and Paramount Television	1966	The television series *Star Trek* debuts
Metro-Goldwyn-Mayer and Stanley Kubrick Productions	1968	The motion picture *2001: A Space Odyssey* debuts
IBM	1969	Developed technique for audio responses from their computers
Bell Labs/Joe Olive	1970s	Worked on concatenative synthesis
IBM	1971	Computers could speak to service technicians
Kurzweil	1974	Kurzweil Computer Products is founded and develops the first Optical Character Recognition (OCR) program that can read all print font styles.
Kurzweil	1975-6	Developed and launched the Kurzweil Reading Machine, which was a bundling of his OCR program with a flatbed scanner and a text-to-speech synthesizer. The machine made it possible for the blind to be able to read all forms of print.
Twentieth Century Fox Film Corp and Lucasfilm	1977	The motion picture *Star Wars* debuts
Texas Instruments	1978	"Speak & Spell, a computerized learning aid for young children…is the first product that electronically duplicates the human vocal tract on a chip" (Kurzweil, 274).
Kurzweil	1978-80	Attracted the interest of Xerox and sold the Kurzweil Computer Products company to them
Twentieth Century Fox Film Corp and Brandywine Productions	1979	The motion picture *Alien* debuts
Kurzweil	1982	Kurzweil started a new company—Kurzweil Applied Intelligence—with dictation software as the primary product
Universal Pictures	1982	The motion picture *E.T.: The Extra-Terrestrial* debuts
IBM	1982	Terminal with audio output for sight-impaired operators
Hemdale Film	1984	The motion picture *The Terminator* debuts
Metro-Goldwyn-Mayer	1984	The motion picture *2010* debuts

Who	*When*	*What Happened*
Apple	1984	The first Mac computer is released and has the computer voice MacInTalk
Honda	1986	Work begins on what will be the first ASIMO robot
IBM	1988	ScreenReader is launched for the IBM PS/2 computer. Enables blind and visually disabled users to have access to text on screen. This also marked the launch of IBM's "Independence Series"--products specifically designed for people with disabilities.
IBM	1992	ScreenReader/2 is launched.
Kurzweil	1996	Founded another reading technology company—Kurzweil Educational Systems. This company had two foci—creating a product for users with reading disabilities (Kurzweil 3000), and creating a reading machine more advanced than the 1970s model.
IBM	1997	Home Page Reader is launched. It is a talking web browser that gives new access to blind and visually disabled users.
Lernout & Hauspie	1997	Buys the Kurzweil Artificial Intelligence company
Microsoft	1997	Internet Explorer 4 is released
Twentieth Century Fox Film Corp and Brandywine Productions	1997	The motion picture *Alien: Resurrection* debuts
Microsoft	1999	Office 2000 is released
Microsoft	2000	Launches Windows 2000 with "Narrator" feature included.
FreedomScientific	2000	This company, the maker of JAWS for Windows, was founded
Texas Instruments	2001	"In 2001 TI left the speech synthesis business, selling it to Sensory Inc. of Santa Clara, CA." (*Texas Instruments*, Wikipedia, retrieved 6/23/09)
Apple	2001	Mac OS X for desktops is released
Microsoft	2001	Windows XP is released
Microsoft	2001	Internet Explorer 6 is bundled with Windows XP and released
Adrianne Wortzel	2001	"Kiru" the robot is on exhibit in the Whitney Museum of American Art
ScanSoft	2001	Acquires some of Lernout & Hauspie's technology during that company's dissolution
Warner Bros, DreamWorks SKG, Stanley Kubrick Productions	2001	The motion picture *AI: Artificial Intelligence* debuts
Microsoft	2001	Windows Vista is released
Ben Rubin and Mark Hansen	2002	"Listening Post" exhibit opens at the Whitney Museum of American Art
Microsoft	2003	Office 2003 is released
Twentieth Century Fox Film Corp	2004	The motion picture *I, Robot* debuts
Nuance	2005	Merges with ScanSoft
Nuance	2006	Dragon NaturallySpeaking 9 is released
Apple	2007	The first iPhone is released.
Pixar Studios	2008	The motion picture *WALL-E* debuts
DreamWorks SKG	2008	The motion picture *Eagle Eye* debuts
Rensselaer Polytechnic Institute/Debbie Rowe	2008	Research on the application of text-to-speech technology in the composition research field proceeds
CBS "60 Minutes"	2008	Airs the segment "Brain Power" discussing the use of brain-computer interfaces
Honda	2009	A brain-machine interface version of ASIMO is introduced
Microsoft	2009	Windows 7 is released

Chapter 3
Digital Speech Technology:
An Overview

H.S. Venkatagiri
Iowa State University, USA

ABSTRACT

Speech generating devices (SGDs) – both dedicated devices as well as general purpose computers with suitable hardware and software – are important to children and adults who might otherwise not be able to communicate adequately through speech. These devices generate speech in one of two ways: they play back speech that was recorded previously (digitized speech) or synthesize speech from text (text-to-speech or TTS synthesis). This chapter places digitized and synthesized speech within the broader domain of digital speech technology. The technical requirements for digitized and synthesized speech are discussed along with recent advances in improving the accuracy, intelligibility, and naturalness of synthesized speech. The factors to consider in selecting digitized and synthesized speech for augmenting expressive communication abilities in people with disabilities are also discussed. Finally, the research needs in synthesized speech are identified.

INTRODUCTION

Talking machines are commonplace. Examples include toys that talk, greeting cards that speak to you, telephones that announce the calling telephone owner's name, elevators and home security systems that give spoken warnings, and, of course, communication and control devices for persons with certain disabilities, which are the subject of this book. Tape recorders, which record and playback speech using magnetic tapes, have been around for more than 75 years. These analog devices have been largely replaced by digital sound devices that store sounds including speech in the form of numbers and convert numbers back into sound waves during playback. Applications that require a small and predetermined number of words or sentences such as a simple toy, a greeting card, or a warning system can use stored digital speech data. However, a different approach needs to be used if an application

DOI: 10.4018/978-1-61520-725-1.ch003

requires a very large number of words or requires words that cannot be fully anticipated ahead of time. Obviously, a telephone that announces the calling telephone owner's name cannot possibly store the spoken forms of the names of all the telephone subscribers in the world. Instead, it should be able to convert text-based names stored in the telephone companies' databases into the spoken form on the fly. Similarly, a person who uses a speech generating device for conversation should not ideally be limited to a small, preselected vocabulary.

Typically, we communicate our thoughts through speech and writing. There is, as yet, no technology that can transform thoughts held in a person's brain directly into speech. We can, however, convert any digitally stored text (a word or a string of words typed at a keyboard or input through other means) into speech. This is known as text-to-speech (TTS) synthesis. Table 1 in the Appendix lists selected applications of TTS synthesis. This chapter will provide a general description of the technology for digital recording and playback of speech and TTS synthesis. The topics covered include an overview of speech technology, a discussion of the technology and uses of digitized speech (digitally recorded speech), a detailed but nonmathematical description of processes involved in converting text into speech, and a discussion of solutions and innovations developed over the years to improve the intelligibility and acceptability of TTS output to listeners. The overall objective is to provide the reader the background information necessary to understand both the potential and the limitations of digital speech technology to meet the complex communication needs of people with disabilities.

Figure 1. The world of speech technology

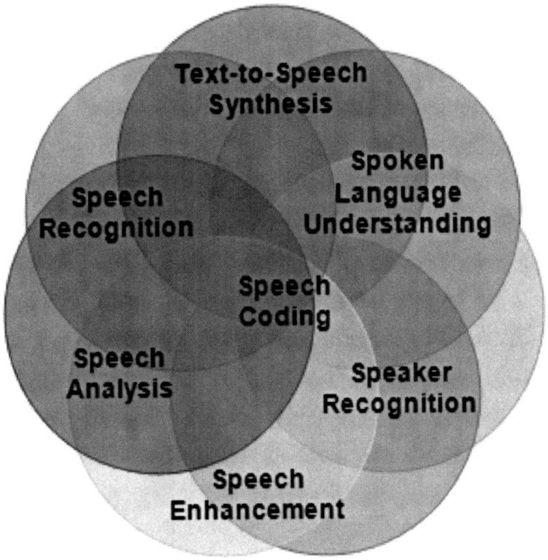

MANY FACETS OF SPEECH TECHNOLOGY

Digital speech technology – the technology that makes talking machines possible – is a burgeoning field with many interrelated applications as shown in Figure 1. The overlapping circles indicate that all these diverse applications share a common knowledge base although each application also requires a set of solutions unique to it. *Speech coding*, which is an essential part of every digital speech application, is the process of generating a compressed (compact) digital representation of speech for the purposes of storage and transmission (Spanias, 1994). The familiar MP3 (MPEG-1 Audio Layer 3; Brandenburg, 1999) is an efficient coding technique for music; some coding techniques used in machine-generated speech will be discussed later in this chapter. Acoustic *speech analysis*, analyzing and graphically displaying the frequency, intensity, and durational parameters of speech (Kent & Read, 1992), has provided the foundational data that are necessary for implementing TTS synthesis, especially a type of synthesis known as the synthesis by rule or formant synthesis (Rigoll, 1987). Formant synthesis is discussed in a later section.

Speech recognition (Holmes & Holmes, 2001; Venkatagiri, 2002) is the opposite of TTS synthesis; it involves converting speech into text. Many real-world applications such as the computer mediated instruction in reading (Williams, Nix, & Fairweather, 2000) require both digitized or synthesized speech and speech recognition technologies. *Spoken language understanding* (Bangalore, Hakkani-Tür, & Tur, 2006) goes beyond speech recognition (i.e. merely converting spoken words into written words) in that it allows a person to have a limited dialog with a computer. Nowadays most U.S. airlines provide arrival and departure information over the phone in response to spoken enquiries and, typically, the telephone directory assistance in the U. S. requires a scripted dialog with a computer. In such a system, the computer "understands" a limited number of spoken queries and retrieves relevant data from its database to provide a spoken response using either TTS synthesis or digitized speech (Zue & Glass, 2000). Humans, with little conscious processing, recognize a familiar speaker's voice. *Speaker recognition* (Campbell, 1997) bestows this ability to computers and is used, among other purposes, for access control and bank transactions over the telephone. Finally, *speech enhancement* (Benesty, Makino, & Chen, 2005) strives to improve the perceptual qualities of speech produced by a speaker so that listeners can better understand speech in difficult listening situations (e.g., battlefield conditions) as well as the speech of individuals with speech disorders. Devices that enhance speech intelligibility (e.g., *Speech Enhancer*; http://www.speechenhancer.com) may be a better alternative to some people who might otherwise need speech-generating devices (SGDs) because it utilizes the natural speaking ability of a person instead of the much slower and more tedious access to digitized or synthesized speech produced by a machine.

BACKGROUND

Digitized Speech

The term "digitized speech," in the present context, is slightly misleading. All speech produced by a computer or any other microprocessor-based device is digitized speech. However, in the literature, it is customary to distinguish between "digitized speech," which is a short form for "digitally recorded human speech" and "synthesized speech," which involves conversion of text into speech through digital processing. Both forms of speech have distinct advantages and disadvantages when used for augmentation of expressive communication in people with disabilities. The selection of either form should be based on a number of factors as discussed later in this chapter.

Analog-to-Digital Conversion

Speech, in its original (analog) form, is a pressure wave in air whose magnitude varies continuously in time. This analog wave is captured by a microphone, which converts it into an analog electrical wave. In order to digitally record these analog electrical signals, two values must be specified: sampling rate and quantization level. The sampling rate determines how often the analog electrical signal is measured and quantization level determines how accurately the measurement is made to derive a set of numbers that represents the analog wave. An *analog-to-digital converter*, a specialized electronic circuitry found in the computer's sound card and in other devices capable of digitally recording sound, samples the electrical signal at user-selected time intervals (sampling rate) to assign it values of magnitude within a user-selected range (quantization).

Natural speech contains significant energy in frequencies up to 8000 hertz (Hz) and beyond (Dunn & White, 1940). A sinusoid ("pure tone") with an upper frequency limit of 8000 Hz has 8000 positive peaks and 8000 negative peaks. A minimum of 16,000 samples (measurements) per second are required to digitally represent the pressure variations of this sound – 8000 for positive peaks and 8000 for negative peaks. The minimum sampling rate, often referred to as the *Nyquist frequency* is, therefore, equal to two times the highest frequency component of the analog signal being digitized. In practice, a sampling rate which is slightly higher than the Nyquist frequency is employed because anti-aliasing (low-pass) filters used to filter out frequencies above the preset upper frequency limit are not perfectly tuned and frequencies slightly above the cutoff frequency of the filter are often found in the filtered signals. If not accounted for, these higher frequencies introduce distortions in the digitized sound.

The analog sound wave varies continuously in pressure (or voltage in the electrical analog) but must be assigned a discrete value when sampled. If the analog-to-digital converter can assign only two values – +1 volt (V) when the peak is positive and -1V when the peak is negative, the quantization level is equal to 1 bit because the values can be coded as a 1 and a 0, respectively, and stored using one bit of memory in a microprocessor. Similarly, a two-bit quantizer has four different discrete output values, and a n-bit quantizer has 2^n output values. In digital sound recording, it is common to set quantization level to 8 (0-255 values), 10 (1,024 values), 12 (4096 discrete values), 14 (16,384 values), or 16 bits (65,536 values).

The signal-to-noise ratio (SNR) of the digitized speech is significantly influenced by the quantization level. Higher bit values result in smaller quantization error and, therefore, larger SNR. Each additional bit (beyond the first one) increases SNR (or reduces noise) by about six decibels (dB) (O'Shaughnessy, 1987). However, the SNR also depends on the average signal amplitude level which, in the case of speech, varies widely because some unvoiced fricatives are inherently very soft while some vowels are relatively quite intense. In order to accommodate the wide dynamic range of speech signal and still obtain a respectable 35 - 40 dB SNR, at least a 12-bit resolution is necessary (O'Shaughnessy, 1987). The amount of data generated per unit time through analog to digital conversion is called the *bit rate* (or data rate) and is measured in bits per second (bps). Bit rate is the product of sampling rate multiplied by the bit value of the quantizer. A sampling rate of 16 kHz (16,000 samples per second) combined with 16-bit quantization produces 256,000 bits of speech data per second and requires 32,000 bytes of memory to store each second of speech.

Speech Coding

Several speech coding techniques have been developed to reduce bit rate and thus the bandwidth required for transmission and the memory required for the storage of the data without significantly reducing intelligibility, naturalness, and SNR. Broadly, speech coding techniques fall into two categories: *waveform coding* and *parametric coding* (or *vocoding*). Waveform coding attempts to preserve the general shape of the original analog waveform in digitized data. Parametric coding, on the other hand, stores the acoustic features (or parameters), such as the fundamental frequency (f_0) and the vocal tract transfer function, in digital form.

Waveform Coding

The output of the analog to digital conversion, as described above, is referred to as the *pulse code modulation* (PCM). PCM requires a minimum of 12,000 bytes of memory to store each second of "telephone" quality speech. (Note: Although it is typical to express coding efficiency in bits per second, which is a measure of information transmission, the readers of this book may be more concerned with the memory requirements for storage expressed in the more familiar bytes per unit of speech). A compression technique known as *log PCM*, which uses a non-uniform step size for quantizing speech and thus boosts the intensity of soft sounds relative to more intense sounds, can produce equivalent SNR while reducing bit rate by a third (8000 bytes of memory for each second of speech) (O'Shaughnessy, 1987). Because most of the acoustic energy is concentrated in the lower frequencies (<1 kHz) in the speech signal, successive samples in PCM-coded data contain a large amount of redundant information. Variations of PCM, *differential pulse code modulation* (DPCM), *adaptive differential pulse code modulation* (ADPCM), *delta modulation* (DM), etc. take advantage of this fact to reduce bit rate and, as a result, the memory requirements of coded speech. For example, memory requirements for storing speech may be halved from 8000 bytes for log PCM to 4000 bytes per second for DM in which a one-bit quantizer is used at a sampling rate of 32 kHz to digitize differences in amplitude between successive samples rather than absolute amplitude values without significantly compromising quality (Alencar & da Rocha Jr. 2005; Jayant & Noll, 1984). Compared to parametric coding discussed below, waveform coding is computationally simpler and has better speech quality. It is used for telecommunication and other purposes in the 16-64 kilobits/second range (between 4 and 8 kilobytes/second). Further compression is not possible without significant distortion in the signal.

Parametric Coding

Waveform coding contains a significant amount of redundant information even when data compression techniques such as DM are employed. Two techniques – *formant coding* and *linear predictive coding* (LPC) – yield a even higher degree of data compression. Unlike waveform coding techniques, which seek to preserve the general shape of the sound wave being digitized, parametric coding techniques digitize only the perceptually important acoustic parameters of speech. The difference between waveform and parametric coding is analogous to storing a scanned somewhat grainy (compressed) picture of a person (waveform coding) versus storing a list of distinguishing features of the person such as the height, weight, hair color, the shape of the face, etc. (parametric coding). In parametric coding, the speech units (speech sounds, syllables, words, or sentences) have to be synthesized (recreated) using the list of parameters extracted from the original signal. Both formant and LPC coding of speech is based on the source-filter theory of speech production (Fant, 1960) and model (recreate) the acoustic output at the lips. For this reason, they are sometimes referred to as *terminal analog synthesizers*.

In formant coding, the source waveform (natural speech) is analyzed to extract up to 60 acoustic parameters such as the center frequencies, bandwidths, and amplitudes of formants, amplitudes of voicing, frication, aspiration, and nasal resonance, etc. (Allen, Hunnicutt, & Klatt, 1987; Witten, 1982). Although formant coding produces highly compressed speech and, when properly implemented, can produce high quality speech, it is not widely used today because synthesis of speech from the acoustic parameters is computationally intensive and it requires considerable trial and error experimentation to develop a working system (Dutoit, 1997). In LPC, the unit of speech to be coded (a speech sound, syllable, word, or sentence) is divided into frames of uniform duration. A frame rate of 30 to 50 per second of speech is sufficient to produce good quality speech. The coding process involves estimating the vocal tract transfer function in each time frame as a set of predictor coefficients, estimating the intensity and frequency of the residue (what remains after the estimated transfer function is filtered out), classifying each frame as either periodic or aperiodic, and specifying a pitch period (fundamental frequency) if the frame is classified as periodic. Bit rates as low as 800 bps are sufficient to crudely model speech using LPC although high quality speech requires rates of 5000 bps or more (Hollingum and Cassford, 1988). The LPC is a computationally efficient coding method and can produce high quality speech. For this reason, many modern telecommunication applications such as the mobile phones and voice over the Internet (VoIP) use variations of LPC to transmit speech. The variants of LPC such as the *code excited linear prediction* (CELP) attempt to optimize the coding of certain perceptually important features of speech while keeping the bit rate low (Yang, 2004). Formant and LPC coding techniques are also used in TTS synthesis although, here too, LPC has a dominating presence.

TTS SYNTHESIS

The conversion of text into speech occurs in at least three different stages: *text processing* (often referred to as *natural language processing* or NLP in the literature), *phonetic transcription of text*, and *speech synthesis* through digital signal processing (DSP). These stages are best described with an example. Henton (2003) describes a "show and tell" session during SpeechTEK 2002 conference where 10 major manufacturers of TTS systems demonstrated their products. One of the requirements of the session was to synthesize the following sentence: "From Laurel Canyon Blvd., turn left onto Mulholland Dr.; Dr. O'Shaughnessy lives at the yellow house on the corner at the first 'Stop' sign: 2529 Wonderland Ave." (Henton, 2003). The target dialect for this sentence was the U.S. General American English.

Text Processing

In this sentence, text processing should correctly expand the abbreviations ("Mulholland Drive" and "Doctor O'Shaughnessy"; "Canyon Boulevard"; "Wonderland Avenue"), format numbers correctly to fit the context ("twenty-five twenty-nine" or, perhaps, "two five two nine" but not "two thousand five hundred [and] twenty nine"), and divide the sentence into intonation phrases (an utterance with a particular pitch pattern and a prominently stressed "nuclear" syllable to convey a single piece of information) based on punctuation marks, morphosyntactic analysis, and heuristics ("Dr. O'Shaughnessy lives at the yellow HOUSE" and "on the corner at the first 'STOP' sign" where capitalized syllables have nuclear accent). Morphosyntactic analysis will be required to correctly pronounce "house" with an /s/ since it is a noun in the present context; it would be pronounced with a /z/ if it were a verb ("We house them in the church"). Although not present in our example sentence, some other aspects of text processing include gemination and homophones. In a word like "unneeded," the /n/ is geminated but not in a word like "funny" in spite of the two "n" letters together (Kaye, 2005). Homophones ("wind" as in "wind is blowing" and "wind up the business") should be correctly recognized. Heuristics and sophisticated syntactic analysis will be needed to pronounce them correctly.

Text processing, therefore, is a crucial step for generating the correct utterance prosody as well as accurate pronunciation of individual words. Broadly, this step involves two processes: text normalization and morphosyntactic processing. During text normalization, abbreviations are expanded and text is reformatted to conform to the spoken form. For example, "$5,000,000" is changed to "five million dollars." Morphosyntactic processing involves identifying parts of speech and intonation phrases using rules of grammar and heuristics. Text processing is, perhaps, the weakest link in today's TTS synthesis. This is, in part, because the process cannot always be neatly divided into text normalization and morphosyntactic processing. Contrast, for instance, "$5" with "$5 bill" (Sproat, Möbius, Maeda, and Tzoukermann, 1998). The first phrase expands to "five dollars" whereas the second, "five dollar bill." The text normalization of the second phrase requires morphosyntactic analysis to recognize that "$5" is functioning as an adjective and plural nouns cannot serve as adjectives in English. Secondly, generating correct utterance prosody frequently requires a knowledge of the meaning or the intention behind the utterance, which goes well beyond morphosyntactic analysis. The analysis of semantics and pragmatics of utterances requires significant amount of time and processing capacity and may impose unacceptable delay in TTS output (Dutoit, 1997). Moreover, computers are not still very good at this type of analysis regardless of time and effort invested.

Phonetic Transcription

Our example sentence about O'Shaughnessy has 128 letters but 142 phonemes excluding spaces and punctuation marks. A complete phonetic transcription, of course, must include information on rate, pauses, stress, and intonation in addition to the specification of phonemes and phonologically significant allophones. In languages such as English and French, converting text into machine-pronounceable phonetic form presents significant challenges because spelling is often unreliable as a guide to pronunciation. Proper names like "O'Shaughnessy" offer the greatest challenge. Apart from the difficulty of transcribing "augh" as /ɑ/ since it takes a different form in common words like "laugh," the designers of the TTS system must also decide whether to use the Irish (/oʃɑknəsi/) or the British (/oʃɑnəsi/ or /ʃɑnəsi/) pronunciation of this name. Typically, modern TTS systems use a combination of rule-based and dictionary-based solutions to derive a phonetic representation of sentences (Dutoit, 1997). Languages that have phonetically consistent spelling such as those spoken in South Asia may largely use rule-based transcription (Choudhury, 2003). Purely rule-based systems cannot adequately account for numerous irregularities in spelling in languages such as English. A dictionary that specifies pronunciation is required to produce high quality TTS output in these languages. Only the frequently used base words and affixes (morphemes) are included in the dictionary to keep it to a manageable size (Coker, 1985). Derived words (those modified with prefixes and suffixes and compound words) are phonetically transcribed combining the pronunciation of the base word(s) and affix(es) retrieved from the dictionary. Levinson, Olive, and Tschirgi, (1993) have described a TTS system that uses a dictionary of 30,000 base words to generate 166,000 different words. Words and proper names not found in the dictionary are transcribed using a set of letter-to-sound rules and by analogy (how a similar group of letters sound in words included in the dictionary).

Speech Synthesis

Phonetic transcription of the text is used to calculate the acoustic parameters necessary to drive a speech synthesizer. Since most languages including English have between 30 and 60 phonemes (including phonologically important allophones), a relatively small amount of memory is sufficient to store the acoustic parameters needed to synthesize all the words in a language. This was the approach used in early speech synthesizers when memory was expensive and memory chips had limited capacity (Green, Logan, & Pisoni, 1986).

Formant Synthesis

Formant coding (Styger & Keller, 1994), described earlier, is one method to convert phonemes into speech sounds. Formant coding is the purest form of machine-generated speech because only the acoustic data for individual phonemes and allophones obtained from a model speaker and gleaned from many years of phonetic research are used to drive a digital signal processor (DSP) to produce speech. The pioneering efforts of Klatt (1987) have shown that formant synthesis can produce high quality speech if sufficient attention is paid to coarticulatory features. It is well known that the articulation of a phoneme is context dependent; in particular, the surrounding sounds, the length of utterance, intonation, sentence stress, and speaking rate affect the acoustic realization of a phoneme (Klatt, 1987). The reasonably intelligible (Drager, Clark-Serpentine, Johnson, & Roeser, 2006; Mirenda & Beukelman, 1987; Ratcliff, Coughlin, & Lehman, 2002) and popular (especially as a device for communication augmentation) DECtalk™ TTS system is a fine example of formant coding.

The development of different voices based on age, gender, and dialect differences is relatively straight forward in formant synthesis because formant trajectories may be adjusted so that they are consistent with changes in pitch (Venkatagiri & Ramabadran, 1995). However, both the development of spectral data for phonemes and allophones and the development of rules and heuristics for spectral smoothing across phoneme and word boundaries require considerable effort making formant synthesis difficult and time-consuming to implement (Dutoit, 1997). Because formant synthesis involves creating speech from acoustic data (rather than from gluing together bits of prerecorded human speech as other methods discussed below do), the voice sounds non-human.

Concatenative Synthesis

Most modern speech synthesizers use concatenative synthesis. They generate speech by concatenating (joining together) small pieces of digitally recorded human speech (Henton, 2002). The units of speech, such as the phonemes or some other similarly short segments of speech that may or may not correspond to traditional linguistic entitities, are modeled by a "voice talent" (a professionally trained speaker) in carefully constructed carrier phrases and stored in a "voice database" either in the form of waveform-coded or parametrically coded signals. Because concatenative synthesis involves using human-generated speech, it has the potential to produce highly intelligible and natural-sounding speech. However, as discussed above, the realization of a phone (speech sound) is significantly affected by the sounds that precede and follow it within an utterance, a phenomenon known as coarticulation (Olive, Greenwood, & Coleman, 1993; Pickett, 1999). Mere concatenation of phones without taking into account coarticulatory features results in discontinuous and nearly unintelligible speech (O'Shaughnessy, et al, 1988; Parsons, 1987). Early concatenative TTS products that used a simple phoneme-based concatenation produced speech of poor intelligibility and naturalness (Green, Logan, & Pisoni, 1986).

While most TTS products have a full inventory of phonemes of the target languages in their voice databases, coarticulatory features are better preserved if the units of concatenation are larger than a phoneme. The *diphone* is a linguistic unit that extends from the center of one phoneme to the center of the next phoneme (Schwartz, et al, 1979) and, therefore, incorporates the crucial interphoneme coarticulation. Diphones are widely used in concatenative speech synthesis (Dutoit, 1997). Most languages have a relatively small number of diphones and it is not necessary to include all possible diphones in a language in the voice database of a TTS product because some pairs of phonemes are relatively devoid of coarticulation (Olive, Santen, Möbius, & Shih, 1998). In the Bell Labs' multilingual TTS product, the number of diphones ranged from 445 for Japanese to 1499 for Russian with a mean of 786 for the eight languages (Olive, Santen, Möbius, & Shih, 1998). How many diphones (or any of the other units of speech discussed below) are used in the voice database of a TTS product is based on a cost benefit analysis. A larger number of units would produce more intelligible and natural-sounding speech but at a higher memory and processing cost. After a certain point, which is determined empirically, the addition of more units would produce negligible gains in the intelligibility and naturalness of speech.

Diphones adequately account for coarticulation that exists at phoneme boundaries. However, coarticulatory influences are not limited to phoneme boundaries; they often extend to whole phonemes as well as to adjacent phonemes within an utterance (Dutoit, 1997; Pickett, 1999). Because nasals, rhotics, and semivowels are especially susceptible to multiple contextual influences, it is important to include special context-sensitive diphones involving these sounds. In addition, to satisfactorily address strong coarticulation beyond diphones within words and at certain word boundaries, a small number of triphones and tetraphones (three- and four- phoneme sequences) may also be included in the database. This polyphone approach to speech synthesis has produced significantly more intelligible speech than a straight diphone-based synthesis (Bigorgne, et al., 1993). Units of speech other than diphones may form the bulk of a voice database for a TTS product. These include demisyllables, the previously mentioned triphones, and half-phones. A demisyllable is one-half of a syllable and is formed by breaking a syllable into two halves with most of the stable portion of the vowel nucleus being in the second half of the syllable (Parsons, 1987). English has about 2000 demisyllables (O'Shaughnessy, et al, 1988). The triphone database can be quite large ranging from about 10,000 (Huang, et al, 1996) to over 70,000 (Olive, Santen, Möbius, & Shih, 1998) in English.

The use of larger units has produced substantial increase in intelligibility and naturalness of synthesized speech but it still significantly lags natural speech in both respects (Schlosser, Blischak, & Koul, 2003; Venkatagiri, 2003). One major obstacle to further improvements in intelligibility and naturalness of TTS synthesis is the "join cost." While diphones, demisyllables, and triphones may adequately model transitions within themselves, spectral and pitch discrepancies occur at the point where two units are joined together contributing to loss of intelligibility and naturalness. *Unit selection synthesis* is a promising approach that seeks to minimize the join cost by selecting the largest available unit (which may span several words) from the acoustic database of a corpus of speech during synthesis (Allauzen, Mohri, & Riley, 2004; Beutnagel, Conkie, & Syrdal, 1998: Möbius, 2003). The availability of fast microprocessors and the negligible cost of computer memory make it possible to select units of optimum size from a large, carefully constructed corpus of speech during concatenation rather than having to work with fixed units. The recent trend in speech synthesis is decidedly in favor of the corpus-based techniques instead of using preset phonetic inventories (of phonemes, diphones, demisyllables, etc.) prepared on the basis of incomplete phonetic-linguistic knowledge. Corpus based techniques better account for coarticulatory influences over larger stretches of speech and, therefore, produce more intelligible and natural-sounding speech. In addition, this trend is facilitated by the development of techniques that automatically label speech data. Several hours of speech provided by a voice talent may be automatically transcribed phonetically using tools that employ hidden Markov models (HMMs) (Makashay, Wightman, Syrdal, & Conkie, 2000; Wightman, Syrdal, Stemmer, Conkie, & Beutnagel, 2000). The resulting transcription is not error-free but compares favorably with those prepared by trained labelers (Makashay, Wightman, Syrdal, & Conkie, 2000).

The hidden Markov modeling, a statistical technique typically used in speech recognition among other real-world applications (Rabiner, 1989), has several advantages when used for speech synthesis. Both the backend development of a database of trained HMMs extracted from a phonetically transcribed corpus of speech as well as the frontend process that actually generates speech from text using that database can be implemented in an efficient and streamlined fashion. The HMMs consist of spectral, pitch, and durational parameters for a set of context-dependent phonemes (or some other sub-word units of speech such as the half-phones). Since the number of detectable context-dependent features is very large, decision trees are used to select the features that are most important for enhancing the intelligibility and naturalness of speech in a language (Tóth, & Németh, 2008). The HMMs may be automatically extracted from a two to four hours long speech corpus provided by a single speaker or several speakers (Masuko, Tokuda, Kobayashi, & Imai, 1997). If HMMs are originally extracted from a multi-speaker speech corpus, the voice characteristics may be adapted to a particular speaker by modifying the HMMs with a five to eight minutes long speech sample obtained from that speaker (Tamura, Masuko, Tokuda, & Kobayashi, 2001).

Specifying Prosody

Prosody is the variations in pitch, amplitude, and duration across units of speech within an utterance and includes syllabic stress (emphasis placed on different syllables within a word), phrasal stress (emphasis placed on different word within an utterance), intonation (variations in pitch over the span of an utterance), duration (duration of syllables within words and of words within the utterance as well as speaking rate), and pausing (at phrase and sentence boundaries). Intelligibility and naturalness of speech are critically dependent on correct prosody. In dictionary-based phonetic transcription of utterances, the syllabic stress is included as part of the pronunciation. Purely rule-based transcription is likely to result in numerous errors in syllable stress assignment in languages such as English because of unpredictability of stress on syllables within words. Punctuation marks serve as a guide for pausing as well as for certain durational differences such as pre-pausal lengthening of syllables in English. Although global changes in speaking rate may be achieved by specifying a rate for a sentence or a range of sentences, appropriate local changes in rate, which are common in natural speech are difficult to produce in TTS output. Phrasal stress and intonation may be incorporated into the utterance by dividing the sentence into intonation phrases using punctuation, morphosyntactic analysis, the knowledge of phonological patterns that exist in a language and heuristics.

At present no completely satisfactory solution exists for inserting an appropriate prosody for different utterances because a knowledge of the context and meaning of and the intention behind an utterance is necessary to derive an appropriate prosody. Most commercially available TTS products use a generic, neutral prosody that may not be fully appropriate but, at the same time, does not sound inappropriate (Monaghan, 1990). Large variations in intonation are possible in formant synthesis because both spectral and source data are specified during synthesis. Large changes in pitch are not possible in LPC-based concatenative synthesis because the spectral data are hard-coded in the LPC data. Dutoit (1997) provides an excellent discussion of many different approaches to the specification of prosody in TTS synthesis.

Generating Speech

Generating speech – either from the acoustic data in the case of formant synthesis or from prerecorded voice data in the case of LPC synthesis – is based on the source-filter theory of speech production (Fant, 1960). Figure 2 shows how the natural speaking process fits into the source-filter model. The larynx is located at the bottom of the pharynx. The pharynx, the oral cavity, and the two nasal passages make up the vocal tract. The source of sound for vowels and sonorants (i.e., nasals and semivowels) is a nearly periodic complex tone generated in the larynx. The source for unvoiced obstruents (i.e., unvoiced fricatives and stops) is a wideband noise generated at the point of constriction in the vocal tract. The constriction occurs when articulators involved in the production of a speech sound come very close to or touch each other. The source for voiced obstruents is a combination of voice produced in the larynx and the noise generated at the point of constriction. The vocal tract acts like a series of acoustic filters and modifies the amplitude spectrum of the source as the sound propagates forward through the vocal tract. The transfer function (the filter characteristics) of the vocal tract changes with changes in the shape of the vocal tract brought about by the different configuration of the articulators. Note that, in Figure 2, the output spectrum shows both resonant peaks called formants and troughs (antiformants).

Figure 2. The source-filter theory of speech production

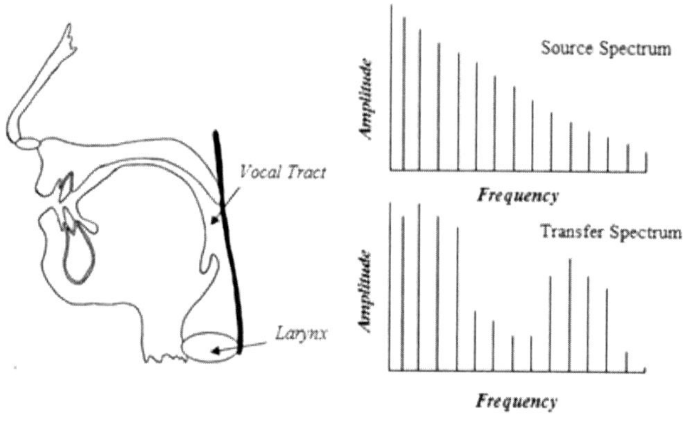

Formant-Synthesized Speech Output

In formant synthesis the source of sound for speech is either a train of periodic pulses simulating voice for the production of vowels and sonorants, a wideband noise for unvoiced obstruents, or a quasi-periodic pulse generator simulating the mixed voice-noise source for voiced obstruents. The digital data representing the voice or the noise or both drive a bank of up to six digital filters dynamically tuned to produce various speech sounds. The filters simulate the transfer function of the vocal tract. The filter bank is organized in parallel or in series depending on the type of speech sound being produced. The cascading filter arrangement (filters arranged in series) more closely resembles the vocal tract without the nasal cavities and, therefore, is a better model for the synthesis of non-nasal voiced sounds. The parallel arrangement yields better results for nasals and unvoiced obstruents (Flanagan, 1957). When we speak, the sound emanating from the lips ("lip radiation") is relatively unconstrained (compared to the enclosed space within the vocal tract), which slightly enhances the amplitude of higher frequency components. The formant synthesizer accounts for this by adding approximately 6 dB/octave to the output. Finally, the output from the formant synthesizer is routed to a digital-to-analog converter which generates the sound waves.

Klatt and Klatt (1990) outlined a number of adjustments that can be made to the simulated glottal source (the periodic pulse train) to improve the naturalness of formant-synthesized speech. The adjustments include adding slight irregularities in the timing of glottal pulses to simulate jitter and diplophonia and adding noise to simulate aspiration and a breathy voice quality. Klatt and Klatt reported that jitter, diplophonia, aspiration on stop sounds, and a breathy voice quality especially towards the end of an utterance as important features of normal voice. They also found that the difference between male and female voices could be heightened by making female voices a little more breathy than male voices. There has not been much additional work done on formant synthesis since the 1990s because LPC- and waveform-based synthesis technologies have been found to produce equivalent or better quality speech at a lower developmental cost.

LPC-Synthesized Speech Output

The LPC synthesis of speech is computationally less complex than formant synthesis because all spectral properties of speech (the transfer function of the vocal tract) are included in the predictor coefficients generated during the coding of the speech unit. Recall that, in LPC, the unit of speech to be coded (a speech sound, syllable, or some other unit) is divided into frames of uniform duration. To recreate each frame, the input to the single digital filter is a train of periodic pulses or a broad-spectrum noise depending on whether the frame was classified as "voiced" or "unvoiced" during the original coding. The parameters that drive the filter include, in addition to the LPC coefficients, the fundamental frequency (if the sound is voiced) and a value representing the overall amplitude of the speech output. The LPC synthesis is based on the "all pole" model, where only the vocal tract resonances (formants) are represented in the output; this fails to adequately account for the presence of perceptually important antiresonances (antiformants) in nasal consonants.

The simple LPC synthesis, as described above, does not allow voice + noise mixed excitation characteristic of voiced obstruents. A single periodic pulse train is used to model these sounds adding to the unnaturalness of speech. Moreover, the use of a purely periodic pulse train to synthesize voiced sounds and the forced binary labeling of each frame of coded speech as either voiced or unvoiced results in a buzzy and unnatural voice quality (Yang, 2004). The voiced segments of natural speech are not completely periodic. The *mixed excitation linear prediction* (MELP) attempts to overcome these drawbacks by using a mix of low-pass filtered periodic pulses and high-pass filtered white noise to synthesize voiced sounds (McCree & Barnwell, 1995).

Waveform-Synthesized Speech Output

Although LPC-based TTS synthesis, a frequency-domain approach, is still popular, the most recent trend in TTS synthesis is to use waveform-based concatenation. Waveform-based methods include the *time-domain pitch-synchronous overlap-add* (TD-PSOLA) (Moulines and Charpentier, 1990) and its variant, the *multiband resynthesis overlap-add* (MBROLA) (Dutoit and Leich, 1993), and the *harmonic-plus-noise model* (HNM) (Stylianou, 2000). These time-domain (waveform-based) concatenative TTS methods afford greater control over prosodic variables such as pitch, duration, and loudness of segments than LPC synthesis. Computationally, they are even more efficient than LPC synthesis although storing waveform-coded speech units requires a large amount of memory. A typical diphone database for a language, which may consist of three to four minutes of speech sampled at 16 kHz with 16 bits resolution, may require about 5 megabytes of memory for uncompressed waveform coding compared to about 200 kilobytes for LPC (Holmes & Holmes, 2001). In HNM, the units of speech that make up the voice database are split into two bands – a low band consisting solely of harmonics and a high band made up of the noise components of speech. The waveform-synthesized speech appears to be slightly more intelligible (Venkatagiri, 2002) and significantly more natural-sounding (Holmes & Holmes, 2001) than either formant-coded or LP-coded speech.

DIGITIZED OR SYNTHESIZED SPEECH?

People who need a speech generating device (SGD) to augment their expressive communication abilities can purchase a dedicated device that produces either digitized speech or synthesized speech or both. They may also use an adapted computer with free or off-the-shelf software and a sound card to produce digitized or synthesized speech. What are the considerations in choosing digitized and synthesized speech? Although digitized speech requires significantly more storage space than synthesized speech, this is no longer an important consideration given that large capacity hard disks and memory chips have become very inexpensive. The advantages of TTS output over digitized speech are mainly two-fold. First, it is relatively easy and quick to program an SGD to produce a TTS message since all that is required is to type in the word or the sentence to be produced.

In contrast, programming a device to produce a digitized speech message requires a sound recording session with a suitable microphone correctly connected to the device, a quiet ambient environment, and a person with an appropriate voice and diction to record the message. Obviously, it would be inappropriate to have a female caregiver serve as a voice source for a male user or an adult to record a message for a child.

Secondly, in TTS systems, novel messages may be created by combining a small number of words in different ways. For instance, if an SGD has "I," "you," "am," "are," "hungry," and "thirsty" displayed on the screen, a TTS system can produce at least six different sentences such as "I am hungry" and "Are you thirsty?" when the user selects these words. Each additional word would allow the production of several more sentences. In a digitized speech system, it is not possible to individually record words and combine them in different ways to produce different messages. Each message such as "I am hungry" and "Are you thirsty?" must be recorded separately and in their entirety. This would, of course, severely limit the number of possible messages that can be displayed on a screen at one time, which, in turn, limits the number of messages that can be accessed at one time. When individual digitized words are combined to form a sentence, they sound more like a list of words than an utterance with a defined prosodic structure. TTS systems automatically impose a prosodic structure on grammatically correct sentences.

Assuming that the recording is done properly, the messages prepared with digitized speech will always have the correct prosody and richly convey the emotional content. In contrast, and as discussed in previous sections, TTS speech output will only approximate the correct prosody for an utterance most of the time and, in many instances, will have a discomfortingly inappropriate prosody. Moreover, the current commercially available TTS systems have no way of incorporating the emotion of an utterance. A sentence such as "I am happy" would sound exactly the same as the sentence "I am angry" as far as the emotional expression is concerned. Thus there are important tradeoffs to consider when choosing digitized and synthesized speech (Cowley & Jones, 1992).

At present, young children, especially those who are of preschool age or younger, are likely to benefit more from digitized speech than synthesized speech. Many commercially available TTS products do not offer a child voice. Clearly, it is inappropriate to use an adult voice for a child. Developing authentic child voices is especially difficult because the high-pitched child voices seem to be much more affected by an interaction between the source and transfer functions than voices that are lower-pitched (Stylianou, 2001). The nature of this interaction is not fully understood at this time. Therefore, the available child voices have proven to be less satisfactory. The DECTalk child voice has been shown to be less intelligible than the adult voices (Mirenda & Beukelman, 1987, 1990). Moreover, a child is likely to be interacting with other children frequently. Studies show that young children do not understand TTS speech as well as digitized speech. Mirenda and Beukelman (1987, 1990) found that 6 to 8 year old children were less accurate in repeating TTS-produced words and short sentences than adults. Similarly, Reynolds and Jefferson (1999) reported that 6-7 and 9-11 years old children had more difficulty understanding the meaning of synthesized speech than digitized speech. Children, much more than adults, are likely to depend on prosodic and emotional cues for understanding the meaning of utterances (Cowley & Jones, 1992). Digitized speech with a prosody appropriate to the intention and emotion of the utterances is highly preferable for younger users of SGDs. A major advantage of the TTS output – the ability to produce many novel utterances by concatenating words in the course of a conversation – is not of critical importance to very young children who need a SGD because they are not usually able to spell words and their vocabulary and knowledge of syntax are likely to be severely limited.

Children as well as adults with significant cognitive deficits may also benefit more from digitized speech. A review of relevant research by Koul (2003) reported that TTS speech was much less intelligible than natural speech to children and adults with developmental disabilities. In spite of advances in acoustic modeling of speech, especially as they relate to coarticulation, the TTS output is significantly less intelligible than natural speech. Listening to speech may be broadly divided into two stages. In the first stage, we analyze the incoming acoustic waveform to extract the phonetic structure of the utterance. In the second stage, the phonetic form of the utterance is analyzed to identify the words and their meanings as well as the meaning of the utterance as a whole. During a typical conversation, we are performing both of these activities simultaneously – even as we are decoding the acoustic-phonetic structure of one portion of an utterance, we are identifying the meaning of words in the portion that preceded it. Duffy and Pisoni (1992) speculated that decoding the acoustic-phonetic structure of even the high quality TTS output may require a substantially greater portion of the available cognitive resources, leaving insufficient resources for higher order linguistic processing. People with cognitive deficits are at a clear disadvantage when listening to TTS output. They may find the high bit rate, uncompressed digitized speech (the closest thing to live speech) more intelligible.

SGDs with TTS output are most appropriate for literate users who require a relatively large vocabulary and the ability to generate novel sentences (i.e., sentences that are not preprogrammed) during discourse. This includes adults with neuromuscular disorders such as amyotrophic lateral sclerosis (ALS). Adult onset neuromuscular disorders may cause severe difficulty with speech production with relatively intact cognition and receptive language ability (Beukelman, Yorkston, & Reichle, 2000). Similarly many older children with neuromuscular (e.g. cerebral palsy) and cognitive (e.g. autism spectrum) disorders will need a TTS-based SGD in school and elsewhere (Glennen & Decoste, 1997). To fully utilize the capabilities of a TTS-based SGD, the user must be able to input text into the device. Preliterate children who are in the process of learning to read and spell words are also good candidates for a TTS-based SGD. Learners with mild educational disabilities appear to benefit from instructional strategies such as a talking word processing software to teach spelling and reading (MacArthur, 2000). Schlosser and Blischak (2001), in their extensive review of research on the use of speech technology with children with autism, found tentative support for its use in the education of children with autism.

FUTURE RESEARCH DIRECTIONS

As discussed above, SGDs for augmented communication use either digitized or synthesized speech. The technology for digitizing and synthesizing speech has come a long way since the days of the slow, 8-bit computers (e.g., Apple II and Commodore 64) with very small memory capacity and no hard disk. With regard to digitized speech, research focused on improving the quality and reducing the bit rate is still a high priority for parametrically coded speech used in telephony and web applications. Digitized speech based SGDs for augmented communication, however, typically use waveform-coded speech. Today's high bit rate, uncompressed digitized speech is virtually indistinguishable from live, natural speech and the use of this type of memory-intensive speech is well within the reach of anyone who can afford a computer. Thus there are no outstanding quality issues with regard to the use of digitized speech for augmented communication. However, there are still other areas of concern that need to be addressed. For instance, even the high quality of digitized speech is less intelligible than live speech because visual cues (facial expression and lip movements), which are an essential part of a dialog (Kim & Davis, 2004), are absent in machine generated speech. Displaying avatars (2-D and 3-D faces) on display screens along with TTS output has been an area of active research in recent years (Tang, Fu, Tu, Hasegawa-Johnson, & Huang, 2008). Synchronizing appropriate facial expressions and lip movements with words is challenging. At present, it depends on marking the text at appropriate points with special codes for different facial expressions. Because digitized speech (unlike synthesized speech) is not based on text, there is no simple way to include the codes for facial expressions.

TTS synthesis is typically evaluated on the basis of accuracy, intelligibility, and naturalness. Accuracy is a measure of how well the text entered into the system is converted into a form suitable for spoken output. Accuracy depends on text processing. In general, current TTS products accurately convert abbreviations, acronyms, numbers, and symbols. Intelligibility is measured by asking listeners to identify words and respond to questions and statements. In ideal listening conditions, the intelligibility of current TTS products is satisfactory (Beutnagel et al., 1999). Word intelligibility scores for the best TTS systems in quiet listening conditions are about 97%, close to what might be expected for live human speech (Kamm, Walker, & Rabiner, 1997). However, in adverse listening conditions of low SNR (Venkatagiri, 2003) and reverberation (Venkatagiri, 2004), the intelligibility of TTS output suffers significantly. Additional research is needed to improve the intelligibility of TTS synthesis in less than ideal listening conditions. Pronunciation of proper names is also a continuing problem for all TTS systems and deserves additional research. Perhaps, the weakest link in the current TTS implementation is the naturalness of speech. Naturalness refers to the degree to which machine-generated speech sounds "human" and is closely related to the prosody (pausing, intonation, stress, and rate of speech) of utterances. Although the current TTS products, especially those that use variable unit concatenation and waveform synthesis, do not suffer from the robotic voice quality, they still tend to have unnatural pauses, word emphases, and intonation (Nass and Lee 2001). Most currently available TTS products more or less correctly model the prosody of simple declarative sentences and questions. However, prosody does more than just convey the basic syntactic structure of a sentence. It differentiates new or important information from "old" or unimportant information, phrase, clause, and utterance boundaries and relations, and how the current sentence relates to previous sentences, and the mood of the speaker (degree of certainty, feelings, and so on). Currently, TTS synthesis is unable to correctly model these subtle, highly variable, and acoustically ill-defined aspects of prosody.

An area of TTS research that is especially relevant to augmented communication for people with disabilities is the development of individualized voice. Each of us has a unique voice and it is a part of our personal identity. The loss of voice not only causes difficulties with communication but is also felt as a loss of a part of one's identity. For individuals with progressive neuromuscular disorders with anticipated loss of speaking ability, it is now possible, on an experimental basis, to design a TTS voice based on a corpus of speech collected from the intended user (Iida & Campbell, 2003). The resulting TTS voice sounds more like the voice of the person who uses it. With additional research and development, we may be able to design a unique voice for each individual user in the future.

REFERENCES

Alencar, M. S., & da Rocha, V. C., Jr. (2005). *Communication systems*. New York: Springer US.

Allauzen, C., Mohri, M., & Riley, M. (2004). Statistical modeling for unit selection in speech synthesis. In *Proceedings of the 42nd Annual Meeting of the Association for Computational Linguistics (ACL'2004)*, (pp. 55-62).

Allen, J., Hunnicutt, S., & Klatt, D. (1987). *From text to speech: The MITalk system.* Cambridge, UK. Cambridge University Press. Bangalore, S., Hakkani-Tür, D., & Tur, G. (2006). Introduction to the special issue on spoken language understanding in conversational systems. *Speech Communication, 48*(3-4), 233–238.

Benesty, J., Makino, M., & Chen, J. (2005). *Speech enhancement.* New York: Springer.

Beukelman, D. R., Yorkston, K. M., & Reichle, J. (2000). *Augmentative and alternative communication for adults with acquired neurological disorders.* Baltimore, MD: Paul H. Brooks Publishing.

Beutnagel, M., Conkie, A., Schroeter, J., Stylianou, Y., & Syrdal, A. (1999). *The AT&T Next-Gen TTS System.* Presented at the Joint Meeting of ASA, EAA, and DAGA, Berlin, Germany.

Beutnagel, M., Conkie, A., & Syrdal, A. K. (1998). Diphone synthesis using unit selection, In *Proceedings of the 3rd ESCA/COCOSDA International Workshop on Speech Synthesis,* (pp. 185-190).

Bigorgne, D., Boeffard, O., Cherbonnel, B., Emerard, F., Larreur, D., Le Saint-Milon, J. L., et al. (1993). Multilingual PSOLA text-to-speech system. In *IEEE International Conference on Acoustics, Speech, and Signal Processing, ICASSP-93,* (Vol.2, pp.187-190).

Brandenburg, K. (1999). *MP3 and AAC explained.* Paper presented at the AES 17th International Conference on High Quality Audio Coding. Retrieved February 23, 2009 from http://iphome.hhi.de/smolic/MMK/mp3_and_aac_brandenburg.pdf

Campbell, J. P. Jr. (1997). Speaker recognition: A tutorial. *Proceedings of the IEEE, 85*(9), 1437–1462. doi:10.1109/5.628714

Choudhury, M. (2003). *Rule-based grapheme to phoneme mapping for Hindi speech synthesis.* A paper presented at the 90th Indian Science Congress of the International Speech Communication Association (ISCA), Bangalore, India.

Coker, C. H. (1985). A dictionary-intensive letter-to-sound program. *Journal of the Acoustical Society of America., suppl. 1, 78*(S1), S7.

Cowley, C. K., & Jones, D. M. (1992). Synthesized or digitized? A guide to the use of computer speech. *Applied Ergonomics, 23*(3), 172–176. doi:10.1016/0003-6870(92)90220-P

Drager, K. D. R., Clark-Serpentine, E. A., Johnson, K. E., & Roeser, J. L. (2006). Accuracy of repetition of digitized and synthesized speech for young children in background noise. *American Journal of Speech-Language Pathology, 15*(2), 155–164. doi:10.1044/1058-0360(2006/015)

Duffy, S. A., & Pisoni, D. B. (1992). Comprehension of synthetic speech produced by rule: A review and theoretical interpretation. *Language and Speech, 35*(4), 351–389.

Dunn, H. K., & White, S. D. (1940). Statistical measurements on conversational speech. *The Journal of the Acoustical Society of America, 11*(3), 278–288. doi:10.1121/1.1916034

Dutoit, T. (1997). High-quality text-to-speech synthesis: An overview. *Electrical and electronics. Engineers Australia, 17*(1), 25–36.

Dutoit, T., & Leich, H. (1993). MBR-PSOLA: Text-to-speech synthesis based on an MBE re-synthesis of the segments database. *Speech Communication, 13*(3-4), 435–440. doi:10.1016/0167-6393(93)90042-J

Fant, C. G. M. (1960). *Acoustic theory of speech production.* The Hague, The Netherlands: Mouton.

Flanagan, J. L. (1957). Note on the design of terminal analog speech synthesizers. *The Journal of the Acoustical Society of America, 29*(2), 306–310. doi:10.1121/1.1908864

Glennen, S. L., & Decoste, D. C. (1997). *Handbook of augmentative and alternative communication.* San Diego: Singular Publishing Group.

Green, B. G., Logan, J. S., & Pisoni, D. B. (1986). Perception of synthetic speech produced automatically by rule: Intelligibility of eight text-to-speech systems. *Behavior Research Methods, Instruments, & Computers*, *18*(2), 100–107.

Henton, C. (2002). Challenges and rewards in using parametric or concatenative speech synthesis. *International Journal of Speech Technology*, *5*(2), 117–131. doi:10.1023/A:1015416013198

Henton, C. (2003). Taking a look at TTS. *Speech Technology*, (January-February), 27-30.

Hollingum, J., & Cassford, G. (1988). *Speech technology at work*. London: IFS Publications.

Holmes, J., & Holmes, W. (2001). *Speech synthesis and recognition* (2nd Ed.). London: Taylor and Francis.

Huang, X., Acero, A., Adcock, J., Hon, H.-W., Goldsmith, J., Liu, J., & Plumpe, M. (1996). Whistler: A trainable text-to-speech system. In *Proceedings of the 4th International. Conference on Spoken Language Processing (ICSLP '96)*, (pp. 2387-2390).

Iida, A., & Campbell, N. (2003). Speech database for a concatenative text-to-speech synthesis system for individuals with communication disorders. *International Journal of Speech Technology*, *6*(4), 379–392. doi:10.1023/A:1025761017833

Jayant, N. S., & Noll, P. (1984). *Digital coding of waveforms*. Englewood Cliffs, NJ: Prentice-Hall.

Kamm, C., Walker, M., & Rabiner, L. (1997). *The role of speech processing in human-computer intelligent communication*. Paper presented at NSF Workshop on human-centered systems: Information, interactivity, and intelligence.

Kaye, A. S. (2005). Gemination in English. *English Today*, *21*(2), 43–55. doi:10.1017/S0266078405002063

Kent, R. D., & Read, W. C. (1992). *The acoustic analysis of speech*. San Diego: Singular Publishing Group.

Kim, J., & Davis, C. (2004). Investigating the audio–visual speech detection advantage. *Speech Communication*, *44*(1-4), 19–30. doi:10.1016/j.specom.2004.09.008

Klatt, D. H. (1987). Review of text-to-speech conversion of English. *The Journal of the Acoustical Society of America*, *82*(3), 737–793. doi:10.1121/1.395275

Klatt, D. H., & Klatt, L. C. (1990). Analysis, synthesis and perception of voice quality variations among female and male talkers. *The Journal of the Acoustical Society of America*, *87*(2), 820–857. doi:10.1121/1.398894

Koul, R. (2003). Synthetic speech perception in individuals with and without disabilities. *Augmentative and Alternative Communication*, *19*(1), 49–58. doi:10.1080/0743461031000073092

Levinson, S. E., Olive, J. P., & Tschirgi, J. S. (1993). Speech synthesis in telecommunications. *IEEE Communications Magazine*, *31*(11), 46–53. doi:10.1109/35.256873

MacArthur, C. A. (2000). New tools for writing: Assistive technology for students with writing difficulties. *Topics in Language Disorders*, *20*(4), 85–100.

Makashay, M. J., Wightman, C. W., & Syrdal, A. K. A. K., & Conkie, A. D. (2000). Perceptual *evaluation of automatic segmentation in text-to-speech synthesis*. A paper presented at the ICSLP 2000 Conference, Beijing, China.

Masuko, T., Tokuda, K., Kobayashi, T., & Imai, S. (1997). Voice characteristics conversion for HMM-based speech synthesis system. In *Proceedings of ICASSP*, (pp.1611–1614).

McCree, A. V., & Barnwell, T. P. III. (1995). A mixed Excitation LPC vocoder model for low bit rate speech coding. *IEEE Transactions on Speech and Audio Processing, 3*(4), 242–250. doi:10.1109/89.397089

Mirenda, P., & Beukelman, D. R. (1987). A comparison of speech synthesis intelligibility with listeners from three age groups. *Augmentative and Alternative Communication, 3*(3), 120–128. doi:10.1080/07434618712331274399

Mirenda, P., & Beukelman, D. R. (1990). A comparison of intelligibility among natural speech and seven speech synthesizers with listeners from three age groups. *Augmentative and Alternative Communication, 6*(1), 61–68. doi:10.1080/07434619012331275324

Möbius, B. (2003). Rare events and closed domains: Two delicate concepts in speech synthesis. *International Journal of Speech Technology, 6*(1), 57–71. doi:10.1023/A:1021052023237

Monaghan, A. I. C. (1990). A multi-phrase parsing strategy for unrestricted text. In *Proceedings of ESCA workshop on speech synthesis*, (pp. 109-112).

Moulines, E., & Charpentier, F. (1990). Pitch-synchronous waveform processing techniques for text-to-speech synthesis using diphones. *Speech Communication, 9*(5-6), 453–467. doi:10.1016/0167-6393(90)90021-Z

Nass, C., & Lee, K. (2001). Does computer-synthesized speech manifest personality? Experimental tests of recognition, similarity-attraction, and consistency-attraction. *Journal of Experimental Psychology. Applied, 7*(3), 171–181. doi:10.1037/1076-898X.7.3.171

O'Shaughnessy, D. (1987). *Speech communication: human and machine*. Reading, MA: Addison-Wesley Publishing Company.

O'Shaughnessy, D., Barbeau, L., Bernardi, D., & Archambault, D. (1988). Diphone speech synthesis. *Speech Communication, 7*(1), 55–65. doi:10.1016/0167-6393(88)90021-0

Olive, J., van Santen, J., Möbius, B., & Shih, C. (1998). Synthesis. In R. Sproat (Ed.), *Multilingual text-to-speech synthesis: The Bell Labs approach*. (pp. 191–228). Dordrecht, The Netherlands: Kluwer Academic Publishers.

Olive, J. P., Greenwood, A., & Coleman, J. (1993). *Acoustics of American English: A dynamic approach*. New York: Springer-Verlag.

Parsons, T. (1987). *Voice and speech processing*. New York: McGraw-Hill Book Company.

Pickett, J. M. (1999). *The acoustics of speech communication*. Boston: Allyn and Bacon.

Rabiner, L. R. (1989). A tutorial on hidden Markov models and selected applications in speech recognition. *Proceedings of the IEEE, 77*, 257–286. doi:10.1109/5.18626

Ratcliff, A., Coughlin, S., & Lehman, M. (2002). Factors influencing ratings of speech naturalness in augmentative and alternative communication. *AAC: Augmentative and Alternative Communication, 18*(1), 11–19.

Reynolds, M., & Jefferson, L. (1999). Natural and synthetic speech comprehension: Comparison of children from two age groups. *Augmentative and Alternative Communication, 15*(3), 174–182. doi:10.1080/07434619912331278705

Rigoll, G. (1987). The DECtalk system for German: A study of the modification of a text-to-speech converter for a foreign language. *Acoustics, Speech, and Signal Processing, IEEE International Conference on ICASSP '87, 12*, 1450-1453. Retrieved on March 14, 2009 from http://ieeexplore.ieee.org/stamp/stamp.jsp?arnumber=1169464&isnumber=26345

Schlosser, R. W., & Blischak, D. M. (2001). Is there a role for speech output in interventions for persons with autism? A review. *Focus on Autism and Other Developmental Disabilities*, *16*(3), 170–178. doi:10.1177/108835760101600305

Schlosser, R. W., Blischak, D. M., & Koul, R. J. (2003). Roles of speech output in AAC. In R. W. Schlosser (Ed.), *The efficacy of augmentative and alternative communication: toward evidenced-based practice*. (pp. 472–532). Boston: Academic Press.

Schwartz, R., Klovstad, J., Makhoul, J., Klatt, D., & Zue, V. (1979). Diphone synthesis for phonetic vocoding. In *Proceedings of IEEE International Conference on Acoustics, Speech, and Signal Processing,* (pp. 891 – 894). New York: IEEE.

Spanias, A. S. (1994). Speech coding: A tutorial review. *Proceedings of the IEEE*, *82*(10), 1541–1582. doi:10.1109/5.326413

Sproat, R., Möbius, B., Maeda, K., & Tzoukermann, E. (1998). Multilingual text analysis. In R. Sproat (Ed.), *Multilingual text-to-speech synthesis: The Bell Labs Approach.* (pp. 31–87). Dordrecht, The Netherlands: Kluwer Academic Publishers.

Styger, T., & Keller, E. (1994). Formant synthesis. In E. Keller (ed.), *Fundamentals of speech synthesis and speech recognition: Basic concepts, state of the art, and future challenges* (pp. 109-128). Chichester, UK: John Wiley.

Stylianou, Y. (2000). *On the Implementation of the Harmonic Plus Noise Model for Concatenative Speech Synthesis*. Paper presented at ICASSP 2000, Istanbul, Turkey. Retrieved on March 14, 2009 from: http://www.research.att.com/projects/tts/papers/2000–ICASSP/fastHNM.pdf

Stylianou, Y. (2001). Applying the harmonic plus noise model in concatenative speech synthesis. *IEEE Transactions on Speech and Audio Processing*, *9*(1), 21–29. doi:10.1109/89.890068

Tamura, M., Masuko, T., Tokuda, K., & Kobayashi, T. (2001). Adaptation of pitch and spectrum for HMM-based speech synthesis using MLLR. In *Proceedings of ICASSP*, (pp.805–808).

Tang, H., Fu, Y., Tu, J., Hasegawa-Johnson, M., & Huang, T. S. (2008). Humanoid audio–visual avatar with emotive text-to-speech synthesis. *IEEE Transactions on Multimedia, 10*(6), 969–981. doi:10.1109/TMM.2008.2001355

Tang, H., Fu, Y., Tu, J., Huang, T. S., & Hasegawa-Johnson, M. (2008). EAVA: A 3D Emotive Audio-Visual Avatar. *IEEE Workshop on Applications of Computer Vision, 2008. WACV 2008,* (pp. 1-6).

Tóth, B., & Németh, G. (2008). Hidden-Markov-Model based speech synthesis in Hungarian. *Infocommunications Journal, 63*, 30-34. Retrieved on June 21, 2009: http://www.hiradastechnika.hu/data/upload/file/2008/2008_7/HT_0807_5TothNemeth.pdf

Venkatagiri, H., & Ramabadran, T. (1995). Digital speech synthesis: Tutorial. *Augmentative and Alternative Communication, 11*(1), 14–25. doi:10.1080/07434619512331277109

Venkatagiri, H. S. (2002). Speech recognition technology applications in communications disorders. *American Journal of Speech-Language Pathology, 11*(4), 323–332. doi:10.1044/1058-0360(2002/037)

Venkatagiri, H. S. (2003). Segmental intelligibility of four currently used text-to-speech synthesis methods. *The Journal of the Acoustical Society of America, 113*(4), 2094–2104. doi:10.1121/1.1558356

Venkatagiri, H. S. (2004). Segmental intelligibility of three text-to-speech synthesis methods in reverberant environments. *Augmentative and Alternative Communication, 20*(3), 150–163. doi:10.1080/07434610410001699726

Wightman, C. W., Syrdal, A. K., Stemmer, G., Conkie, A. D., & Beutnagel, M. C. (2000). *Perceptually based automatic prosody labeling and prosodically enriched unit selection improve concatenative text-to-speech synthesis*. A paper presented at the ICSLP 2000 Conference, Beijing, China.

Williams, S. M., Nix, D., & Fairweather, P. (2000). Using speech recognition technology to enhance literacy instruction for emerging readers. In B. Fishman & S. O'Connor-Divelbiss (Eds.), *Fourth international conference of the learning sciences*. (pp. 115-120). Mahwah, NJ: Erlbaum.

Witten, I. H. (1982). *Principles of computer speech*. London: Academic Press.

Yang, M. (2004). Low bit rate speech coding. *IEEE Potential*, *23*(4), 32–36. doi:10.1109/MP.2004.1343228

Zue, V. W., & Glass, J. R. (2000). Conversational Interfaces: Advances and Challenges. *Proceedings of the IEEE*, *88*(8), 1166–1180. doi:10.1109/5.880078

ADDITIONAL READING

Allen, J., Hunnicutt, S., & Klatt, D. (1987). *From text to speech: The MITalk system*. Cambridge, UK. Cambridge University Press.

Beutnagel, M., Conkie, A., & Syrdal, A. K. (1998). Diphone synthesis using unit selection, In *Proceedings of the 3rd ESCA/COCOSDA International Workshop on Speech Synthesis*, pp. 185-190.

Henton, C. (2002). Challenges and rewards in using parametric or concatenative speech synthesis. *International Journal of Speech Technology*, *5*(2), 117–131. doi:10.1023/A:1015416013198

Henton, C. (2003). Taking a look at TTS. *Speech Technology*, January-February. 27-30.

Klatt, D. H. (1987). Review of text-to-speech conversion of English. *The Journal of the Acoustical Society of America*, *82*(3), 737–793. doi:10.1121/1.395275

Moulines, E., & Charpentier, F. (1990). Pitch-synchronous waveform processing techniques for text-to-speech synthesis using diphones. *Speech Communication*, *9*(5-6), 453–467. doi:10.1016/0167-6393(90)90021-Z

O'Shaughnessy, D. (1987). *Speech communication: Human and machine*. Reading, MA: Addison-Wesley Publishing Company.

Stylianou, Y. (2000). On the Implementation of the Harmonic Plus Noise Model for Concatenative Speech Synthesis. Paper presented at *ICASSP 2000*, Istanbul, Turkey. Retrieved on March 14, 2009 from: http://www.research.att.com/projects/tts/papers/2000–ICASSP/fastHNM.pdf.

Syrdal, A. K., Bennett, R. W., & Greenspan, S. L. (1995). *Applied speech technology*. Boca Ratan, FL. CRC Press.

Venkatagiri, H. S. (2003). Segmental intelligibility of four currently used text-to-speech synthesis methods . *The Journal of the Acoustical Society of America*, *113*(4), 2094–2104. doi:10.1121/1.1558356

Yang, M. (2004). Low bit rate speech coding. *IEEE Potential*, *23*(4), 32–36. doi:10.1109/MP.2004.1343228

APPENDIX

Table 1. Some uses of text-to-speech synthesis technology

"Read" text on the computer screen and in the digital books	People with visual impairment may need "screen readers" to access computer screen contents and digital books.
Augmentative communication devices	Computer programs or dedicated devices that augment expressive communication abilities of individuals with certain disabilities.
Access to emails	People who are away from home or workplace can access email over the phone.
Educational activities	Computers and sophisticated educational toys that use speech as part of the multimedia instruction.
Voice response systems	Customer service over the telephone or at self-service kiosks in shopping centers, airports, etc..
Automated broadcasts	Informing and alerting the public about breaking news through general broadcasts or subscribers through telephones calls.

Section 2
Emerging Technologies

Chapter 4
Humanizing Vox Artificialis:
The Role of Speech Synthesis in Augmentative and Alternative Communication

D. Jeffery Higginbotham
University at Buffalo, USA

ABSTRACT

In this chapter, the authors will discuss the use of speech synthesis as a human communication tool in what is now referred to as Augmentative and Alternative Communication (AAC). The authors will describe the history and use of speech synthesis in AAC, relevant stakeholders, a framework for evaluating speech synthesis in AAC and relevant research and development with respect to intelligibility, comprehension, social interaction, emotional expressivity and personal identity potential of current implementations of speech synthesis into SGD technologies. Throughout the chapter recommendations will be made for making SGDs more effective and appropriate for social interaction and emotional expression. This chapter will also provide 1st person accounts of relating to SGD use in order to provide a stakeholder perspective.

INTRODUCTION

What has happened to the human voice. Vox Humana. Hollering, shouting, quiet talking, buzz. I was leaving the airport, it's in Atlanta. You know you leave the gate, you take a train that took you to concourse of your choice, and I get in to this train. Dead silence, Few people are seated or standing. Up above you hear a voice that once was human voice, but no longer, now it talks like a machine - "Concourse 1, Fort Worth, Dallas, Lubbock" - that kind of voice. And just then the doors are about to close - pneumatic doors - one young couple rush in and push open the doors and get in. Without missing a beat, that voice above says, "Because of late entry, we're delayed 30 seconds". The people looked at that couple as if that couple just committed mass murder, you know. And the couple are shrinking like this, you know... I'm known for my talking . I'm gabby. And so I say, "George Orwell, your time has come and gone!" I expect a laugh - dead silence. And now they look at me and I'm

DOI: 10.4018/978-1-61520-725-1.ch004

with the couple, the three of us are at the Hill of Calvary on Good Friday. And then I say, "My God, where's the human voice"? And just then there's a little baby - maybe the baby is about a year or something. And I say, "Sir or Madam" to the baby. "What is your opinion of the human species"? Well what does the baby do? baby starts giggling. I said, "Thank God! The sound of a human voice." [Terkel (2008)].

Studs Terkel's soliloquy on the human condition sets the stage for this chapter on the use of synthesized speech in computerized Speech Generating Devices (SGD) by individuals with Complex Communication Needs (CCN). For more than any other application of this technology, speech synthesis (and supporting computer tools) is charged with the responsibility to serve as a major expressive modality during social interactions. As argued in this chapter, this responsibility goes beyond that of merely being a tool to convey information, it also serves importantly as an interactive tool for achieving common ground and as a means for conveying a speaker's, health, attitude, affiliations, emotion, meaning and identity. What can be done to humanize speech synthesis for individuals who use SGDs as their *social voice*? What is it about the vox artificialis that keeps it from being *one's voice*?

In the course of this chapter, we will discuss the use of speech synthesis as a human communication system in what is now referred to as Augmentative and Alternative Communication (AAC)[1]. We will describe 1) how speech synthesis is currently used in Speech Generating Devices (SGDs); 2) the stakeholders in AAC; 3) a history of speech synthesis in AAC, 4) frameworks for evaluating the Augmented Voice. We will then cover AAC research and development in areas of speech intelligibility, sentence and discourse comprehension, social interaction, and emotion and identity. Throughout the chapter, recommendations are presented for improving speech synthesis devices to make them more effective and appropriate for interaction and expression. That is to say, we will be responding to Terkel's plea to humanize vox artificialis.

SYNTHETIC SPEECH AND AAC TECHNOLOGIES: SPEECH GENERATING DEVICES

Over the past three decades, major technological advances in AAC area have resulted in special purpose computerized communication aids and improved microcomputer access for those individuals with significant communication and physical access challenges. These advances include customized input and computer interfaces, sophisticated vocabulary databases and search algorithms, synthetic speech output, as well as new ways to access to standard computers and the internet.

Two forms of speech output used in past and current AAC are text-to-speech synthesis and digitized speech. We will focus here on those SGDs that utilize some form of text-to speech synthesis. Speech synthesis is inextricably linked with the SGD platform in which it is employed. The SGD features influence the output method used to speak a message (e.g., speak after each sentence, speak after each word, speak after each keypress), the prosodic capabilities and flexibility associated with message production (e.g., utterance intonation, word emphasis) and the speech modifications available to the user during face-to-face interaction (i.e. ability to change volume, speed, voice settings in real-time).

The form-factor for the modern SGD varies from handheld PDA's, laptop PCs, and specialized platforms dedicated to AAC use (Figure 1). Users of AAC technologies produce speech output by selecting a pre-stored message or by constructing a message through individual letters and stored words and phrases. Message construction can be facilitated through word prediction,

Figure 1. Four contemporary speech generating devices (SGDs)

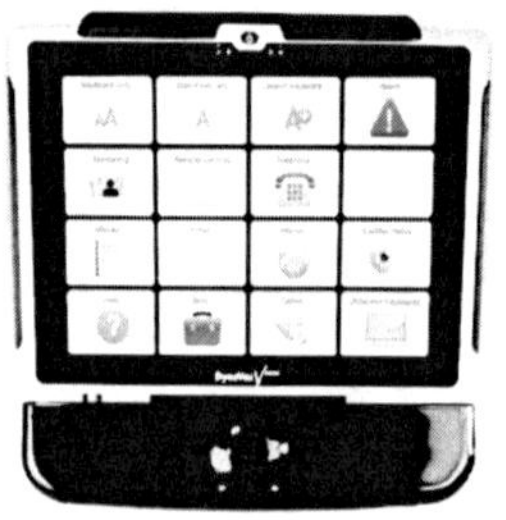

DynaVox Series 5

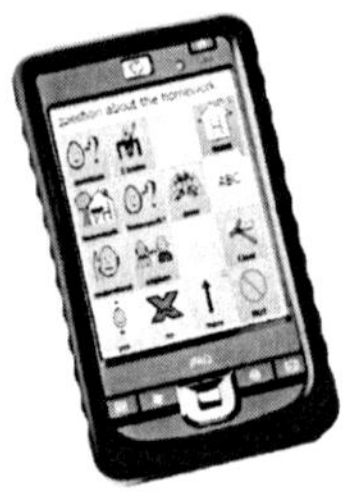

Saltillo Chat PC Silk (handheld)

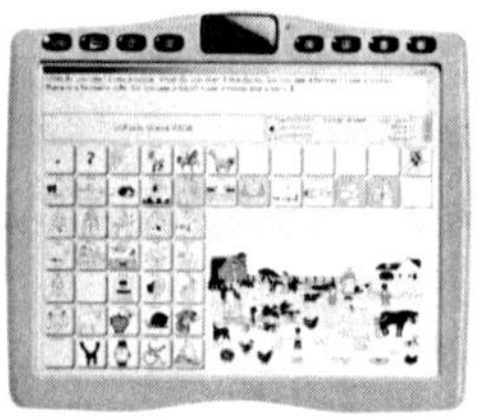

Prentke Romich ECO-14

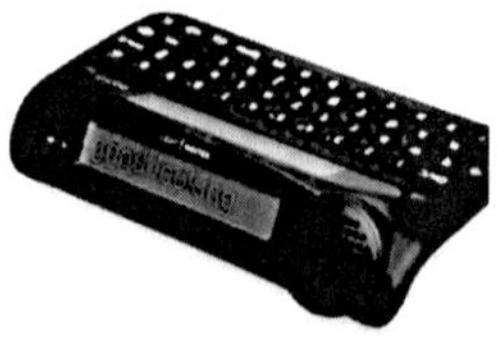

Toby Churchill Lightwriter SL-40

letter abbreviations or iconic codes (Beukelman & Mirenda, 2005)

The speed with which spoken messages are produced varies considerably, depending upon the individual's cognitive/linguistic and physical abilities, their means of device access and the selection efficiency of the device, as well as the communication task and context (Demasco, 1994; Higginbotham, Shane, Russell & Caves, 2007). For individuals directly accessing their SGD using their hands, feet, headstick, or electronic pointing system, output speeds during spontaneous communication average 8 - 15 words per minute (Higginbotham, Shane, Russell & Caves, 2006, 2007). Such speeds are considerably slower in comparison with spoken speech rates, which averages about 160 words per minute (Higginbotham, et al., 2007; Hill, 2001). Slow speech production rates place significant burdens on listener attention and comprehension during face-to-face and telephone interactions, and constitute a major challenge for AAC research and development – not to mention its successful use (Higginbotham, et. al., 2007). Recently, efforts have been made to speed up message production through the use of pre-stored utterance constructions that can be delivered at speaking rates between 20 and 60 words per minute (Todman, 2000; Todman, Alm, Higginbotham & File, 2008; Wilkins & Higginbotham, 2005).

AAC STAKEHOLDERS

Device Users

More than 3.5 million persons in the United States have CCN that cannot be remediated through traditional speech and language therapy. Individuals with CCN may possess one or more of a variety of disabling conditions, including: 1) those with developmental origins such as cerebral palsy, mental retardation, autism; 2) those occurring from injuries such as head injury, spinal injury, stroke, 3) and those resulting from degenerative diseases such as Alzheimer's, multiple sclerosis, Amyotrophic lateral sclerosis (ALS) and cancer (Beukelman & Mirenda, 2005). The ratio of adults to children (under 21) with CCN is approximately 4 to 1, largely due to the disproportionate number of injuries and degenerative diseases acquired by adults. The term CCN is a functional classification, not tied to a specific etiology. It is used to describe diverse groups of individuals in terms of their social, cognitive, communication and physical needs and skills. Because of their impairments and the societal response to their differences, many of these individuals are at great risk for obtaining adequate education, finding and keeping a job, maintaining self esteem and being socially isolated and losing communicative competencies.

Scientists and Clinicians

The AAC field began to emerge in the late 1960's and early 1970's, drawing from such diverse areas as electrical engineering, child language, linguistics, speech-language pathology and special education (see Vanderheiden (2002) and Zangari,

Lloyd & Vicker (1994) for detailed histories of the discipline). AAC has become both a scientific and clinical specialty recognized by the American Speech-Language and Hearing Association. Research in AAC has been funded for the last three decades by the National Institutes of Health (NIH) and the National Institute on Disability and Rehabilitation Research (NIDRR). Clinical services in AAC are typically provided by speech-language pathologists, as well as, special educators, occupational and physical therapists and rehabilitation engineers. University and graduate research centers that now have specialty training in AAC include the University of Nebraska, Pennsylvania State University, Purdue University, and SUNY Buffalo.

Manufacturers

There has also emerged a vital manufacturing community that designs and produces a variety of SGDs, communication software and device access technologies. The Assistive Technology Industry Association (http://atia.org) is the primary AAC professional organization for manufacturers. It provides an important networking context for research, clinical and manufacturing communities.

HISTORY OF SPEECH SYNTHESIS IN AAC

In 1984, I began to work with a young man with severe head and spinal injuries due to an auto accident which left him paralyzed and without a functional means of communication. Supported by the client's insurance company we purchased one of the first AAC devices with an Echo text-to-speech synthesizer. After approximately 150 hours of device programming and training, my client called his insurance agent over the phone to show her how well he was doing. Shortly after that phone call, the insurance agent cancelled my service contract with the client because she could not understand the synthesized voice (Higginbotham, 1997).

Several experimental AAC devices were developed during the mid-1970s, the first commercial mass-marketed communication aid with speech synthesis was the Phonic Ear Handivoice™ developed in 1978, which utilized Votrax™ speech synthesis from Federal Screw Works (Vanderheiden, 2002).

The original Handivoice™ provided the user with approximately 1000 spoken utterances, words, letters and phonemes. Novel words were generated by combining phoneme units. Other SGDs, such as the Echo™ speech synthesizers utilized early text-to-speech systems such as Echo and Real-Voice synthesizers. Speech intelligibility of these early devices was typically poor, and with the exception of ACS's Real Voice™ – which used an early speech concatenation approach - speech sounded robotic. As evidenced in the clinical account above, the speech qualities of these early synthesizers were unacceptable to many individuals who struggled with understanding these machine-mediated vocalizations.

In the mid-1980's speech intelligibility took a major leap forward with the commercial availability of the DECTalk™ speech synthesizer. Originally marketed by the Digital Equipment Cooperation to provide text-to-speech output for banking transactions, a hardware version of this synthesizer was licensed to Boston Children's Hospital for manufacturer. This and a later software version became the default speech synthesis system for over a decade, with word and intelligibility levels in quiet conditions rivaling natural speech (Shane, 2009).

With the advent of software-based speech synthesis and increasing demands for computer and internet voice response systems, a number of natural sounding voices have become commercially available in recent years. However, despite the advances in speech synthesis, their implementation on current SGDs is still problematic for social communication, for expressing emotional content and for expressing personal identity.

FRAMEWORKS FOR EVALUATING THE AUGMENTED VOICE

Three complementary frameworks are proposed for evaluating the human communication capabilities of current speech synthesis systems and their SGD counterparts. One is drawn from the work of Steven Connor that presents the idea of voice as a whole body phenomenon, another from the functional taxonomy proposed by Roman Jakobson, and a third is an adaptation of the Maslow hierarchy by an augmented speaker, Colin Portnuff.

Connor's Idea of Voice as Gesture

Steven Connor (2009) has recently proffered a notion of voice as being inseparable from the whole body:

Nor is the production of the voice limited to the physical production of sound or those parts of the body that are capable of producing sound. For the voice also induces and is taken up into the movements of the body. The face is part of the voice's apparatus, as are the hands. The shaping of the air effected by the mouth, hands, and shoulders marks out the lineaments of the voice-body (which is to be distinguished from the voice in the body). When one clicks one's fingers for emphasis, claps one's hands, or slaps one's thigh, the working of gesture is being taken over into sound, and voice has migrated into the fingers. (p. 300 – 301).

Connor's description of the voice-as-gesture encourages us to consider how the augmented speaker's other communication modalities, such as limb gesture and facial expression are coordinated and integrated with synthesized speech and with SGD.

Jakobson's Verbal Functions

A second framework considers how synthesized is designed and used to accomplish the verbal functions associated with everyday human activity. Jakobson (1960) provides six functions served by verbal language:

Jakobson's six functions are the 'expressive function' (speaker's emotion, attitude is expressed); the 'directive (conatative) function' (speaker uses utterance to get interlocutor to do something); the 'social function' (speaker uses utterance to signal social relation and social information); the 'referential function' (speaker uses utterance to describe states of affairs and objects); the 'poetic function' (the speaker's utterance shows creative elements like wordplay, humor etc.) and the 'metalinguistic' function (the speaker's utterance refers reflexively to language structures and use – e.g. "Speak more slowly please") (Wilkins, 2006).

How are these functions facilitated or impeded by current speech synthesis technologies or by their technological infrastructures? If the purpose of SGDs is to enable individuals, without the ability to speak – to be able to more fully and independently participate in society, then all of Jakobson's communicative functions should be supported by the SGD.

Portnuff's Hierarchy of Needs

A third framework has been proposed by Portnuff (2006), an individual with ALS and an augmented speaker, who addressed his expectations for his synthesized voice, in the form of a hierarchy of speech synthesis needs:

Based loosely on Maslow's (1943) *Hierarchy of Needs*, Portnuff provides a wide range of feature requirements in order to meet his expectations of

Table 1. Portnuff's (2006) hierarchy of speech synthesis feature requirements

Features	Portnuff's Comments
1. Sapi 5 compatibility	*If I can't use the voice on my system, it is of no use to me.*
2. Intelligibility & pronunciation editing	*I spoke articulately ... before last year and I want that capability now.*
3. Pitch and speed Controls	*A natural human speaker can vary the pitch and speed without sounding like a machine.*
4. Socially interactive[2]	*Group conversation... is very difficult to participate when my pace is so much slower than the group.*
5. Expressiveness	*I want a question to sound like a question and an exclamation to sound like an exclamation.*
6. Multilingual Capability	*I used to speak reasonably fluent and perfectly accented French... I want to be able to speak other languages than English and in my selected voice.*
7. Loudness	*I want a "shout" capability that is not the volume control of my speaker*
8. Talk to animals	*I want to talk to animals... they do not associate my synthesized voice with me.*
9. Ability to sing	*I used to sing with perfect pitch.*

himself as a communicator (Table 1). Portnuff's hierarchy is valuable because it addresses a wide range of human communication needs (i.e., information, social, emotional, identity) applied to the use of speech synthesis in SGDs. And except for Feature 4 (socially interactive) that was added by this author, this framework reflects the perspectives and experience someone who speech synthesis and SGD technologies on a daily basis. Along with Connor's voice-as-gesture and Jakoboson's taxonomy of verbal functions, Portnuff's speech synthesis needs hierarchy provides a means for evaluating the sufficiency of the current generation of speech synthesis and SGDs and their ability to provide an integrated, functional and comprehensive voice for the individual with CCN.

SPEECH SYNTHESIS RESEARCH

Research in the speech synthesis has being going on for nearly three decades. The research has covered a number of areas, with most being dedicated to studying the intelligibility of speech produced by SGDs, how well the speech output can be understood, how well the devices serve during social interactions, and for expression of emotion and social identity. We will detail some of the research and end with some recent new directions that appear to have promise.

Intelligibility Studies

Beginning in the mid-1980's the fledgling AAC research community began to investigate the intelligibility levels and social acceptability of various speech synthesizers by different listener groups (children versus adults, females versus males, persons with disabilities) (Hoover, Reichle, Van Tasell & Cole, 1987; Mirenda & Beukelman, 1987; Mitchell & Atkins, 1989) (see Mullennix & Stern (this issue) for a review of social acceptability research). The overarching purpose of these studies was to determine which speech synthesis technologies were intelligible enough to be used for communication.

Using a variety of single word and sentence-level intelligibility tasks, the intelligibility of DECTalk™ speech was found to be comparable to natural speech in quiet conditions and more intelligible than most other commercially available speech synthesizers such as MacinTalk™, Votrax™ and Echo™ text-to-speech synthesis. Also, the male DecTalk™ voice (Perfect Paul) was more intelligible than the DecTalk™ female (Betty) or child's voice (Kit) (Hoover, Reichle, Van Tasell & Cole, 1987; Hustad, Kent & Beukelman, 1998; Mirenda & Beukelman, 1987,

1990; Mitchell & Atkins, 1989). Perception and comprehension of synthetic speech was found to be more susceptible to a variety of factors including noise and divided attention tasks than was to natural speech. Further, perception and comprehension appear to be significantly affected by listening experience, linguistic context, and listener variables such as age, and disability status. (Drager & Reichle, 2001a, 2001b; Drager, et al., 2007; Hustad, Kent & Beukelman, 1998; Koul & Allen, 1993; Koul, 2003). Although the newer high quality voices being used in SGDs have not been thoroughly evaluated, Venkatagiri (2004) found that the AT&T high quality text-to-speech system was significantly less intelligible in reverberant and noisy conditions compared to lower quality synthesizers (IBM Via Voice™, Festival™). From this author's informal clinical observations, the intelligibility of high quality voices still suffer in noisy situations compared to natural speech. This can be especially problematic for female synthesized voices.

Sentence and Discourse Comprehension

Although intelligibility studies provided initial comparative information about speech synthesis, they failed to take into account many of the real-world factors that affected the effectiveness of speech synthesis in AAC. Such factors included the effect of background noise and output methods, and discourse context. Starting in the 1990's AAC researchers began to look at sentence and discourse comprehension of synthetic speech.

Using sentence and discourse level stimuli, researchers have found synthetic speech to be adversely affected under reverberant and background noise conditions (Drager et al., 2007; Koul & Allen, 1993; Venkatagiri, 2004). Drager and Reichle (2001a) examined the differences in natural versus synthetic speech. They used a divided attention task, studying its effects on story comprehension of speech produced by younger and older adults (mean CA 21 vs. 70 years). Both groups performed significantly better when listening to natural speech versus synthetic speech, and when the task was focused versus divided. Younger adults performed better than older adults in all task conditions.

Several studies found that listener ability to accurately summarize paragraph level spoken texts were affected by the method of speech output (word-by-word > sentence > words mixed with spelled out words) as well as the quality of speech synthesis (Echo vs. Dectalk™) (Higginbotham, Drazek, Kowarsky, Scally & Segal, 1994; Higginbotham, Scally, Lundy & Kowarsky, 1995). When speech was harder to understand, listeners relied on their own knowledge about the assumed topic and the linguistic environment to fill the informational gaps caused by the problematic discourse (Higginbotham & Baird, 1995). Drager et al. (2007) found a similar ordering for communication output mode. The addition of a video of the augmented speaker formulating the message in the Drager study did not significantly improve sentence transcription performance.

To determine the impact of speech production rate in AAC on listener comprehension, Kim (2001) inserted pauses of varying lengths between words within synthetic speech narratives, producing overall speech production output rates between 8.8, 17.5, 35, 70 and 140 wpm. She found significant improvements in discourse comprehension at each increment in production rate except for 140 wpm which was marginally worse than 70 wpm. Since typical communication rates for current AAC systems range between 5 and 15 words per minute, they fall at the lower end of the output rate spectrum – the end that Kim found to be associated with the most comprehension problems. Kim also developed a communication competence rating scale based on Grice's (1975) work on conversational maxims. Subjective ratings of speaker competence were significantly correlated with speech production rate and listener discourse comprehension ratings.

In summary, research on the intelligibility and comprehension of synthesized speech used in AAC has shown it to be of sufficient intelligibility for communication–although limited by environmental factors. Listener comprehension is also limited by the ways in which speech synthesis is produced via the SGD. At slow output rates - under 35 words per minute - comprehension is compromised. At higher output rates listener comprehension improves as well as subjective evaluations of the speakers' communication competence. The challenge for researchers, clinicians and manufacturers is to find technologies and strategies which minimize the real-world constraints on successful AAC communication. Based on Portnuff's hierarchy, the more human sounding high quality voices like AT&T's Natural Voices™, may not offer the expected intelligibility performance in everyday acoustic environments.

SPEECH SYNTHESIS RESEARCH IN SOCIAL INTERACTION

The institutionalized, naturalized, socially consensual order of conversation has a time order, a rhythm that assumes an intersubjective coordination of physical human bodies. Having a body which could not inhabit this time order was a breach of the normalized conversational environment. (Robillard, 1994)

Timing is a pragmatic that a polite augmented communicator is aware of and adapts his or her conversations around. By timing, I do not mean rate of speech. What I mean is being conscious of how much time the other person has to talk and adjusting the conversation accordingly. (Creech, 1996)

Over the last decade there has been an increasing awareness of the importance of the sequential and temporal aspects of augmentative communication that bear on social interaction success (Higginbotham, Shane, Russell & Caves, 2007; Koester & Levine, 1997; Shane, Higginbotham, Russell & Caves, 2006; Todman et al., 2008). As indicated by Robillard and Creech, communication with an impaired body and via augmented means is not simply a message production task. Utterances need to be constructed and be issued in time and be jointly coordinated with one's communication partner in order to be relevant and successful (Bloch & Wilkinson, 2007; Clarke & Wilkinson, 2007, 2008; Higginbotham & Wilkins, 1999; Sweidel, 1991/1992). While Creech (who uses an AAC device) regards timing as a conscious and important consideration, Robillard (who doesn't use any AAC) considers performing communicatively relevant interactions in an able-bodied world a near impossibility because of timing issues.

In order to better understand how individuals communicate in face-to-face contexts, researchers have begun to develop and test models of language and interaction usage that attempt to account for the social interactive performance of its participants (Clark, 1996; Clark & Brennan, 1991; Clark, Horn & Ward, 2004; Higginbotham & Caves, 2002; Higginbotham & Wilkins, 1999, 2009). There is considerable descriptive evidence from sociolinguistics and an increasing number of experimental studies demonstrating the collaborative nature of communication. In the AAC field a number of research studies have provided accounts of the collaborative social interactions involving AAC device use (Blau, 1986; Buzolich & Wiemann, 1988; Clarke & Wilkinson, 2007, 2008; Higginbotham, 1989; Higginbotham and Wilkins, 1999, 2009).

Higginbotham and Wilkins (1999) and Higginbotham and Caves (2002) provided a set of tenets for conducting social interactions using augmented means:

- Produce semantically pragmatically interpretable utterances (single words, single phrases, longer phrasal constructions) appropriate to participant roles and the communication task at hand. The standing goal of interaction is to achieve a reciprocal level of mutual understanding or common ground.
- Produce utterances via multiple communication modalities (e.g., speech, gesture, device) appropriate for the communication task. For example, deictic and spatially descriptive tasks are often accomplished more efficiently with gesture accompanies spoken words.
- Jointly coordinate with one's interlocutor within a socially appropriate temporal-attentional frame. Typically the coordination of content and process happens synchronously and immediately upon utterance completion. Conversational turns must occur within a second or two of the last speaker's utterance or the speaker's intentions and/or abilities will be held suspect by their interlocutor.
- When utterances incorporate signals unfamiliar to one's interlocutor or when signals are produced asynchronously in time, the joint achievement of common ground is delayed, resulting in misunderstanding and jeopardizing interaction success.

Higginbotham and Caves (2002) argue that following the above interaction tenets can be particularly challenging for augmented speakers, as most SGDs are designed to promote utterance construction through spelling or via a coding system, and not within a time-frame acceptable in typical spoken interaction. Currently, most AAC technologies have not been explicitly designed to facilitate utterance production in real-time social interaction. There has been relatively little engineering directed toward the producing socially pragmatic or temporally appropriate utterances.

We have tried to address the paucity of research in this area. For example, in a study done in our laboratory in Buffalo, (Higginbotham, Kim & Scally, 2007) we showed that when faced with slow speech output rates (< 10 wpm) most traditional AAC devices can be modified to maintain the interlocutor's attention and improve collaborative communication. The device modifications involve adjusting the communication output to speak each letter or word selection that the user makes on his device. Participants who used the mixed words and letters output method produced utterances at a significantly faster rate, were more collaborative in their message constructions, used a wider range of communication strategies and preferred the "mixed" communication output mode to one which only output whole words. These findings are supported by a other descriptive evidence pointing out comprehension problems related to message preparation delays. Our research and that of others has also revealed the interactive adaptations made by participants to overcome these problems (Blau, 1986; Clark & Wilkinson, 2007, 2008; Higginbotham & Wilkins, 1999; 2009; Sweidel, 1991/1992)

Recently we have begun to study the interactions of individuals with late stage amyotrophic lateral sclerosis a progressive neurodegenerative disease which results in movement and vocal paralysis (Luo, 2009; Luo, Higginbotham & Cornish, 2008. We found that individuals with no functional speech still used voice and gesture to deliver approximately 50 percent of their communications. These findings are striking given the level of limb and/or vocal paralysis experienced by these individuals. A close inspection of our videos revealed that vocalizations and gestures were frequently used during situations that demanded a rapid response or topic shift involving a problem requiring an immediate solution (e.g, fixing misunderstandings, gaining attention, physical repositioning, device malfunctioning). That is, the ALS speakers selected communication modalities that were most likely to be effective within the temporal mandates of the situation at hand. The SGDs used by the ALS participants are developed for constructing utterances and not issuing quick responses. Speech synthesis output was not readily available for temporally demanding communications.

The "acid test" for testing the real-world social communication adequacy of speech synthesis in AAC is the telephone call. In this temporally demanding context only device output and vocalizations are available to the augmented speaker. Portnuff (2006) has indicated that phone conversations are among the most challenging of contexts. Using a high quality female Dectalk™ voice, Hanson and Sudheimer (2009) placed 100 phone calls to randomly selected businesses in two different geographically distinct cities. In each call the speaker asked the same information ("what are your hours"). In half the calls the question was issued immediately, in the other half, a 3 second delay preceded the question. Also, half of the requests were preceded by a floorholder ("Please wait, I'm using a computer to talk"), half were not. Their results showed that less than 50% of the calls were successfully transacted in any condition, with the floorholder/no-delay condition being the most successful at 46% and no-floorholder/no-delay at 29%, floorholder/delay at 26% and no-floorholder/delay at 4%. The use of floorholder utterances appeared particularly effective in preventing telephone hang-ups which occurred in the majority of no-floorholder calls. Follow-up interviews indicated that a large number of persons regarded the telephone transaction either as a prank or joke call, weird, an automated solicitation, or incomprehensible - particularly if the call was not preceded by the floorholder.

With the importance and frequency of use of telephone communication in our culture, Hanson and Sudheimer's findings are of particular significance for our understanding of the real world impact of the acoustic and temporal characteristics of speech synthesis use in everyday conversations.

Recent Developments

Over the last few years researchers and manufacturers have begun to develop SGD technologies that are designed to promote social interaction. Two recent developments are reviewed here, Visual Scenes Displays and Utterance-based systems.

Visual Scenes Display

In an attempt to reduce the cognitive linguistic loads associated with traditional AAC interfaces, researchers have utilized personalized photographic and graphic materials in digitized Visual Scenes Displays (Beukelman, et al., 2007; Light & Drager, 2007). Designed for young children just acquiring language and for individuals with acquired language impairments (e.g., aphasia, closed head injury), Visual Scenes Displays integrate pictures, which typically provide narrative support for life events with relevant text messages and/or speech output (Figure 2). By overtly involving both partners with the Visual Scenes Display the social dynamic of communication is transformed from one person sending a message to their partner, to that of two individuals engaged in multimodal, joint interactions around visual materials. In the Visual Scenes Display situation, speech synthesis output provides one of several modalities that the augmented speaker can use for their communication. At the time of publication, at least 7 AAC manufacturers have provided VS software for young children and/or adults with significant cognitive/linguistic impairments.

Utterance-Based Systems

Another area that has been under study has been that involving utterance-based systems. These are AAC technologies that provide storage and organization of pre-constructed words, phrases and whole utterances available for rapid interaction (Todman, Alm, Higginbotham & File, 2008). Research by

Figure 2. Visual scenes display

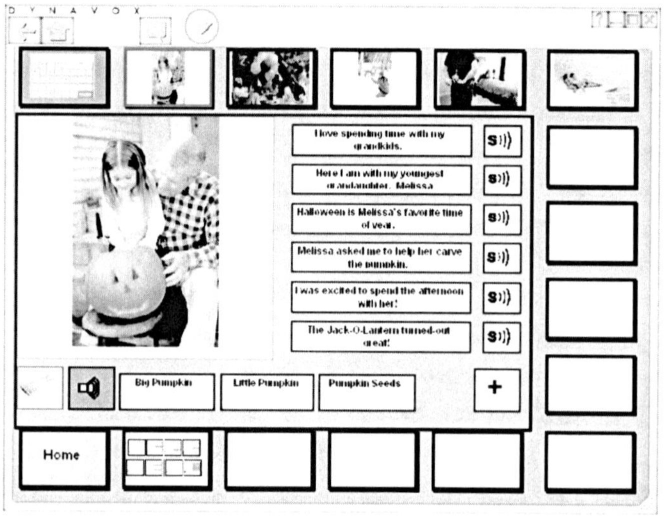

John Todman and his colleagues at the University of Dundee has demonstrated the facilitative effects of reducing the message preparation time for synthesized speech-mediated interactions. Todman (2000) videoed an adult with complex communication needs learning to use an utterance-based SGD. Over the course of the experiment, Todman taught the augmented speaker how to use an utterance-based system. At the end of each session the augmented speaker, her interlocutors, and observers rated each interaction using a questionnaire designed by the authors to evaluate social communication competence and enjoyment. With median speech production rates ranging between 36 and 74 words per minute, Todman demonstrated a significant relationship between the reduction of pre-utterance preparation pause times and the participants' and observers' perceptions of communication competence and enjoyment.

Todman and Rzepecka (2003) altered the pre-utterance pause lengths (2s,6s,10s,16s) of speech synthesis utterances spoken by 3 AAC users using an SGD while engaging in a series of introductory conversations with their communication partners. By having a group observers rate each of the 9 conversations using a version of a social competence and questionnaire. They found a significant linear relationship between the length of pre-utterance pauses and higher communication competence ratings. This suggests that that the reduction in pre-utterance pause times results in improved perceptions of the speaker's communication competence. Based on these findings, the authors argue for providing utterance-based components for AAC devices in order to support temporally demanding social exchanges: "In the future, Voice Output Communication Aids that do not provide for a dynamic balance between competing demands for speed and accuracy will not be serving their potential users well" (Todman & Rzepecka, 2003, p. 233).

Through independent and collaborative ventures between Todman's group at the University of Dundee, our own lab in Buffalo, and commercial AAC manufacturers (Wilkins & Higginbotham, 2005; Todman, 2000; Todman, Alm, Higginbotham & File, 2008); we have developed utterance-based technologies providing rapid access to word, phrasal and sentence-level utterances, organized by topic or context.

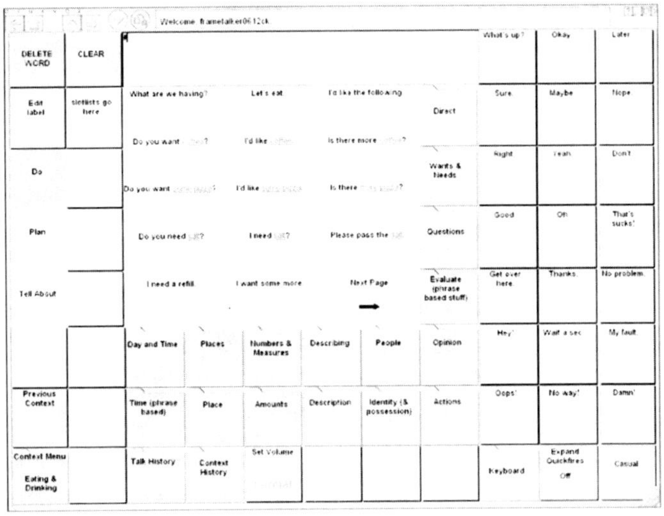

Figure 3. Frametalker utterance-based system

Figure 3 shows our latest development efforts. The 3 columns of single words (right side) are designed to provide the speaker rapid access to wide range of highly pragmatic utterances that can be used to maintain one's turn in conversation. Quick access to specific topics or communication contexts can be achieved using the utterances in the center portion of the interface which provides up to 28 utterances for "Planning", "Doing", and "Telling About" (accessed by the three buttons to the left of the context area). Individual utterances may be modified by selecting items from slotlists. Surrounding the context area are buttons which, when touched, replace the context area with more generic word and phrasal constructions relating to time, places, numbers, directions, wants & needs, etc. Finally a keyboard with word prediction is available for slower, but more precise message formulations.

Making a More Functional SGD for Social Interaction

A number of significant problems remain to be studied in order to design Speech Generative Devices that will result in satisfying social interactions.

First, much more work needs to be done to develop AAC technologies that help augmented speakers control and maintain the temporal flow of their social interactions. Augmented speakers need to be able to issue temporally responsive utterances in order to be pragmatically appropriate and effective and to avoid the social repercussions and questions about one's competence that is associated with mis-timings and perceived non-responsiveness (Higginbotham and Wilkins, 1999; Robillard, 1994).

Second, The prosodic capabilities of most commercially available speech synthesis technologies are limited with respect to the extensive and complex manipulation of pitch, loudness, speed and timing required for spoken language use during social interactions. In currently available systems, prosody is lightly modulated, satisfactory for polite voice response systems, and serviceable for listening to longer texts (emails, papers, books). The lack of sufficient intonation for interactive vocal communication is a particularly critical issue for speech synthesis in AAC. Many Augmented speakers are physically limited with respect to their gestural expressiveness and could significantly benefit from a prosodically expressive synthesis system. Portnuff (2006) calls for his speech synthesizer to be able to yell above the surrounding din. However, few systems provide for immediate changes in volume level or voice (e.g., yelling, whispering). Nor can automatically compensate for changes in ambient noise levels, as does natural speech.

Finally, no current commercial AAC technology provides for nonspeech vocal sounds and speech qualities (e.g., audible inspiration, expiration, variable articulation precision, breathiness) that could be used to prompt a listener's attention and provide additional pragmatic support, such as expressing exasperation with a loud exhalation (Kim, 2001; Higginbotham, Shane, Russell, & Caves, 2007). The ability to issue both speech and non-speech sounds in a timely manner takes on considerable importance when trying to address the multimodal speech as gesture, pragmatic diversity and speech synthesis criteria set forth by Connor (2009), Jakobson (1960) and Portnuff (2006).

SPEECH SYNTHESIS PERSPECTIVES ON EMOTION AND IDENTITY

If people told me if I was going to make it in college...I'd have to master the computer voice. But I hated the damn thing. Nobody knows the real man, not even my mom. I'm worried that people will not talk to me, but to the computer. There is no way in hell a computer voice can express the emotion I have inside of me. (Dan Keplinger, in Whiteford, 2000)

The challenge comes when there is strong emotional context to the conversation. First of all the speech system always has the same, sometimes slightly peculiar intonation. So the listener has to listen to the actual words and ignore the intonation. This is difficult for some people to do. By the same token, there are times when intonation would help greatly to soften the impact of words. I have gotten into hot water a few times saying something that I might have gotten away with by moderating my tone of voice I am learning to try to use facial expression and gesture to help with communication, and as much as possible to maintain some eye contact and not look at the screen or keyboard while I am typing, although that is difficult (Portnuff, 2006).

My Voice

The term "voice" has several different meanings. So far when discussing speech synthesis, voice has been used to denote the speech synthesizer, its acoustic properties, intelligibility and use as a tool for interaction. But the notion of voice goes far beyond that to address issues of emotional expression and identity. For Terkel (2008) the sound of a human voice represents our humanity. In the movie, *King Gimp*, Keplinger's critiques his "computer voice" exemplifying the distinction between the external "computer voice" and "his voice". The inability of synthesized speech systems to portray one's self is a fundamental problem for many augmented speakers. For example, Portnuff (2006) finds that the automated intonation interferes with his communication partner's ability to understand the meaning and intention of his communications.

Current speech synthesis technology is geared to providing voices representing an "other" person, that is, the narrator of a story, computerized email speaker, digital bank or travel assistant. In these cases, the synthesized voice portrays a pleasant, intelligible speaker from one's general linguistic community. Personality is non-individualized and typically pleasant. Korzeniowski (2008) indicates that the speech synthesis industry has traditionally shied away more emotional voices due to the challenges associated with their proper use in automated business systems. However, when the voice is "one's own", the speaker may want to identify with his or her voice. The acoustic-linguistic characteristics of the synthesized voice need to represent one's personality. The variety of past and current voices is limited, impacting an individual's ability to identify with their synthesized voice and to provide a personalized acoustic vocal signature when interacting with others. Because the AAC manufacturing community must rely on commercial speech synthesis manufacturers who provide cost-effective speech, consumers are typically limited to a restricted number of commercially available voices.

In the 80's and 90's most speakers used DECTalk™, which provided 3 male, 3 female and one child's voice for functional communication purposes[3]. Although the number of different new, high quality voices has been growing over the past decade, the variety is still quite restricted. Table 2 provides a list of different "high quality"[4] synthetic voices offered by 5 major AAC manufacturers. From the table below (Table 2) one can see that 4 different speech synthesis companies have licensed their products for use by AAC manufactures, with AT&T Natural voices being offered by every manufacturer as a default voice. Each company offers two to four adult male and four to six female voices, and two child voices. Most companies still provide lower quality Microsoft and/or DECtalk™ voices. Also, most manufactures provide additional high quality foreign voices. Although it is encouraging that current SGDs offer more than one manufacturer's voice, the diversity in voice quality is still quite limited, with no provision for voice personalization or dialect variation.

Because of the artificial and restricted sound of synthesized voices, it is not surprising that many augmented communicators do not view their SGD voice as representing their authentic "voice". One individual who has used synthesized speech for decades, named her AAC system "Jimmy". Although using an adult female voice of high acoustic quality, she relegates her device and synthesized voice to being an assistant, one that helps her to communicate, but not one who represents her personality. The lack of voice personalization is also exemplified by the lack of voice diversity. At the 2009 Conference on evidence-based practice in AAC, 5 long-time AAC users attended the conference, gave presentations and/or entered into conference discussions. The lack of voice diversity was apparent. Among the 5 speakers, three speakers used the same AT&T male voice, one speaker used a DECtalk™ male voice and another used a DECtalk™ female voice.

Although the augmented speaker can carefully construct utterances to convey aspects of one's personality and interpersonal stance (e.g., the strategic use of politeness markers, profanity, idiosyncratic vocabulary), reliance on particular linguistic constructions for these purposes in everyday communication, particularly in time-constrained contexts like in-person conversation is limited.

The lack of vocal identity and emotion expressiveness in AAC is not just a problem at the manufacturing level. There is no empirical research published in AAC on these topics. In a recent paper, Blackstone & Wilkins (2009) introduced the topic of emotion to the AAC community, noting that many individuals who use AAC lack the body-based and technical "tools" needed to express themselves emotionally. She

Table 2. Synthetic speech voices used by 4 major SGD manufacturers

SGD Manufacturer	TTS Voice Manufacturers used	Total Number of Voices
DynaVox, LLC	AT&T, Acapella	4 male, 5 female, 2 child
Prentke Romich Company	AT&T, Scansoft	4 male, 6 female, 2 chld
Tobii / ATI	AT&T, Acapella	2 male, 3 female, 2 child
Words Plus	AT&T, Neospeech	4 male, 4 female

spells out the problems faced by individuals with CCN in communicating emotional content and how such problems impact on development and quality of life.

Recent Advances in Personalized and Emotive Voices

There are three recent developments advancing the potential for personalized and emotive voices. These include the ModelTalker,Loquendo speech synthesis technologies, and the innovations of experienced and talented augmentative speakers, especially as professional speakers and performers.

ModelTalker

ModelTalker (http://www.modeltalker.com) is a speech synthesis software package designed to generate a SAPI 5.0 compatible synthesized voices based on voice samples provided by individuals who are in the early stages of losing their voices due to ALS or other medical conditions. It has emerged through a collaborative effort between AgoraNet Inc. and Nemours Speech Research Laboratory at the University of Delaware, Unlike commercially available synthesized voices, the ModelTalker voice preserves identifying vocal characteristics of the speaker. Voices are based on approximately 1600 sentences recorded by the system. In our own lab at UB we were able to create a remarkably realistic voice for an ALS client with moderate intelligibility, based on only 400 sentences.

Loquendo Text-to-Speech

Loquendo(tm) has produced a commercially available set of high quality, multilingual voices, that are designed with pragmatic and emotional expression capabilities. The expressive elements of the Loquendo voice can be controlled via VoiceXML. Currently Loquendo is being used by the Saltillo Corporation for their handheld SGD.

Augmented Speakers as Professional Presenters

Over the last decade, a number of augmented speakers have begun to give presentations at professional conferences and to make video and audio recordings of their lectures and creative performances. What distinguishes these individuals is the creative manner in which they employ their speech synthesizers.

Michael Williams, for example, is a long-time leader in the AAC and disability movements, and the editor of Alternatively Speaking, a newsletter on AAC issues. He speaks regularly at scientific conferences on a variety of AAC issues and has been involved with different professional video productions (e.g., Blackstone & Hunt-Berg, 2004). Recently Williams posted a video lecture about his life and the involvement in the disability movement (http://aac-rerc.psu.edu/index-11439.php.html). A highly skilled orator, Williams prepares his lectures with different DECtalk™ voices and vocal stylings in combination with highly individual linguistic style. In combination with precisely coordinated gestural displays, Williams works his audience, emphasizing important points, cracking jokes and producing biting sarcasm.

Another presenter, Snoopi Botten (http://www.jukeboxalive.com/snoopi) is a musician and performing artist. Most notably, Botten programs his DECtalk™ to sing. Like lecturing, the song must be prepared prior to its performance, and Botten accompanies his musical performances with synchronized gesture. Currently, Botten has made several musical recordings and recently published an instructional video on programming the DECtalk™ to sing. The Prentke Romich Company has integrated some of Botten's music programming techniques into their line of SGDs.

The AAC field is just beginning to address the issues of representing personal identity and expressing emotion through SGDs. The lack of integration, timing and voice modulation controls hampers the augmented speaker's ability to speak with their own *voice*. The emergence of professional speakers and technical developments in voice personalization and more emotional speech synthesis signal the potential for more personally representative voices.

CONCLUSION

This chapter has presented different aspects of this highly complex problem of providing synthesized voices for individuals with complex communication needs. By drawing on the experiences and suggestions of augmented speakers one can get a good picture of the current challenges they face when using speech synthesis with their SGDs.

Terkel's (2007) feelings about artificial voices and his call for voices that are human sounding lays out the predicament for AAC. Currently, speech synthesis provides many of the informational capabilities, providing a sometimes polite, sometimes cold, inflexible voice that has an impact on its audience. The lack of human voice qualities can have negative consequences, like impeding one's ability to maintain normal human relationships or to engage in successful social and business transactions..

Speech synthesis can be used with varying degrees of success in AAC. However, both the research and the words of the augmented speakers presented here suggest that success is mitigated by the inability of synthesized speech to be integrated into one's rhythm and movements, to fully express the complexities of one's intentions, and to meet the personal needs of the augmented speaker. The details of speaker needs and recommendations for further development have been offered as a plea for more and better research and technology development in this area.

Portnuff (2006) challenges the scientific & technical community to carefully consider who we see and hear when we talk to an individual using an SGD:

It is only natural to associate voice with identity, but I think the professionals doing, and guiding, research should be cautious about the flip side. Do you really hear the individuality of each speaker who uses the same voice? As scientists, I know you hear the words and analyze content, but how readily can you see through the artificial characteristics of our voices to the reality of our character and the emotions that we try to express. Can you distinguish clearly between on the one hand, how articulate we are and how much like you we sound, and on the other hand, the actual words and ideas we express? That is, to separate out the quality of the voice from the speech it enables.

Can we, as scientists, see the person behind the synthesized voice? If so, then we need to determine the technical solutions that will make the barrier between synthesized speech and one's voice disappear. From the review of research and development presented here, three goals immediately come to mind. First, speech synthesizers need to be more emotionally expressive. They need to allow augmented speakers to yell, sing, talk to animals, etc. Second, synthetic voices need to be individualized. The ModelTalker technology brings us part way there, but practically speaking, we either need a very large bank of voices for potential speakers to use, or a means of voice blending so that the desirable features of several voices can be "morphed" into a single unique synthesized voice. Finally, we need to develop some semblance of "real-time" expressive control over utterance productions. One means of providing control may be to determine what ancillary, volitional movements can be tapped to control one or more prosodic dimensions. Another option may be to increase the number of communicatively functional "pre-packaged" prosodic variations, providing speakers with different ways *intone* their utterances.

At its best, temporal control over expressive productions would begin to address Connor's assertion that the human voice is part of one's multimodal, temporally integrated communication apparatus and would provide the speaker with the ability to communicate in multiple ways such as those rendered by Roman Jakobson and Colin Portnuff.

ACKNOWLEDGMENT

Portions of this work has been funded in part by the National Institute on Disability and Rehabilitation Research (NIDRR) under Grant #H133E030018. The author would like to express his thanks to Judith Duchan for helping with editing and humanizing this paper.

REFERENCES

American Speech-Language-Hearing Association. (2005). *Roles and Responsibilities of Speech-Language Pathologists With Respect to Augmentative and Alternative Communication: Position Statement*. Available from www.asha.org/policy.

Beukelman, D., Fager, S., Ball, L., & Dietz, A. (2007). AAC for adults with acquired neurological conditions: A review. *Augmentative and Alternative Communication*, *23*, 230–242. doi:10.1080/07434610701553668

Beukelman, D. R., & Mirenda, P. (2005). *Augmentative & alternative communication: Supporting children & adults with complex communication needs* (3rd ed.). Baltimore: Paul H. Brookes Publishing Company.

Blackstone, S., & Hunt-Berg, M. (2004). *Social networks: A communication inventory for individuals with complex communication needs and their communication partners.* Verona, WI: Attainment Company.

Blackstone, S., & Wilkins, D. P. (2009). Exploring the Importance of emotional competence in children with complex communication needs. *Perspectives on Augmentative and Alternative Communication*, *18*, 78–87. doi:10.1044/aac18.3.78

Blau, A. F. (1986). Communication in the backchannel: social structural analyses of nonspeech/speech conversations (augmentative communication, discourse analysis). Ph.D. dissertation, City University of New York, New York. Retrieved August 10, 2009, from Dissertations & Theses: Full Text.(Publication No. AAT 8629674).

Bloch, S., & Wilkinson, R. (2007). The understandability of AAC: A conversation analysis study of acquired dysarthria. *Augmentative and Alternative Communication*, *20*, 272–282. doi:10.1080/07434610400005614

Buzolich, M. J., & Wiemann, J. W. (1988). Turn taking in atypical conversations: The case of the speaker/augmented-communicator dyad. *Journal of Speech and Hearing Research*, *31*, 3–18.

Clark, H., Horn, L. R., & Ward, G. (2004). Pragmatics of language performance. In *Handbook of Pragmatics* (pp. 365-382). Oxford: Blackwell.

Clark, H. H. (1996). *Using language*. Cambridge, UK: Cambridge University Press.

Clark, H. H., & Brennan, S. E. (1991). Grounding in communication. In *Perspectives on socially shared cognition* (pp. 127-149). Washington, DC: American Psychological Association.

Clarke, M., & Wilkinson, R. (2007). Interaction between children with cerebral palsy and their peers 1: Organizing and understanding VOCA use. *Augmentative and Alternative Communication*, *23*, 336–348. doi:10.1080/07434610701390350

Clarke, M., & Wilkinson, R. (2008). Interaction between children with cerebral palsy and their peers 2: Understanding initiated VOCA-mediated turns. *Augmentative and Alternative Communication*, *24*, 3–15. doi:10.1080/07434610701390400

Connor, S. (2009). The strains of the voice. In K. Izdebski (ed.), *Emotions in the human voice, volume 3: Culture and perception* (1st ed.), (pp. 297-306). San Diego, CA: Plural Publishing Inc.

Creech, R. (1996) *Extemporaneous speaking: Pragmatic principles*. Paper Presented at the 4th. Annual Pittsburgh Employment Conference, Pittsburgh, PA.

Demasco, P. (1994). Human factors considerations in the design of language interfaces in AAC. *Assistive Technology, 6*, 10–25.

Drager, K. D. R., Anderson, J. L., DeBarros, J., Hayes, E., Liebman, J., & Panek, E. (2007). Speech synthesis in background noise: Effects of message formulation and visual information on the intelligibility of American English DECtalk. *Augmentative and Alternative Communication, 23*, 177–186. doi:10.1080/07434610601159368

Drager, K. D. R., & Reichle, J. E. (2001a). Effects of age and divided attention on listeners' comprehension of synthesized speech. *Augmentative and Alternative Communication, 17*, 109–119.

Drager, K. D. R., & Reichle, J. E. (2001b). Effects of discourse context on the intelligibility of synthesized speech for young adult and older adult listeners: Applications for AAC. *Journal of Speech, Language, and Hearing Research: JSLHR, 44*, 1052–1057. doi:10.1044/1092-4388(2001/083)

Grice, H. P. (1975). Logic & conversation. *Syntax & Semantics, 3*, 41–58.

Hanson, E. K., & Sundheimer, C. (2009). Telephone talk: Effects of timing and use of a floorholder message on telephone conversations using synthesized speech. *Augmentative and Alternative Communication, 25*, 90–98. doi:10.1080/07434610902739926

Higginbotham, D.J. (1997). Class Lecture.

Higginbotham, D. J., & Baird, E. (1995). Discourse analysis of listeners' summaries of synthesized speech passages. *Augmentative and Alternative Communication, 11*, 101–112. doi:10.1080/07434619512331277199

Higginbotham, D. J., & Caves, K. (2002). AAC performance and usability issues: the effect of AAC technology on the communicative process. *Assistive Technology, 14*(1), 45–57.

Higginbotham, D. J., Drazek, A. L., Kowarsky, K., Scally, C., & Segal, E. (1994). Discourse comprehension of synthetic speech delivered at normal and slow presentation rates. *Augmentative and Alternative Communication, 10*, 191–202. doi:10.1080/07434619412331276900

Higginbotham, D. J., Kim, K., & Scally, C. (2007). The effect of the communication output method on augmented interaction. *Augmentative and Alternative Communication, 23*, 140–153. doi:10.1080/07434610601045344

Higginbotham, D. J., Scally, C., Lundy, D., & Kowarsky, K. (1995). The effect of communication output method on the comprehension of synthesized discourse passages. *Journal of Speech and Hearing Research, 38*, 889–901.

Higginbotham, D. J., Shane, H., Russell, S., & Caves, K. (2007). Access to AAC: Present, past, and future. *Augmentative and Alternative Communication, 23*, 243–257. doi:10.1080/07434610701571058

Higginbotham, D. J., & Wilkins, D. (2009). In-person interaction in AAC: New perspectives on utterances, multimodality, timing and device design. *Perspectives on Augmentative Communication.*

Higginbotham, D. J., & Wilkins, D. P. (1999). Slipping through the timestream: Time and timing issues in augmentative communication. In J. Duchan, D. Kovarsky & M. Maxwell (eds.), *The social construction of language incompetence*, (pp. 49-82). Mahwah, NJ: Lawrence Erlbaum Publishing.

Hill, K. J. (2001). *The development of a model for automated performance measurement and the establishment of performance indices for augmented communicators under two sampling conditions.* Ph.D. dissertation, University of Pittsburgh, Pennsylvania. Retrieved August 10, 2009, from Dissertations & Theses: Full Text. (Publication No. AAT 3013368).

Hoover, J., Reichle, J., Van Tasell, D., & Cole, D. (1987). The intelligibility of synthesized speech: Echo II versus Votrax. *Journal of Speech and Hearing Research, 30*, 425–431.

Hustad, K. C., Kent, R. D., & Beukelman, D. R. (1998). DECtalk and MacinTalk speech synthesizers: Intelligibility differences for three listener groups. *Journal of Speech, Language, and Hearing Research: JSLHR, 41*, 744–752.

Jakobson, R. (1960). Linguistics and poetics. In T. A. Sebeok, (Ed.), *Style in language*, (pp. 350-377). Cambridge, MA: MIT Press.

Kim, K. (2001). *Effect of speech-rate on the comprehension and subjective judgments of synthesized narrative discourse.* University at Buffalo, Communicative Disorders and Sciences.

Koester, H. H., & Levine, S. P. (1997). Keystroke-level models for user performance with word prediction. *Augmentative and Alternative Communication, 13*, 239–257. doi:10.1080/07434619712331278068

Korzeniowski, P. (2008). An Emotional Mess. *SpeechTechMag.com*, Retrieved March 30, 2009. http://www.speechtechmag.com/Articles/Editorial/Cover-Story/An-Emotional-Mess-51042.aspx

Koul, R. (2003). Synthetic speech perception in individuals with and without disabilities. *Augmentative and Alternative Communication, 19*, 49–58. doi:10.1080/0743461031000073092

Koul, R. K., & Allen, G. D. (1993). Segmental intelligibility and speech interference thresholds of high-quality synthetic speech in the presence of noise. *Journal of Speech and Hearing Research, 36*, 790–798.

Light, J., & Drager, K. (2007). AAC technologies for young children with complex communication needs: State of the science and future research directions. *Augmentative and Alternative Communication, 23*, 204–216. doi:10.1080/07434610701553635

Luo, F. (2009). *Personal narrative telling by individuals with ALS who use AAC devices.* Ph.D. dissertation, State University of New York at Buffalo, New York. Retrieved August 10, 2009, from Dissertations & Theses: Full Text. (Publication No. AAT 3342143).

Luo, F., Higginbotham, D. J., & Cornish, J. (2008). *Personal Narrative Telling of AAC Users with ALS.* American Speech Language and Hearing Association, Chicago, IL, November 21, 2008.

Maslow, A. H. (1943). A theory of human motivation. [Retrieved from: http://www.emotionalliteracyeducation.com/abraham-maslow-theory-human-motivation.shtml]. *Psychological Review, 50*, 370–396. doi:10.1037/h0054346

Mirenda, P., & Beukelman, D. (1990). A comparison of intelligibility among natural speech and seven speech synthesizers with listeners from three age groups. *Augmentative and Alternative Communication, 6*, 61–68. doi:10.1080/07434619012331275324

Mirenda, P., & Beukelman, D. R. (1987). A comparison of speech synthesis intelligibility with listeners from three age groups. *Augmentative and Alternative Communication, 3*, 120–128. doi:10.1080/07434618712331274399

Mitchell, P. R., & Atkins, C. P. (1989). A comparison of the single word intelligibility of two voice output communication aids. *Augmentative and Alternative Communication*, *5*, 84–88. doi:10.1080/07434618912331275056

Portnuff, C. (2006). *Augmentative and Alternative Communication: A Users Perspective*. Lecture delivered at the Oregon Health and Science University, August, 18, 2006. http://aac-rerc.psu.edu/index-8121.php.html

Robillard, A. (1994). Communication problems in the intensive care unit. *Qualitative Sociology*, *17*, 383–395. doi:10.1007/BF02393337

Shane, H. (2009, April 3). Telephone Interview.

Shane, H., Higginbotham, D. J., Russell, S., & Caves, K. (2006). *Access to AAC: Present, Past, and Future*. Paper presented to the State of the Science Conference in AAC. March, Los Angeles.

Sweidel, G. (1989). Stop, look and listen! When vocal and nonvocal adults communicate. *Disability & Society*, *4*, 165–175. doi:10.1080/02674648966780171

Sweidel, G. (1991/1992). Management strategies in the communication of speaking persons and persons with a speech disability. *Research on Language and Social Interaction*, *25*, 195–214.

Terkel, S. (2008). Looking for the human voice. *NPR Morning Edition*, Nov. 07, 2008. Retrieved Nov. 10, 2008 from http://www.npr.org/templates/story/story.php?storyId=96714084&ft=1&f=1021.

Todman, J. (2000). Rate and quality of conversations using a text-storage AAC system: Single-case training study. *Augmentative and Alternative Communication*, *16*, 164–179. doi:10.1080/07434610012331279024

Todman, J., Alm, N., Higginbotham, D. J., & File, P. (2008). Whole utterance approaches in AAC. *Augmentative and Alternative Communication*, *24*, 235. doi:10.1080/08990220802388271

Todman, J., & Rzepecka, H. (2003). Effect of pre-utterance pause length on perceptions of communicative competence in AAC-aided social conversations. *Augmentative and Alternative Communication*, *19*, 222–234. doi:10.1080/07434610310001605810

Vanderheiden, G. (2003). A journey through early augmentative communication and computer access. *Journal of Rehabilitation Research and Development*, *39*, 39–53.

Venkatagiri, H. S. (2004). Segmental intelligibility of three text-to-speech synthesis methods in reverberant environments. *Augmentative and Alternative Communication*, *20*, 150–163. doi:10.1080/07434610410001699726

Whiteford, W. A. (2000). *King Gimp*. VHS Tape, HBO.

Wilkins, D. (2006). *General Overview Linguistic and Pragmatic Considerations in the Design of Frametalker/Contact*. Unpublished manuscript. University at Buffalo, Department of Communicative Disorders and Sciences, Buffalo, NY.

Wilkins, D. P., & Higginbotham, D. J. (2005). The short story of Frametalker: An interactive AAC device. *Perspectives on Augmentative and Alternative Communication*, *15*, 18–22.

Zangari, C., Lloyd, L., & Vicker, B. (1994). Augmentative and alternative communication: An historical perspective. *Augmentative and Alternative Communication*, *10*, 27–59. doi:10.1080/07434619412331276740

ENDNOTES

1 Augmentative and alternative communication (AAC) refers to an area of research, clinical, and educational practice. AAC involves attempts to study and when necessary compensate for temporary or per-

manent impairments, activity limitations, and participation restrictions of individuals with severe disorders of speech-language production and/or comprehension, including spoken and written modes of communication. (ASHA, 2005)

2 This item was added by the author to highlight the important social interaction functions carried via speech synthesis and noted by Portnuff as well as other augmented speakers. The comment was taken from Portnuff's (2006) presentation.

3 DecTalk also presented a few other specialty voices (whispering female, hoarse female).

4 High quality speech utilizes a 16k or greater bit rate, lower quality speech uses an 8k bit rate.

Chapter 5
Advances in Computer Speech Synthesis and Implications for Assistive Technology

H. Timothy Bunnell
Alfred I. duPont Hospital for Children, USA

Christopher A. Pennington
AgoraNet, Inc., USA

ABSTRACT

The authors review developments in Computer Speech Synthesis (CSS) over the past two decades, focusing on the relative advantages as well as disadvantages of the two dominant technologies: rule-based synthesis; and data-based synthesis. Based on this discussion, they conclude that data-based synthesis is presently the best technology for use in Speech Generating Devices (SGDs) used as communication aids. They examine the benefits associated with data-based synthesis such as personal voices, greater intelligibility and improved naturalness, discuss problems that are unique to data-based synthesis systems, and highlight areas where all types of CSS need to be improved for use in assistive devices. Much of this discussion will be from the perspective of the ModelTalker project, a data-based CSS system for voice banking that provides practical, affordable personal synthetic voices for people using SGDs to communicate. The authors conclude with consideration of some emerging technologies that may prove promising in future SGDs.

INTRODUCTION

Assistive technology (AT), broadly defined, includes any device designed to assist individuals with disabilities to perform tasks they might not otherwise be able to perform. One area in which AT devices have been used is in providing communication capabilities for non-speaking individuals. In this context, AT devices can range from very simple boards with pictures or letters (or both) to which the user points, to complex electronic devices that accept keyboard or switch input, use word prediction algorithms to enhance input rate, and render output in the form of an acoustic speech signal. For AT devices using speech output (commonly referred to as Speech Generating Devices or SGDs), the quality of the speech is crucial to the user's ability to communicate. One approach to speech output is

DOI: 10.4018/978-1-61520-725-1.ch005

to record a set of pre-selected words and phrases that can be played back on demand. Assuming the quality of the recordings and the playback equipment are high, this approach ensures the speech output will be of high quality, intelligible, and natural sounding. Unfortunately for many SGD users, a fixed set of prerecorded utterances is inadequate for communication. According to the AAC Institute, language activity monitoring of SGD users with high communication skills suggests that less than 2% of communicative output comprises prerecorded utterances. To express themselves fully, skilled communicators must have the ability to convey most or all of the words and phrases of their language. Clearly, it is impractical to provide this ability through a fixed set of stored utterances.

The alternative to fixed sets of prerecorded utterances is unrestricted computer speech synthesis (CSS). With CSS, input in the form of text is processed through a series of steps to create an audible speech signal. The CSS technology that is most widely in use today has been developed over the past 40 to 50 years along two parallel paths. These paths represent two distinct ways of approaching the problem: one, a more pragmatic engineering approach, will be termed *data-based synthesis* because it relies on managing large amounts of recorded speech data; the other, a more theory-driven approach, will be referred to as *rule-based synthesis* since it relies on the discovery of principles or rules that describe the structure of human speech. Both approaches have advantages and disadvantages, and development along both paths has been heavily influenced by changes in computer hardware capabilities.

In the following section, we review the development of current CSS technology, with particular emphasis on one system, the ModelTalker TTS system that was developed in the Speech Research Laboratory at the Alfred I. duPont Hospital for Children. The ModelTalker TTS system is one component of the broader ModelTalker project, which has the goal of providing highly intelligible and natural sounding personal synthetic voices for users of SGDs. The ModelTalker software allows people to "bank" their voice by recording speech to create a personalized CSS system that has their own voice quality.

BACKGROUND

Figure 1 illustrates the three primary stages of processing that are necessary for CSS. When starting with English text, the first stage of processing, *Text normalization* is required to convert the text to a sequence of words or tokens that are all "speakable" items. In the figure, this is illustrated by a simple address wherein several abbreviations and numbers must be interpreted to determine exactly what words one would use if the address was to be read aloud. First, "Dr." must be read as "doctor" (and not "drive"). The street address 523 is usually spoken as "five twenty-three" and not "five hundred and twenty three." The street name should probably end in "drive" (and not "doctor"), and so forth.

Then, given the normalized text, the *Text to Phonemes* stage converts the English words to an appropriate sequence of speech sounds or phonemes. These are represented in Figure 1 (and within the ModelTalker system) using text symbols like "DD" (for the /d/ phoneme), "AA1" (for the /a/ phoneme with primary stress), "KK" (for the unaspirated /k/ phoneme), and so forth. While the phoneme and other codes illustrated in Figure 1 are specific to the ModelTalker system, they are similar to codes used in many other CSS systems. Note that in this stage, too, there are potential problems that must be addressed. For example, the word "reading" used here as a proper noun is more likely to be pronounced /ɹɛdiŋ/ (as in the railroad and towns in Pennsylvania and Massachusetts), but would more likely be pronounced /ɹidiŋ/ if it was identified as a verb. In addition to the basic phonetic segment sequence as illustrated in Figure 1, a full description of the intended ut-

Figure 1. Typical CSS processing stages. Input text passes through a normalization stage that converts all non-word input to words, then through a process that converts words to a phonetic representation. The phonetic representation is then converted to sound.

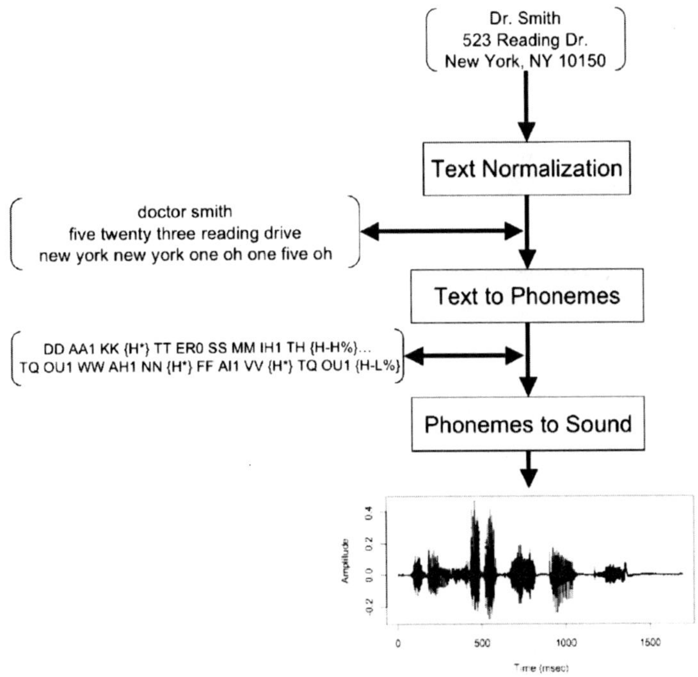

terance requires specification of the utterance's prosodic structure to indicate the relative strength or stress of each syllable, the locations and types of important boundaries, and intonational features. Some of these are illustrated in Figure 1 as, for example, the digits following vowel symbols that indicate the lexical stress level associated with syllable nuclei, and intonational markers based loosely on the ToBI system (Silverman, et al., 1992) such as {H*} (a high pitch accent) that are associated with some stressed syllables, and complex tones such as {H-H%} and {H-L%} that flag intonational features associated with the ends of phrases.

Although quite detailed in terms of both phonetic segments and prosodic properties, the output of the text to phoneme stage is nonetheless a symbolic linguistic description of the utterance to be synthesized. This symbolic description contains no information that would necessarily distinguish one talker from another. Thus, the final stage of processing, *Phonemes to Sound* takes this general linguistic description and from it renders an acoustic speech signal that has all the talker- (or synthesizer-) specific properties of recognizable speech. Methods of achieving this acoustic rendering from a symbolic linguistic description differ widely among CSS systems. So, while all CSS systems that accept unrestricted text as input must employ a similar series of processing stages to produce synthetic speech, the stage that accounts for most of the differences between different CSS systems is this final stage. It is that stage of processing on which we now focus.

Although there are historical examples of speech synthesis—loosely defined—dating back to mechanical talking heads in the 18th century, modern computer speech synthesis is mainly rooted in research from the 1950's onward. Much of the modern speech synthesis research has been motivated by a desire to better understand human speech production and perception. Early work by Stevens and House (1955) and Fant (1960), among others, established the basic relationships between the shape of the human vocal tract as controlled by the position of articulators such as the lips, tongue, jaw, and velum and the steady-state acoustic structure of vowel and consonant sounds. This work characterized speech sounds as the product of a sound-source representing the sound generated by the vocal folds or turbulent airflow fed through a filter whose response characteristics were determined by the shape of the vocal tract in front of the sound source. This work led to the development of analog, and later digital models of sound production in the vocal tract.

While some investigators extended this theoretical work in an effort to develop "articulatory synthesizers" (e.g., Mermelstein, 1973) that numerically modeled the dynamic behavior of speaking, the difficulty of developing effective and efficient control algorithms to describe articulator motion over time rendered the resulting synthetic speech relatively poor in quality and computationally impractical. Articulatory synthesis remains a laboratory tool for exploring theories of speech production (e.g., Magen, Kang, Tiede, & Whalen, 2003; Whalen, Kang, Magen, Fulbright, & Gore, 1999), but has not been used as the phoneme to sound stage in practical text to speech systems.

By contrast, synthesizers that use source-filter theory to directly model the acoustic end-product of articulation, rather than articulation itself, developed rapidly from the 1960's onward and gave rise to numerous research as well as commercial text to speech systems (see Klatt, 1987, for an extensive review). These systems functioned by specifying the acoustic characteristics of the source function in terms of a time-varying waveform and the filter characteristics of the vocal tract in terms of the time-varying parameters for a set of vocal tract resonant frequencies or formants. Klatt (1980) published the Fortran source code for one such synthesizer along with some general rules/guidelines for synthesizing English vowels and consonants by specifying target values for 39 control parameters at several points in time.[1] This synthesizer and its descendents (Klatt and his colleagues modified the system several times after its initial publication) became the laboratory standard for generating synthetic speech stimuli for use in speech perception studies.[2]

By using tables of target parameter values of each phoneme and rules for interpolating variations in parameter values over time as they changed from one target to the next, digital formant synthesis systems required relatively small amounts of memory and placed light demands on computer processors. This allowed rule-based formant synthesis to create intelligible continuous speech in better than real time on 1980's computer systems. Systems such as DECTalk (a direct descendent of the Klatt (1980) system), Prose 2000 and 3000 systems from Speech Plus Inc, Infovox, Votrax, and others were all popular and relatively intelligible rule-based synthesis systems. Some of these units remain in use today in SGDs. For instance, DECTalk continues to ship as the default voice in many devices, and physicist Stephen Hawking is a well-known user of a Prose 3000 unit.

Despite their considerable success, rule-based synthesis systems share several unfortunate characteristics. First and foremost, rule-based synthesis requires rules that must be painstakingly developed by people with expert knowledge of several areas of linguistics (e.g., phonology and phonetics) as well as a good understanding of programming and the capabilities and limitations of computer technology. The rules themselves are sufficiently complex that some researchers have developed the equivalent of computer programming languages capable of accepting high-level rule descriptions and compiling them into the lower level, more finely detailed rules that are actually needed by the synthesis system (Hertz & Huffman, 1992). Other investigators have attempted to exploit redundancy among the parameters of formant synthesis systems to reduce the control space to a smaller number of higher-level parameters (Hanson & Stevens, 2002; Stevens & Bickley, 1991).

Even with the finest of rule systems developed, the speech output by rule-based systems is not truly natural in quality. In fact, while intelligible, most rule based synthetic speech is notably unnatural sounding. Listeners virtually never mistake rule-based synthetic speech for natural speech. Additionally, rule-based synthesizer voices tend to be very generic; they do not sound much like any given talker. Neither of these latter problems is an inherent shortcoming of formant synthesis per se. Holmes (1961; 1973 referenced in Klatt, 1987) demonstrated that with sufficient care it is possible to make a formant synthesis copy of natural utterances that are very close replicas of the original utterances, sounding both natural and recognizably like the talker whose utterance is being copied. Thus, the unnaturalness of rule-based synthesis reflects weakness in our understanding of what the rules should be. This becomes an even more glaring weakness when we try to extend rule systems to capture not only the general phonetic properties of human speech, but also the fine-grained talker-specific detail that lends both naturalness and a sense of talker identity to speech.

An alternative to rule-based synthesis that aims to avoid these problems is data-based synthesis. For data-based synthesis, a talker records a corpus of speech from which regions of natural speech (concatenation units) can be extracted and stored. These units can then be concatenated in novel sequences (i.e., sequences that were not originally recorded) to produce "synthetic" speech that retains the voice quality of the talker who recorded the corpus from which the units were extracted. Obviously, using this approach, it is unnecessary for an expert to deduce rules that describe the acoustic structure of speech since the rules are implicitly part of the natural speech concatenation units.

The fundamental assumption behind unit concatenation synthesis is that natural speech can be broken down into a set of basic waveform units that can be concatenated to form continuous utterances in much the same way that letters can be concatenated to form words, and words to form sentences. A seemingly obvious choice for concatenation units would be phonemes or a somewhat extended set of phonetic segments that include acoustically distinct allophones of some phonemes (e.g., aspirated versus unaspirated stops, syllable-initial versus syllable-final liquids, etc.). For most languages, the number of such segments would be substantially fewer than 100, making for a very compact inventory of concatenation units. However, no successful synthesizer has been designed using such phonetic units. In continuous speech, the structure of every phoneme varies substantially as a function of its immediate phonetic context due to physical constraints on the way our articulators must move continuously from one segment to the next (Harris, 1955). These constraints, termed coarticulation, entail a blending of the articulatory gestures associated with adjacent segments and lead to smooth and continuous acoustic variation as each segment blends into the next. This acoustic continuity is typically violated for any phonetic segment that is not placed in the same phonetic context from which it was originally extracted.

Recognizing the crucial role that coarticulation plays in determining the acoustic structure of continuous speech, it is obvious that the choice of concatenation units must respect coarticulatory influences. Since the strongest influence of coarticulation is observed at the boundary between adjacent phonemes, one potential unit is the diphone, a segment of speech that extends from the center of one phoneme to the center of an adjacent phoneme (Peterson, Wang, & Siversten, 1958). If we assume there are roughly 60 phonetic segments of English (including allophones), then there are potentially 3600 unique diphones that can be formed from those 60 phonetic segments. However, not all of these are likely to occur due to phonotactic constraints on the language. In the first version of the ModelTalker system, which used diphone synthesis, we determined that about

2400 diphones were adequate for synthesis of most American English utterances. This set covered all the words in a large dictionary and most inter-word boundaries.

While the diphone is the smallest concatenation unit that has consistently been shown to produce acceptable synthetic speech, it has several clear drawbacks. Most prominently, the assumption that all coarticulatory effects are always restricted to a span of approximately half a phoneme is demonstrably wrong. Coarticulation has been shown to span multiple segments (e.g., Fowler, 1980; Goffman, Smith, Heisler, & Ho, 2008) and its effects have been shown to be perceptually significant over these extended spans (e.g., Lehiste & Shockey, 1972; Martin & Bunnell, 1981, 1982; Öhman, 1966). To account for these longer-range effects, investigators have proposed the use of triphones (Wicklegran, 1969), syllable dyads (Sivertsen, 1961), and other mixed units (O'Shaughnessy, 1992). Of course, with all these extended units, the number of units that must be used for synthesis increases geometrically. Using 60 phonetic segments as the basic number of singleton units, a complete inventory of English triphones (there is a distinct different version of each triphone segment for every possible combination of preceding and following phonetic segments) would theoretically require more than 200,000 units, although many of those would either never occur, or would occur very infrequently. Unfortunately, as van Santen (1992) has pointed out, there are a very large number of very infrequently occurring units in natural speech, and consequently, the odds of needing *some* infrequent unit in any given utterance are actually quite high. This means that one cannot significantly prune the number of units by removing infrequently occurring units without impacting the quality of the synthetic speech.

In addition to the problem of determining the number and precise composition of concatenation units for fixed-unit concatenation, there is the problem of locating and extracting the units from recorded natural speech. For early diphone concatenation synthesizers, this was done by hand and involved many hours of an expert's time to select the best beginning and ending locations for each unit. If these locations were not chosen carefully, perceptually jarring discontinuities could arise at concatenation joints when constructing synthetic speech. One response to this problem was an effort to develop effective algorithms for automatic diphone extraction that would simultaneously minimize the amount of manual effort involved in building a diphone synthesis system and optimize the concatenation boundary locations to minimize the amount of perceptually salient discontinuity when units are concatenated for synthesis (e.g., Conkie & Isard, 1994; Yarrington, Bunnell, & Ball, 1995).

However, there is a fundamental difficulty with diphone (or any fixed-unit) synthesis and that is the notion that exactly one "ideal" instance of each fixed unit can be preselected and saved for use in synthesis. If instead, multiple versions of each nominal unit (drawn from different utterance contexts) were saved, it might be possible at the time of synthesis to select a specific version of the unit that would be a "best fit" for the precise utterance context in which it was needed. Because it is a direct extension of diphone synthesis, this is the approach we pursued for the second version of the ModelTalker system (Bunnell, Hoskins, & Yarrington, 1998). Rather than store single diphones in its unit database, ModelTalker stored every instance of each *biphone* (two complete adjacent phonetic segments) that was recorded by the talker as part of the speech corpus. Then during synthesis, a complex search strategy was used to select both the specific instance of each biphone and the locations of diphone boundaries within each biphone that would minimize concatenation discontinuities. In effect, much of the task of selecting diphones was postponed until an utterance was actually being synthesized. Then it was possible to select specific units that minimized the distortion due to mixing segments from different coarticulatory contexts.

The approach used for ModelTalker, while an extension of diphone synthesis, is effectively equivalent to another approach termed non-uniform unit selection (Sagisaka, 1988; Takeda, Abe, & Sagisaka, 1992). This approach is now simply referred to as unit selection and contrasts with diphone synthesis or other fixed-unit concatenation synthesis where the units are preselected. In unit selection, phonetic segments (and typically subsegments) from recorded utterances are identified and indexed in a database that includes all or most of the phonetic content in every utterance that the talker recorded. For synthesis, this database is searched to locate potential concatenation units that satisfy a set of target constraints (e.g., a specific phonetic segment from a specific phonemic context, from a specific prosodic context, at a specific phrasal location). Candidate units are assigned a target cost that reflects how well they meet these constraints and are then further compared to find the specific combination of units that minimizes both the target costs and the acoustic phonetic discontinuities (join costs) in the concatenation process.

One of the great advantages of the algorithms used by ModelTalker and other unit selection systems is the tendency to find the longest possible sequences of recorded natural speech when constructing synthetic utterances. That is, when a unit selection synthesizer is asked to create an utterance containing words or phrases that match those recorded for the database, its search algorithm tends to find and play back those words or phrases as intact stretches of natural speech. The larger the original corpus of natural speech used to create the unit selection database, the greater will be the likelihood of finding relatively long stretches of natural speech or composite sequences of shorter stretches of speech that are so well-matched to the needed context as to be nearly indistinguishable from longer stretches of natural speech. Not surprisingly, this has led developers of unit selection synthesis systems to move in the direction of recording larger and larger speech corpora in pursuit of increasingly natural-sounding CSS systems. A number of the best sounding commercial and laboratory unit selection systems now require several tens of hours of continuous natural speech to achieve the very high degree of intelligibility and naturalness that they exhibit.

To summarize, the two dominant approaches to CSS in wide use today are (a) rule-based formant synthesis, and (b) data-based waveform unit concatenation synthesis. Rule-based systems use tables of acoustic parameter "target" values associated with each phonetic segment, and a system of rules that model how these parameters vary over time from one target to the next. To synthesize an utterance, the rules are used to generate a time-varying sequence of parameters that, in turn, control software that generates a time-varying source waveform and digital filter function through which the source waveform is passed to create output waveforms that resemble human speech. The contrasting approach to CSS, data-based synthesis, starts with a corpus of natural speech recorded by one individual and divides the recordings into selectable units that are stored in a database. Synthetic speech output is then formed by searching the database to find appropriate units given the desired phoneme sequence and concatenating them to form speech waveforms that, in the best cases, closely resembles the natural speech of the individual who recorded the corpus, and even in the worst cases, typically preserves the voice quality of that individual.

With rule-based synthesis, prosodic features like utterance intonation and timing must be modeled in the synthesis process along with the phonetic information. For data-based synthesis, this is not necessarily the case. Systems that use a sufficiently large database of natural speech that has been tagged or indexed with information about prosodic features, can make prosody part of the unit selection search criteria, favoring selection of those phonetic units that are also consistent with a desired prosodic structure. However, for fixed-unit concatenation systems such as diphone synthesizers or for variable unit selection systems that use a small database of recorded speech, it is unlikely that all of the units needed to create natural-sounding prosody will be present in the database. In that case, the system may use methods to alter prosodic features in the originally recorded speech to force it to match a specific prosodic structure. That is, while phonetic content is concatenated, the prosodic structure of the utterance is synthesized by altering the naturally recorded speech.

There are a variety of methods that have been used to allow data-based systems to superimpose synthetic prosody onto concatenated units. These include using Linear Predictive (LP) coding (Atal & Hanauer, 1971) to model the speech, Pitch Synchronous Overlap Add (PSOLA) coding (Moulines & Charpentier, 1990), and several others. Unfortunately, all of these methods necessarily involve altering the natural speech in one way or another, and consequently, entail adding distortion to the natural speech, making it sound less natural. Thus, for data-based synthesis, there is a complex interplay involving the size of the database, prosodic control, and naturalness. With small databases, the system must either forgo allowing control of intonation to avoid distorting the speech and giving it a more synthetic quality, or allow prosodic control at the expense of less natural-sounding speech with more appropriate intonation. In the ModelTalker system this mode of operation is optional, allowing users to switch between using synthetic prosody and using only those prosodic features that are actually available within the database. In ModelTalker, even when synthetic prosody is enabled, the system attempts to locate concatenation units that most closely approach the desired prosody and therefore, only alter the natural speech in places where it is necessary to do so.

APPLICABILITY FOR ASSISTIVE TECHNOLOGY

The applicability of various types of CSS systems to assistive devices depends on three broadly defined characteristics: intelligibility; naturalness; and technical considerations. Obviously, intelligibility of the CSS system is crucial to its usefulness in an SGD. Naturalness, broadly defined, is a multifaceted attribute that includes both the extent to which the voice resembles a human talker (perhaps a specific human talker), and also the extent to which the CSS system is able to impart human-like expressiveness to the synthetic speech. Expressiveness would mean, at a minimum, an ability to render the prosodic features of an utterance to reflect the different meanings talkers might want to convey with exactly the same phonetic content. Consider, for example, the different meanings one might intend by "Yes." or "Yes?" or "Yes!" and the associated prosody for each. Expressiveness can also mean an ability to impart more global emotional qualities such as happiness, sadness, or anger to synthetic speech. Finally, the CSS system must be implemented within the technical constraints of the SGD in which it is to be used. In the following, we consider each of these factors as they apply to present generation CSS technology generally, and the ModelTalker system specifically.

Intelligibility

Users of SGDs depend heavily upon the quality of their synthetic speech. Foremost, of course, is the concern that the synthetic speech be intelligible. For many years, the DECtalk systems were regarded as the most intelligible systems on the commercial market. For example, Perfect Paul—the most intelligible DECTalk voice—provides sentence-level intelligibility of 86-95% words correct in meaningful sentences, and single-word intelligibility of about 87% correct for isolated words in an open response set (Greene, Manous,

& Pisoni, 1984; Logan, Greene, & Pisoni, 1989). Other voices built into DECTalk (there are 9 in all) provide slightly lower intelligibility (Logan, et al., 1989). Such results led to DECtalk being the CSS system of choice in many SGDs.

However, there have been significant advances in unit concatenation systems since the time of the extensive studies conducted by Pisoni and his colleagues and most of those studies focused on rule-based formant synthesis systems. More recently, we compared five female CSS voices (ModelTalker Kate, AT&T Crystal, Microsoft Mary, Cepstral Linda, and DECtalk Betty) using semantically unpredictable sentence (SUS) material (see Benoît, Grice, & Hazan, 1996 for a description of SUS tests; Bunnell, Pennington, Yarrington, & Gray, 2005 for the comparison of ModelTalker and other systems). All of these systems except DECtalk are unit concatenation systems developed or refined within the last 10 years. The AT&T and Cepstral voices use strict unit concatenation in which only phoneme timing is controllable by the synthesizer; intonation in the synthetic utterances depends entirely upon finding appropriate units that follow a desired intonation pattern. The Microsoft voice uses units stored as parameterized speech in a way that permits control of intonation and timing in the synthetic speech. In this experiment, the ModelTalker system was operated with prosodic control enabled, resulting in appropriate intonation patterns at the expense of some naturalness in voice quality.

The SUS test materials are sentences that adhere to acceptable English grammatical structure with randomly selected words constrained by their part of speech. For example, "The search hired the pool that stood." The SU sentences we used further challenged the listeners and CSS systems by using only one-syllable words that contained many consonant clusters. This placed strong emphasis on the ability of the CSS system to correctly render word boundary cues and the relatively low frequency transitions that are likely to occur between the final consonant(s) of one word and the initial consonant(s) of the next. Some early use of SU sentences in evaluating CSS intelligibility ignored word boundary errors, however, there is now a consensus that doing so results in unrealistically high intelligibility scores. Hence, if a sentence contained a sequence such as "gray day" but a listener reported hearing "grade A," this would be considered two incorrect words.

In our experiment, 25 listeners heard and transcribed 100 SU sentences (20 from each of the five systems being compared). Every sentence was rendered by each of the five CSS systems so there were 500 sentences in all, divided into five balanced sets of 100 sentences, with five listeners assigned to each set. Listeners heard a sentence only once and were then required to type what they heard into a computer. In our original analysis (Bunnell, et al., 2005) we scored each response as the proportion of key words that were correctly reported by each subject for each sentence. More recently, we have shifted to using an "edit distance" measure that counts the number of word or phoneme insertions, deletions, and substitutions that would be necessary to map the listener's response onto the intended utterance. To maintain word boundary information in phoneme-level analyses, we use a special "phoneme" to mark the location of each word boundary. Misplacing a word boundary thus incurs two edit errors at the phonemic as well as word level, however, because there are normally many more phonemes per sentence than words, the overall proportion of errors associated with misplacing a word boundary is substantially smaller.

Figure 2 shows the overall results of this experiment in terms of mean phoneme-level edit distance for each CSS system. Perhaps the most important observation to make regarding the results of this experiment is the striking difference in mean edit distance between the DECtalk Betty voice and all of the unit concatenation systems. This difference was highly significant statistically, indicating that listeners found the DECtalk voice much harder to understand. Neither the DECtalk system, nor the

Figure 2. Mean phonemic edit distance between listener responses and intended utterances for each of five CSS systems

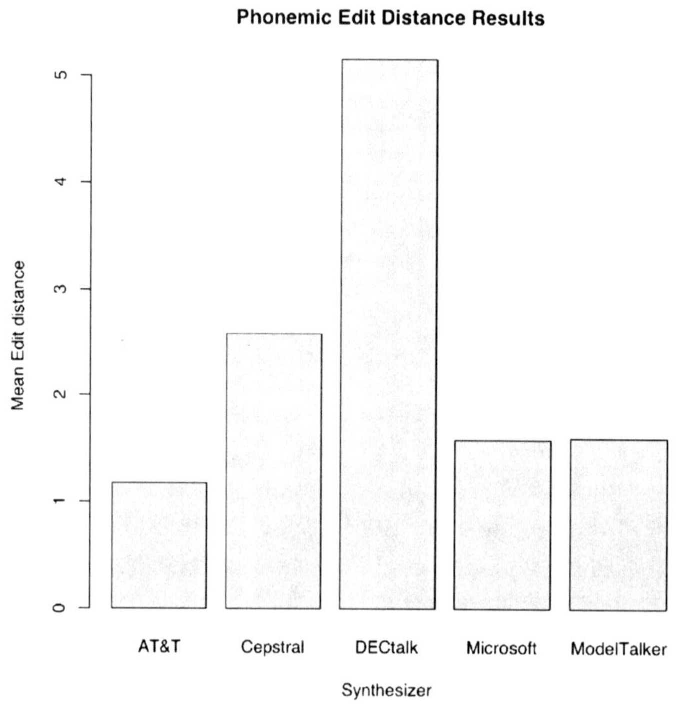

Microsoft Mary voice have been changed since this study was conducted. Although we have not conducted a follow-up study, it is highly probable that ongoing work by developers with AT&T, Cepstral, and ModelTalker since the time of the study has led to further improvements in the quality of those systems and the voices associated with them. Thus, it seems clear that even the best of the available rule-based systems cannot rival recent data-based systems for intelligibility.

This is not to say that all data-based synthesis systems are necessarily more intelligible than rule-based systems. It is both a virtue and a potential shortcoming of data-based synthesis that every new synthetic voice carries with it the features of the talker who recorded the data upon which the voice is based. There is measurable variation in intelligibility from one talker to another with the speech of some talkers being easier to perceive in quiet or with competing background noise (e.g., Cox, Alexander, & Gilmore, 1987; Nabelek, Czyzewski, Krishnan, & Krishnan, 1992). This natural variation in intelligibility should be expected to carry through to the intelligibility of voices created from the recordings of individuals for data-based synthesis. Moreover, there is reason to believe that some talker-specific properties that do not in themselves necessarily affect intelligibility could significantly influence the intelligibility of synthetic voices created from their speech. For example, if the speech within a corpus is highly variable in factors like speaking rate, voice quality, loudness, and pitch range, it will be extremely difficult to locate units that can be concatenated smoothly. Thus, talkers who tend to introduce more variability into their speaking rate, loudness, and style, may be poor target speakers for data-based synthesis.

Beyond variation in voice quality that is due to the talker, data-based systems are also susceptible to variation due to audio recording quality such as signal to noise ratio, microphone and transmission channel characteristics, digital sampling rate, and others. For commercial CSS systems, voice data is always recorded under studio conditions with professional-grade equipment. However, for systems like the ModelTalker system that are designed to be used "in the field" there is often greater variability in the basic audio quality of the corpus, and this may further affect the intelligibility of synthetic voices.

In most current data-based CSS systems the actual *system*—all the rules and logic needed to convert text to phonemes and the signal processing software needed to convert phoneme strings to sound by concatenating speech units—is completely divorced from the speech data that constitutes the voice. For example, the ModelTalker system is designed so that specific "voices" are literally just a few data files that need to be dropped into a directory for ModelTalker to find them. All the other properties of the system remain the same, no matter what voice is being used. This separation of the CSS system from a specific "voice" means that one cannot readily compare CSS systems per se. The fact that the AT&T system was best and Cepstral system worst of the four data-based systems in our experiment cannot be generalized beyond the specific voices we used in this experiment. To be comparable with the commercial systems, the voice we used for the ModelTalker system in the experiment was based on speech we recorded under studio/laboratory conditions using a professional radio announcer as the talker.

Finally, these SUS results are specific to *intelligibility* as opposed to other properties of the CSS voices such as perceived naturalness. In the experiment described above, we asked listeners to rate the naturalness of each sentence in a 5-point scale after they finished transcribing the sentence. The five voices differed significantly in naturalness ratings as well, and again, the AT&T voice was rated most natural while the DECtalk voice was rated least natural. However, the rankings of the other three systems did not reflect the intelligibility rankings. The Cepstral voice was ranked a close second to the AT&T voice for naturalness, while the Microsoft and ModelTalker voices were again very similar in ranking, but between the Cepstral and DECtalk voices.

This difference in intelligibility versus naturalness was also illustrated by additional data reported in Bunnell et al. (2005) that was based on results obtained in the 2005 Blizzard Challenge (Black & Tokuda, 2005). The Blizzard challenge is organized by the CSS research community to allow labs to compare their system to those of other labs under carefully controlled conditions. In the Blizzard challenge, systems are compared for intelligibility using SUS materials, and for naturalness using meaningful sentences drawn from newspapers and other sources. Naturalness ratings are in terms of a mean opinion score (MOS) wherein listeners rate each sentence for naturalness on a scale from one (unnatural) to five (natural). In the 2005 challenge—the last one in which a ModelTalker system participated—the ModelTalker system came out second overall for intelligibility among the 6 systems that took part in the challenge; only one other system had a lower overall word error rate in the SUS tests. However, the same ModelTalker voices were rated as next to worst for naturalness in the MOS tests. This disparity between measures of naturalness and intelligibility leads directly to consideration of the importance of several facets of naturalness in assistive technology.

Naturalness

As previously mentioned, synthetic speech produced by rule-based systems typically does not sound as natural as synthetic speech produced by data-based systems. However, there is wide variation in how natural data-based systems sound, and within a single system, there can be wide variability in how listeners rate the naturalness of individual voices. As with intelligibility, at the "system" level, this variation is due to the size and composition of the speech corpus on which the data-based system relies,[3] the nature of the speech coding strategies it uses for storing and reconstructing the speech, and the extent to which the system attempts to alter speech, as in systems that actively synthesize prosody. At the level of individual voices, naturalness, like intelligibility, can vary depending upon such talker-specific factors as voice quality, consistency, and accuracy.

To illustrate how important the talker is for data-based synthesis, we conducted a study in which we compared ModelTalker CSS "voices" generated with data from 24 different talkers. This experiment held all the system-level factors constant across the talkers. However, the talkers were a very diverse group. They ranged in age from young adults to people in their 60's. One talker had experience as a radio announcer and several of the talkers had mild dysarthria or poor phonatory control or both due to ALS. All talkers recorded the same set of about 1650 utterances that comprise the standard speech corpus used to create ModelTalker voices. The recordings were made in the talkers' homes using their own computers and a variety of audio interfaces ranging from inexpensive consumer-grade to nearly studio-quality hardware. Using the resulting 24 ModelTalker voices, we synthesized 20 Harvard sentences for each voice and presented these to 14 listeners who were asked to rate the naturalness of each sentence on a scale ranging from 1 (synthetic) to 5 (natural). Average ratings for each talker are shown in Figure 3 where the error bars illustrate the 95% confidence intervals for each average; data points for which the error bars do not overlap would be significantly different in a simple t-test (we did not apply any correction for multiple test). As the figure illustrates, some voices are rated much more natural sounding than others despite the fact that all voices were based on the same amount of natural speech data and synthesized by the same CSS system under the same conditions.

One of the things that makes natural speech sound natural is that it contains identity-bearing acoustic cues that allow listeners to recognize

Figure 3. Mean opinion scores for a sample of 24 ModelTalker voices

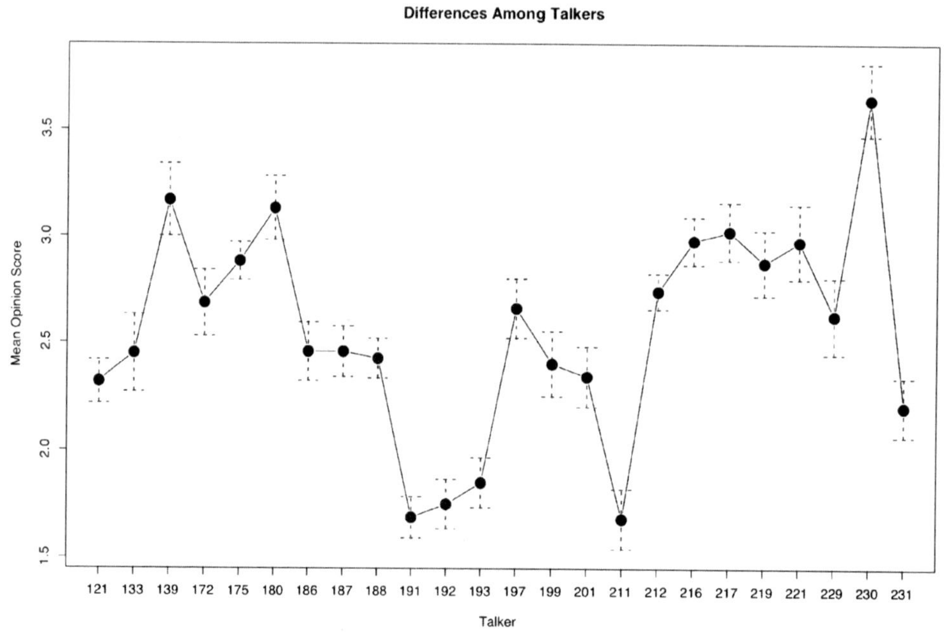

the speaker. While we do not know precisely what all the identity-bearing features of speech are, it is clear that they include phonatory features (related to the structure of the individual's glottal source waveform), resonance properties that are due to vocal tract anatomy such as the length of the talker's vocal tract and the size and shape of structures throughout the supraglottal vocal tract, and behavioral factors that relate to the way an individual would articulate a specific utterance ranging from the fine-grained details of how individual phonemes are (co)articulated to prosodic factors like speaking rate, patterns of emphasis, and how the individual chooses to instantiate intonational features (Kreiman & Papcun, 1991; Walden, Montgomery, Gibeily, Prosek, & Schwartz, 1978).

In our experiment on naturalness, we did not ask listeners to judge how well the talkers' identity was preserved. Had we, it is unlikely that the ratings would be highly correlated with those seen in Figure 3. As Kreiman and Papcun (1991) note, talkers may vary considerably in the distinctiveness of their speech. Voices that are highly distinctive (for whatever reason) probably deviate more than non-distinctive voices from listeners' internal idealized model for natural speech and consequently may be judged "less natural." Many of the synthetic voices in our naturalness experiment were associated with talkers who had quite distinctive natural voices and whose speech would readily have been recognized from their synthetic voices. In some cases, the distinctiveness of the talker's speech may have led to lowering its average "naturalness" rating. This was particularly the case for some of the talkers with mild ALS-related dysarthrias.

Technical Constraints

SGDs are typically built on laptop or mobile computer technology. As such, the speech synthesis system is only one component of a more complex system that must also handle input from one or more interfaces and allow other software such as letter- and word-prediction functions to run simultaneously with applications such as word-processors, email clients, and web browsers. System resources, notably dynamic memory, processor cycles, and file storage space must be shared by all of these system components. Historically, limitations in both device memory and processor capability meant that SGDs were often custom designed proprietary systems with very limited storage capabilities in terms of both the dynamic memory space in which software executes and the long-term file storage space (typically disk or solid state "memory card") in which programs and data must be permanently stored. Consequently, early SGDs required CSS systems with small memory requirements and this in turn favored rule-based systems like DECtalk, or small data-based systems such as limited diphone synthesizers. Moreover, the CSS software had to be tailored specifically to the device so that every device needed a unique version of the CSS software.

Within the last decade, two factors have converged to relieve the constraints. First, memory and storage space has increased significantly as the cost of memory chips has decreased and their density (the amount of memory per chip) has increased. Second, CPU capabilities have expanded greatly, allowing the processor to handle many more programs of much larger size without difficulty. These advances in computer technology have relaxed the size and processor constraints on CSS systems to the point that there is no longer an advantage for rule-based or very small data-based systems. Moreover, advances have made it possible for AT device manufacturers to implement their devices as software applications running on standard laptop or mobile devices that use standard operating systems (most commonly, Windows XP or Windows CE). With the shift to predominantly Windows-based SGDs, any Windows-compatible CSS software can be used to render speech, opening AT devices up to a wide range of possible CSS systems.

To illustrate in practical terms what these advances mean, the present version of the ModelTalker system requires about 200 MB of permanent storage for the program itself and all of the data it uses. When the system is running, a significant amount of this data must be held in dynamic memory. These memory requirements would have made the ModelTalker system completely impractical for early SGDs, but present virtually no problem for current hardware.

PERSONAL VOICES FOR ASSISTIVE TECHNOLOGY

In terms of intelligibility, naturalness, and technical considerations, it is clear that data-based synthesis represents the current best available technology. Despite these clear advantages, users of SGDs have, based on anecdotal evidence, tended to use older rule-based CSS technology for their voices. Partly, this usage pattern may reflect nothing more than the prevalence of those older systems in SGDs that were on the market until quite recently. Further, clinicians who prescribe SGDs for clients were guided by published studies that indicated high intelligibility for some of the rule-based systems, perhaps leading them to recommend the use of those systems over newer technology that has not been so extensively studied. Finally, one can speculate that in the absence of a voice that is truly personal, users of SGDs may prefer to use a somewhat artificial-sounding voice to one that sounds more distinctly like some other real person.

It was with several of these possibilities in mind that we undertook the ModelTalker project with the intent of making high quality personalized voices available to users of SGDs. The goal of the ModelTalker project has been to develop not only CSS software, but more importantly, to develop the software and procedures needed to automate the creation of personal voices. This would allow current users of SGDs to select from a potentially large array of "donated" voices so that each individual could have a personal voice that was not used by other augmented communicators. Moreover, people diagnosed with neuro-degenerative diseases such as ALS would be able to record or "bank" their own voice and from those recordings create a personal synthetic voice that was recognizably their own.

At present, the complete ModelTalker system comprises a program called the ModelTalker Voice Recorder (MTVR for short), software for converting raw speech recordings made by MTVR into a speech synthesis database, and the ModelTalker CSS program itself, which uses the speech synthesis database to produce synthetic speech from English text input. These software components are further supported by a centralized server that communicates with remote copies of the MTVR program so users can download inventories (collections of utterances to record), and upload their recorded speech for analysis and conversion. Once uploaded speech has been converted to a ModelTalker speech database, users are able to download a Windows installer package that will install the voice data files and TTS engine on a computer or SGD as a Microsoft SAPI 5.1 synthetic voice.

As discussed above, concatenative synthesis depends crucially upon the integrity of the speech data it uses. Existing speech technology companies that produce and sell concatenative synthesis products invest tens and even hundreds of thousands of dollars in the development of a single "voice" to ensure optimum quality for the speech database. The costs of developing a voice are associated with (a) recording hours of running speech from professional speakers under studio conditions, (b) automatically labeling and hand-correcting the recorded utterances to see that every phonetic segment is accurately identified, (c) examining and hand-correcting pitch tracking data, and (d) extensively testing the resulting synthetic speech to further identify and repair errors in the labeling, pitch tracking, or original recordings. Much of this work requires access to sophisticated computer software for speech processing and a significant investment of time on the part of one or more individuals with expert knowledge of speech acoustic structure.

The major challenge for the ModelTalker project has been to circumvent this time-consuming and costly voice development process, substituting good consumer-grade audio hardware for professional audio hardware, homes or speech clinics for recording studios, novice users for professional voice talent, and software screening techniques for speech experts. While meeting this challenge is an ongoing process, the current software is being used widely and with generally good success, both by individuals acting on their own, and increasingly by patients working with the assistance of Speech Language Pathologists and AT specialists to develop voices for their SGDs. This latter approach, since it provides users with immediate hands-on support and training in the best use of the software, is the approach that we most strongly recommend.

In our experience with generating personal voices using MTVR and its predecessor software that was called InvTool, two broad areas stand out as being most challenging for users: audio signal quality and speaking style. Problems with audio signal quality can arise from many factors, including environment (people do not realize how loud their refrigerators, fans, air conditioners, and kids can be), microphone (for highly consistent mouth-to-mic distance, we strongly encourage users to purchase a head-mounted microphone), and sound card (many inexpensive sound cards or on-board chips add distortion or noise such as 60 Hz hum). To minimize problems with audio signal quality, we require users of MTVR to record a series of screening sentences and upload them to our central server so that project staff can verify that the signal quality is acceptable for generating a synthetic voice.

Speaking style is the other area of concern for users of MTVR. Good synthetic voices result for corpora that are recorded with very consistent speaking rate, loudness, voice quality, and intonation range. It is also important to speak in a fluent, connected-speech manner. MTVR uses a measure of pronunciation accuracy to screen user recordings on the fly and requests that the user redo any utterance that fails the pronunciation screen. It is very common for users, when asked to redo an utterance, to repeat the utterance in "clear speech" mode as though repeating the utterance for a hearing impaired individual who failed to understand them. Unfortunately, clearly spoken utterances are likely to contain inter-word silences that are undesirable in a corpus designed for continuous speech synthesis, and are likely to be inconsistent with other utterances in factors like speaking rate, loudness, and voice quality. Moreover, because the MTVR pronunciation measure is designed to give the highest scores to utterances that exactly match a template with no inter-word silences, repeating the utterance with silence between each word will typically only serve to further lower the pronunciation rating. As with potential audio problems, the screening sentences users record and upload provide an opportunity for project staff to notice these speaking style pitfalls. Staff can then provide feedback to help users correct style problems so they are more likely to successfully record a corpus.

Obviously, because this process does involve interaction with trained project staff, we have not totally achieved our original goal of an automated process that anyone can use without assistance. We estimate that on average each ModelTalker voice we create requires approximately four hours of staff time. This includes time to review and respond to screening sentences (typically more than once per voice) as well as time to check the pronunciation of user-defined text (typically names of places or people) in the final corpus, run and verify the voice creation process, and build the final voice installer package. Very few of the potential users of this technology have an adequate background in audio electronics, computers, and linguistics to make effective use of MTVR without some expert assistance. Consequently, it is unlikely that it will be possible to significantly reduce the amount of assistance that is needed whether that assistance is provided by ModelTalker project staff as it now is, or the assistance is provided by an AT specialist in a clinical setting as we intend ultimately for this system.

While MTVR and the overall corpus recording process has reached a relatively mature state and is nearly ready to become a commercial package, we continue with basic research related to improving the quality and applicability of synthetic voices to AT. We turn finally to a brief discussion of what directions this CSS technology might take in the future.

FUTURE DIRECTIONS

Despite all the advances in data-based synthesis over the past two decades, there remain areas for improvement. This is especially true for CSS used in SGDs as can be seen by contrasting CSS usage in applications such as an automated call center with CSS usage in SGDs. In the former, the domain of discourse is typically very constrained (e.g., time schedules for trains or flight schedules for planes), and the underlying semantics are "known" to the system. This allows designers for call centers to (a) select inventories of utterances to record that will provide deep coverage of the phonetic content that will be needed for the discourse domain, and (b) apply task-specific knowledge to enhance the text input to the CSS system with markup tags that provide additional pragmatic information such as where focus (placing special emphasis on the most important word in a sentence) should be placed. By contrast, an SGD has as its domain of discourse anything the assisted communicator wants or needs to talk about. This means that in designing the inventory of utterances to be recorded, it is not feasible to trade breadth of phonetic coverage for depth in a specific domain; one must plan for adequate depth in all possible domains. Because a human user rather than a computerized discourse script or agent is providing text to be spoken, the text will probably not contain a rich set of markup tags that allows the system to place pragmatic features correctly, nor would most SGD users be able to provide these tags without special training. Moreover, unlike a call center, SGD users need to express a wide range of feelings and emotions in communicating with others.

Ideally, SGD users should be able to make their voice sound happy, sad, or angry. They should be able to express surprise or doubt not only with words, but also with "tone of voice." At present, the only viable method for producing these effects in data-based synthesis (without significantly reducing naturalness) is to expand the inventory of recorded speech to include utterances spoken in a happy, sad, angry, etc. voice. This is one approach being taken by researchers who are developing large-scale commercial CSS systems (Pitrelli, et al., 2006).

Unfortunately, for individuals who are recording their own speech with MTVR to create a personal CSS voice, greatly increasing the diversity and size of the speech inventory to be recorded is impractical or even impossible. First, not everyone can read utterances that convincingly convey any particular emotion on demand. So, merely adding utterances where the user is asked to sound happy or sad or whatever, is not guaranteed to achieve the desired result. Further, if anything, the existing ModelTalker inventory of about 1650 utterances is already too long for some users (e.g., children or ALS patients). Adding more utterances would likely raise the "entry bar" too high for the users to whom we would most like to apply this technology. This brings us to what is really the fundamental problem that must be solved to make personalized voices for SGDs: reducing the amount of data needed to create a high quality voice that also retains the identity bearing features of an individual's speech.

A number of research groups are actively exploring this issue, primarily within a framework that is evolving from present data-based approaches to use statistically trained parametric representations of an individual's speech (for an excellent technical review, see Zen, Tokuda, & Black, 2009). In this approach, machine-learning techniques, typically using Hidden Markov Models (HMMs), are employed to "train" context-dependent models of phonetic segments in terms of time-varying sequences of vocoder parameters. This approach alone does not solve the corpus size problem. These statistical machine learning techniques require at least as much data as current unit selection systems to derive stable models of an individual's speech. However, because the statistical models are parametric descriptions of an individual's speech, it is possible to apply systematic transformations to the parameters so that speech reconstructed from the parameters is quite different in quality than the speech of the talker who originally recorded the corpus. Carrying this one step further, if one could determine a mapping from the parameter space of the talker who recorded the corpus to that of a different target talker, perhaps using only a small sample of the target talker's speech, the mapping could be applied to all parameters of the statistical phonetic models thus converting the models to generate speech that more closely resembles that of the target talker. This approach is being actively explored in a number of research laboratories (e.g., Roux & Visagie, 2007; Zen, et al., 2009; Zen, Tokuda, & Kitamura, 2007).

In one recent report, Watts, Yamagishi, Berkling, and King (2008) used this approach to create a synthetic voice from recordings of a child. They tried both creating a voice using only recordings from the child (using about 90 minutes of speech), and also using the talker adaptation technique to map a larger adult voice onto the parametric space of the target child talker. However, their results in the latter case revealed relatively poor voice quality, particularly when only a small amount of speech (15 minutes) was used to estimate the mapping. Results of the Watts et al. study underscore another general finding related particularly to children's speech: it is often quite 'fragile' under standard signal processing techniques used for vocoders and parametric synthesis engines even if those techniques are found to work well when applied to adult speech. The most realistic sounding children's voices will result from speech that undergoes the least amount of signal processing.

Even adult voices created with HMM-based parametric systems are subject to the same problems that one encounters whenever the raw speech of the target talker is manipulated in one way or another. While these systems do capture the talker identity, and produce speech without the sorts of discontinuities often associated with waveform concatenation systems, the voices have a somewhat 'buzzy' sound that is typical of impulse-excited LPC synthesis. Moreover, because the parameters from which the synthesis models are derived represent averaged acoustic data, HMM-based synthesis tends to have flat and unexpressive characteristics.

This brings us almost full-circle. Rule-based systems employ a compact and efficient description of speech in terms of a set of parameters and rules for how those parameters vary over time. However, they suffer from the fact that we do not have a sufficiently detailed understanding of how best to parameterize speech and what the rules should be; that is, we lack a deep understanding of what makes speech sound natural or how to capture the identity of an individual talker. This has led to the emergence of data-based synthesis as the dominant approach in the current generation of CSS systems, since with data-based systems, the elements that convey naturalness and talker identity are implicit in the recorded speech data. However, to extend the data-based approach to produce synthetic speech that truly rivals natural speech in all ways, notably expressiveness, we have found that it may be necessary to increase the amount of recorded speech to nearly prohibitive levels (tens of hours of continuous speech in multiple speaking modes). This in turn has led researchers to apply machine-learning techniques to infer synthesis rules from parameterized speech corpora. Once these rules are inferred from a very large corpus produced by one (source) talker, they can be applied to synthesize speech from multiple other (target) talkers using only enough data to estimate features that are systematically different between the source and target talkers. Unfortunately, in this process some of the naturalness and talker identity are lost because we still do not have a sufficiently deep understanding of what features make speech sound natural or what features convey talker identity to design parameter sets and rules that fully capture these features.

For the ModelTalker project, we will continue to employ unit selection synthesis while striving to reduce as far as possible the number of utterances that a user must record to create an acceptable personal voice. In the laboratory, we are actively exploring ways to improve the audio quality of our voices by changes to the way speech is coded in the voice database (equivalent to designing a better parameter set). Simultaneously, we are continuing to use similar machine learning techniques to those described by Zen (2009) in an effort to discover and remove redundant material in the inventory of utterances we ask users to record (Bunnell & Lilley, 2008).

Ultimately, we expect that research will provide solutions to the problems of creating fully natural sounding and expressive synthetic speech. Probably as part of those solutions, we will also learn how to capture the voice quality of an individual from a relatively small but representative sample of their fluent speech whether the individual is an adult or a child. Moreover, it is possible that this will allow us to go one step further and generate realistic natural-sounding voices for dysarthric individuals who presently cannot produce anything more than a few isolated vowel sounds. In fact, in conjunction with a colleague at Northeastern University, we are already exploring how some data-based CSS technology might be used to achieve this (Jreige, Patel, & Bunnell, 2009). There is much work ahead, but there is also great promise in the future for CSS in Assistive Technology.

ACKNOWLEDGMENT

Development of the ModelTalker system has been supported by grants from the US Department of Education and the National Institutes of Health. We are also deeply indebted to Nemours Biomedical Research for ongoing programmatic support. The authors gratefully acknowledge the assistance and support of all members of the ModelTalker project development team, particularly, Jim Polikoff, John Gray, Jason Lilley, Debra Yarrington, Kyoko Nagao, Bill Moyers, and Allegra Cornaglia.

REFERENCES

Atal, B. S., & Hanauer, S. L. (1971). Speech analysis and synthesis by linear prediction of Speech Wave. *The Journal of the Acoustical Society of America*, *50*(2b), 637–655. doi:10.1121/1.1912679

Benoît, C., Grice, M., & Hazan, V. (1996). The SUS test: A method for the assessment of text-to-speech synthesis intelligibility using Semantically Unpredictable Sentences. *Speech Communication*, *18*(4), 381–392. doi:10.1016/0167-6393(96)00026-X

Black, A., & Tokuda, K. (2005). The Blizzard Challenge - 2005: Evaluating corpus-based speech synthesis on common datasets. *INTERSPEECH-2005*, 77-80.

Bunnell, H. T., Hoskins, S. R., & Yarrington, D. M. (1998). A biphone constrained concatenation method for diphone synthesis. *SSW3-1998*, 171-176.

Bunnell, H. T., & Lilley, J. (2008). Schwa variants in American English. *Proceedings: Interspeech, 2008*, 1159–1162.

Bunnell, H. T., Pennington, C., Yarrington, D., & Gray, J. (2005). Automatic personal synthetic voice construction. *INTERSPEECH-2005*, 89-92.

Conkie, A., & Isard, S. (1994). Optimal coupling of diphones. *SSW2-1994*, 119-122.

Cox, R. M., Alexander, G. C., & Gilmore, C. (1987). Intelligibility of average talkers in typical listening environments. *The Journal of the Acoustical Society of America, 81*(5), 1598–1608. doi:10.1121/1.394512

Fant, G. (1960). *Acoustic theory of speech production*. The Hague, The Netherlands: Mouton & Co.

Fowler, C. A. (1980). Coarticulation and theories of extrinsic timing. *Journal of Phonetics, 8*, 113–133.

Goffman, L., Smith, A., Heisler, L., & Ho, M. (2008). The breadth of coarticulatory units in children and adults. *Journal of Speech, Language, and Hearing Research: JSLHR, 51*(6), 1424–1437. doi:10.1044/1092-4388(2008/07-0020)

Greene, B. G., Manous, L. M., & Pisoni, D. B. (1984). *Perceptual evaluation of DECtalk: A final report on version 1.8* (Progress Report No. 10). Bloomington, IN: Indiana University Speech Research Laboratory.

Hanson, H. M., & Stevens, K. N. (2002). A quasiarticulatory approach to controlling acoustic source parameters in a Klatt-type formant synthesizer using HLsyn. *The Journal of the Acoustical Society of America, 112*(3), 1158–1182. doi:10.1121/1.1498851

Harris, Z. S. (1955). From phoneme to morpheme. *Language, 31*(2), 190–222. doi:10.2307/411036

Hertz, S. R., & Huffman, M. K. (1992). A nucleus-based timing model applied to multi-dialect speech synthesis by rule. *ICSLP-1992*, 1171-1174.

Holmes, J. N. (1961). Research on Speech Synthesis Carried out during a Visit to the Royal Institute of Technology, Stockholm, from November 1960 to March 1961. *Joint Speech Resear4ch Unit Report JU 11.4, British Post Office, Eastcote, England.*

Holmes, J. N. (1973). The influence of the glottal waveform on the naturalness of speech from a parallel formant synthesizer. *IEEE Trans., AU-21*, 298–305.

Jreige, C., Patel, R., & Bunnell, H. T. (2009). VocaliD: Personalizing Text-to-Speech Synthesis for Individuals with Severe Speech Impairment. In *Proceedings of ASSETS 2009.*

Klatt, D. H. (1980). Software for a cascade/parallel formant synthesizer. *The Journal of the Acoustical Society of America, 67*(3), 971–995. doi:10.1121/1.383940

Klatt, D. H. (1987). Review of text-to-speech conversion for English. *The Journal of the Acoustical Society of America, 82*(3), 737–793. doi:10.1121/1.395275

Kreiman, J., & Papcun, G. (1991). Comparing discrimination and recognition of unfamiliar voices. *Speech Communication, 10*(3), 265–275. doi:10.1016/0167-6393(91)90016-M

Lehiste, I., & Shockey, L. (1972). On the perception of coarticulation effects in English VCV syllables. *Journal of Speech and Hearing Research, 15*(3), 500–506.

Logan, J. S., Greene, B. G., & Pisoni, D. B. (1989). Segmental intelligibility of synthetic speech produced by rule. *The Journal of the Acoustical Society of America, 86*(2), 566–581. doi:10.1121/1.398236

Magen, H. S., Kang, A. M., Tiede, M. K., & Whalen, D. H. (2003). Posterior pharyngeal wall position in the production of speech. *Journal of Speech, Language, and Hearing Research: JSLHR, 46*(1), 241–251. doi:10.1044/1092-4388(2003/019)

Martin, J. G., & Bunnell, H. T. (1981). Perception of anticipatory coarticulation effects. *The Journal of the Acoustical Society of America, 69*(2), 559–567. doi:10.1121/1.385484

Martin, J. G., & Bunnell, H. T. (1982). Perception of anticipatory coarticulation effects in vowel-stop consonant-bowel sequences. *Journal of Experimental Psychology. Human Perception and Performance, 8*(3), 473–488. doi:10.1037/0096-1523.8.3.473

Mermelstein, P. (1973). Articulatory model for the study of speech production. *The Journal of the Acoustical Society of America, 53*(4), 1070–1082. doi:10.1121/1.1913427

Moulines, E., & Charpentier, F. (1990). Pitch-synchronous wave-form processing techniques for Text-to-Speech synthesis using diphones. *Speech Communication, 9*(5-6), 453–467. doi:10.1016/0167-6393(90)90021-Z

Nabelek, A. K., Czyzewski, Z., Krishnan, L. A., & Krishnan, L. A. (1992). The influence of talker differences on vowel identification by normal-hearing and hearing-impaired Listeners. *The Journal of the Acoustical Society of America, 92*(3), 1228–1246. doi:10.1121/1.403973

O'Shaughnessy, D. (1992). Recognition of hesitations in spontaneous speech. *Proceedings of the IEEE Conference on Acoustics, Speech, and Signal Processing*, 521-524.

Öhman, S. E. G. (1966). Coarticulation in VCV Utterances: Spectrographic Measurements. *The Journal of the Acoustical Society of America, 39*(1), 151–168. doi:10.1121/1.1909864

Peterson, G., Wang, W., & Siversten, E. (1958). Segmentation techniques in speech synthesis. *The Journal of the Acoustical Society of America, 30*, 739–742. doi:10.1121/1.1909746

Pitrelli, J. F., Bakis, R., Eide, E. M., Fernandez, R., Hamza, W., & Picheny, M. A. (2006). The IBM expressive text-to-speech synthesis system for American English. *IEEE Transactions on Audio Speech and Language Processing, 14*(4), 1099–1108. doi:10.1109/TASL.2006.876123

Roux, J. C., & Visagie, A. S. (2007). Data-driven approach to rapid prototyping Xhosa speech synthesis. *SSW6-2007*, 143-147.

Sagisaka, Y. (1988). Speech synthesis by rule using an optimal selection of non-uniform synthesis units. *IEEE ICASSP1988*, 679-682.

Silverman, K., Beckman, M. E., Pitrelli, J., Ostendorf, M., Wightman, C., Price, P., et al. (1992). ToBI: a standard for labeling English prosody. *Proceedings of the Second International Conference on Spoken Language Processing*, 867-870.

Sivertsen, E. (1961). Segment inventories for speech synthesis. *Language and Speech, 4*(1), 27–90.

Stevens, K. N., & Bickley, C. A. (1991). Constraints among parameters simplify control of Klatt formant synthesizer. *Journal of Phonetics, 19*, 161–174.

Stevens, K. N., & House, A. S. (1955). Development of a quantitative description of vowel articulation. *The Journal of the Acoustical Society of America, 27*(3), 484–493. doi:10.1121/1.1907943

Takeda, K., Abe, K., & Sagisaka, Y. (1992). On the basic scheme and algorithms in non-uniform unit speech synthesis. In G. Bailly, C. Benoît & T. R. Sawallis (Eds.), *Talking machines: Theories, models, and designs* (pp. 93-105). Amsterdam, The Netherlands: North-Holland Publishing Co.

van Santen, J. P. H. (1992). Deriving text-to-speech durations from natural speech. In G. Bailly, C. Benoît & T. R. Sawallis (Eds.), *Talking machines: Theories, models, and designs* (pp. 275-285). Amsterdam, The Netherlands: North-Holland Publishing Co.

Walden, B. E., Montgomery, A. A., Gibeily, G. J., Prosek, R. A., & Schwartz, D. M. (1978). Correlates of psychological dimensions in talker similarity. *Journal of Speech and Hearing Research, 21*(2), 265–275.

Watts, O., Yamagishi, J., Berkling, K., & King, S. (2008). HMM-Based Synthesis of Child Speech. *1st Workshop on Child, Computer and Interaction (ICMI'08 post-conference workshop).*

Whalen, D. H., Kang, A. M., Magen, H. S., Fulbright, R. K., & Gore, J. C. (1999). Predicting midsagittal pharynx shape from tongue position during vowel production. *Journal of Speech, Language, and Hearing Research: JSLHR, 42*(3), 592–603.

Wicklegran, W. A. (1969). Context-sensitive coding associative memory and serial order in (speech) behavior. *Psychological Review, 76*, 1–15. doi:10.1037/h0026823

Yarrington, D., Bunnell, H. T., & Ball, G. (1995). Robust automatic extraction of diphones with variable boundaries. *EUROSPEECH, 95*, 1845–1848.

Zen, H., Tokuda, K., & Black, A. W. (2009). Statistical parametric speech synthesis. *Speech Communication, 51*(11), 1039–1064. doi:10.1016/j.specom.2009.04.004

Zen, H., Tokuda, K., & Kitamura, T. (2007). Reformulating the HMM as a trajectory model by imposing explicit relationships between static and dynamic feature vector sequences. *Computer Speech & Language, 21*(1), 153–173. doi:10.1016/j.csl.2006.01.002

ENDNOTES

1. Some phonemes, such as fricatives and nasals, have relatively stable and constant target values throughout their duration and need only one set of target values. Others, such as stop consonants, glides, and diphthongs, have more complex time-varying structure and require multiple sets of target values associated with different regions of the phoneme. In these cases, it is also necessary to specify rules for how parameter values change over time as they vary from one set of target values to another.
2. A web-based implementation of the Klatt (1980) synthesizer is available for educational use at http://www.asel.udel.edu/speech/tutorials/synthesis/index.html.
3. This assumes that each system uses its own standard, possibly proprietary, inventory of utterances that are used for every voice.

Chapter 6
Building Personalized Synthetic Voices for Individuals with Dysarthria Using the HTS Toolkit

Sarah Creer
University of Sheffield, UK

Phil Green
University of Sheffield, UK

Stuart Cunningham
University of Sheffield, UK

Junichi Yamagishi
University of Edinburgh, UK

ABSTRACT

For an individual with a speech impairment, it can be necessary for them to use a device to produce synthesized speech to assist their communication. To fully support all functions of human speech communication: communication of information, maintenance of social relationships and displaying identity, the voice must be intelligible and natural-sounding. Ideally, it must also be capable of conveying the speaker's vocal identity. A new approach based on Hidden Markov models (HMMs) has been proposed as a way of capturing sufficient information about an individual's speech to enable a personalized speech synthesizer to be developed. This approach adapts a statistical model of speech towards the vocal characteristics of an individual. This chapter describes this approach and how it can be implemented using the HTS toolkit. Results are reported from a study that built personalized synthetic voices for two individuals with dysarthria. An evaluation of the voices by the participants themselves suggests that this technique shows promise for building personalized voices for individuals with progressive dysarthria even when their speech has begun to deteriorate.

DOI: 10.4018/978-1-61520-725-1.ch006

INTRODUCTION

Adult speech impairment can be congenital, caused by conditions such as cerebral palsy or acquired through conditions such as motor neurone disease (MND), stroke or traumatic head injury. In some acquired conditions, such as MND, diminishing neurological function contributes to a progressive loss of speech ability. Such neurologically-based motor speech impairments are known as *dysarthria* and are characterized by impaired movement of the articulators and control of respiration (Duffy, 2005). In the case of acquired conditions such as MND and Parkinson's disease (PD), the progressive loss of speech motor control results in increasingly severe impairment.

Synthesized voices currently available on communication aids are highly intelligible and can approach human-like naturalness, but there are limited opportunities to personalize the output to more closely match the speech of an individual user. However, recent advances in technology offer the prospect of using probabilistic models of speech to generate high quality personalized synthetic speech with minimal input requirements from a *participant speaker*.

The aim of this chapter is to describe the need for the personalization of speech synthesis for use with communication aids; to set out currently available techniques for personalization and their limitations for people with speech disorders; to assess whether personalized voices can be built successfully with probabilistic models for individuals whose speech has begun to deteriorate and finally to implement this technique for those individuals and allow them to evaluate the personalized synthetic voices.

BACKGROUND

Why is a Personalized Speech Synthesizer Necessary?

For individuals with severe speech impairment it may be necessary for them to use alternative and augmentative communication (AAC) methods to support their communication. This may be a 'low-tech' solution such as an alphabet board, or may be a 'high-tech' solution such as a *voice output communication aid* (VOCA). An individual can compose a message on a VOCA device using a keyboard or touch screen and this message is then 'spoken' by a speech synthesizer.

People who still have some speech ability often use VOCAs to augment their communication (Bloch and Wilkinson, 2004). With a progressive condition an individual's speech ability will deteriorate, and it may eventually become very difficult for them to efficiently communicate with unfamiliar communication partners. It is therefore possible that the output from the VOCA can become the individual's primary mode of communication. The output from the speech synthesizers becomes the 'voice' of the individual.

Locke (1998) defines two purposes of communication: the transmission of impersonal facts and the construction, maintenance and enjoyment of social relationships. When the communication is verbal, speech has a secondary role in conveying individual characteristics of the speaker. Ideally, the many roles of speech output should be retained in the output of the VOCA.

In speech communication the spoken message has to be intelligible to the receiver of the message. Intelligibility is defined as the accuracy with which an acoustic signal is conveyed by a speaker and recovered by a listener (Kent, Weismer, Kent and Rosenbek, 1989). High levels of intelligibility ensure that the transmission of impersonal facts takes place successfully.

For a VOCA to facilitate social interaction, and to enable the user to create, maintain and use social relationships, the speech output must be highly intelligible and it is also desirable for the output to be natural-sounding to promote understanding and increase motivation for both conversational partners to interact. As social closeness is developed through frequency of interaction rather than content of communication, regular communication should be promoted by a VOCA to avoid social withdrawal of the user (Light, 1988; Murphy, 2004; O'Keefe, Brown and Schuller, 1998).

It is known that negative experiences caused by difficulties in communication for an individual with a speech disorder will reduce motivation to interact with others (Kemp, 1999; Miller, Noble, Jones and Burn, 2006). If the preferences of both speakers and their conversational partners can be met with appropriate speech output from a VOCA it is likely to increase motivation. There is evidence to suggest that positive attitudes toward non-speaking individuals are influenced by the use of voice output in their VOCA rather than other communication devices (Gorenflo and Gorenflo, 1991; Lilienfeld and Alant, 2002). These high-tech devices replicate more closely oral communication that conversation partners are more accustomed to using. Limitations of the technology still place restrictions on how far the interaction will reproduce normal conversation due to the time taken to compose and produce responses on a VOCA. However, in relation to how the output is comprehended, if the output is easy to listen to and understand, it will provide motivation for further interaction for both conversational partners.

People often attach human-like attributes and associations to synthetic speech just as they do to natural speech and this can also affect their attitude towards the VOCA user as well as the message being conveyed (Nass, Moon and Green, 1997; Stern, Mullennix, Dyson and Wilson, 2002). Participants in Stern, Mullennix, Dyson and Wilson's (1999) experiment perceived a speaker with a synthetic voice as less truthful, knowledgeable and involved in the interaction compared to a speaker with natural speech. The synthetic speech rated as having a higher quality was perceived to be closer to the natural speech for these factors than the lower quality synthetic speech. These results imply that the quality of synthetic speech is related to the positivity of a listener's attitudes towards the individual using it.

It is known that the possibility of the listener having a negative attitude is reduced if the speaker is known to be speech-impaired and therefore has no other choice but to use the synthesized voice (Stern, 2008; Stern, Mullennix and Wilson, 2002; Stern, Mullennix and Yaroslavsky, 2006). Attitudes from a listener's point of view are non-negative towards the individual who is using a communication aid. However, these results rely on the voice being high quality, easily comprehensible and pleasant sounding. Having a better quality, natural-sounding voice is also likely to reduce listener fatigue due to the cognitive load placed on the listener to understand the speech that is being presented to them.

People usually adapt their speech dependent on who they are communicating with, a process referred to as speech accommodation theory (Street and Giles, 1982). There is evidence that this type of behaviour also occurs in human-computer interaction, which has implications for interaction with artificial dialogue systems (Coulston, Oviatt and Darves, 2002; Darves and Oviatt, 2002; Moore and Morris, 1992). An unnatural sounding voice could be an obstacle to having a usual human-to-human conversational interaction rather than a human-to-computer interaction and a higher quality synthesis could help to reduce this obstacle.

A more natural-sounding voice in a VOCA may promote easier association of the device with the individual and the social distance imposed by using the device as an intermediary in a conversation is lessened. Social closeness is more likely to be preserved through increased interaction using a more accepted, natural voice by the speaker and the encouragement to interact in a human-like way for the listener. This provides evidence that highly natural-sounding speech synthesizers can be used to substitute the ability to create, maintain and enjoy social relationships through speech by increasing motivation for interaction and more closely replicating human speech communication.

To be able to convey identity in the same way a natural voice does, a VOCA needs to represent the individual through the characteristics of the output voice. The voice provides information about the sex, age, size, ethnicity and geographical identity of that individual (Chambers, 1995; Wells, 1982). Losing this ability to represent individuality through the voice means a lack of ability to be represented as the individual who was previously identified by that voice.

If a voice does not contain appropriate information that matches an individual's identity, it may restrict an individual's ability to form associations with others through voice communication. Using an inappropriate voice may also lead to disassociations with a group and lead to a lack of motivation for the speaker to interact. This can be detrimental where group membership is particularly important, for example, for cultural associations (Angelo, Kokosa and Jones, 1996; Hetzroni and Harris, 1996; Parrette and Huer, 2002) and within age group, specifically adolescents (Smith, 2005).

Synthesized voices themselves display non-neutral vocal identity which may or may not overlap with those of the VOCA user. The features the voice displays may or may not have negative associations and provoke negative attitudes for the user. If the individual does not want to associate with the voice and the features it conveys, they will not be willing to use it. For example, anecdotal evidence suggest that the most popular voice chosen by users in Northern England is a US English voice, as British English synthetic voices have a Southern English accent. To understand this decision means taking into account the social background of the individual, their own and their community's attitudes and associations made with that voice. It suggests that there is an awareness of the presentation and inference of identity through the voice and the implications of using a voice that is not well matched to the individual involved. This is a personal choice and will depend on the views and associations of that particular individual as well as their group membership.

When listeners are asked to express a preference reveal a preference for gender-appropriate and age-appropriate voices (Crabtree, Mirenda and Beukelman, 1990) in addition to intelligence- and socially-appropriate voices (O'Keefe et al., 1998). Listening to matched voices and users led to a more positive attitude towards interaction with the VOCA user. These results are echoed with participants in Crabtree et al., (1990) matching the most highly rated natural-sounding and gender-appropriate voice to themselves when asked which voice they would prefer if they were to use a VOCA. This relates to suggestions of how assistive technology should be designed, indicating that individuals would prefer to have a voice output that matches the characteristics of the person who was using it (Light, Page, Curran and Pitkin, 2007). It is also suggested that any communication aid should be highly customizable for the wants and needs of users (Allen, 2005). Crabtree et al. (1990) and Light et al. (2007)'s evaluations used participants who were not speech-impaired. The lack of available resources to currently personalize communication aids restricts the ability to provide empirical evidence for these types of evaluations based on actual VOCA users.

A personalized VOCA where the synthetic voice has characteristics of the user could reduce the social distance imposed by this mode of communication by re-associating the output content with the user through use of vocal identity. This argument also implies that if social distance is reduced by using a personalized output, conversely distance from the device would be imposed by using a non-personalized voice. This may be preferable if the individual was still using his or her own voice as a primary mode of communication and used a VOCA as a supplementary aid.

It therefore seems possible for VOCAs to replace all three functions of speech communication if the voice output is highly intelligible, natural-sounding and has some similarity to the individual user.

It may be that the individual feels that a personalized voice is not appropriate and wish to have a voice output that does not match what was previously their own. If they wish to disassociate themselves from that voice then it is unlikely that they would be de-motivated by a lack of personal identity with the voice. However, individuals should be presented with a choice of how they wish to represent themselves through the synthetic voices that are available, including one based on their own speech characteristics.

Current Personalization Techniques

Pre-Recorded Output

Many currently available VOCAs provide a synthesized output and pre-stored digitized recorded speech output. A level of personalization can be achieved by using pre-stored utterances recorded by either an individual with a similar accent, age and the same sex or by using phrases previously stored by the VOCA user. This technique restricts the user to a limited pre-defined set of communication utterances. To be able to produce any novel utterance, the choice of voices is restricted to those few impersonal off-the-shelf voices available with the VOCA.

Voice Banking

An alternative for personalization of synthetic voices is to 'bank' recordings from an individual. *Voice banking* is the process of making recordings from which to build a personalized voice prosthesis that is able to produce any novel utterance and can be used either on a home computer or ported onto a communication aid. This process is most suitable for those individuals at the onset of a progressive condition while their speech is sufficiently unaffected to be able to be captured in the banking process. Currently available methods for producing personalized synthetic voices using concatenative and parametric synthesis are described below.

Concatenative Synthesis

The currently available techniques for building a new synthetic voice require large amounts of recorded speech to construct a voice of reasonable quality. This requirement for large amounts of speech data stems from the fact that the synthetic voices constructed are based on concatenative synthesis. This is a technique in which recordings of speech are segmented into small time units which can then be recombined to make new utterances. Concatenation is more than simply joining one unit to another - the listener must not be able to perceive the 'join'. This is conventionally done with using a signal manipulation technique such as PSOLA (Pitch Synchronous Overlap and Add) to reduce the differences between neighbouring joined units (Moulines and Charpentier, 1990). Festvox, (Black and Lenzo, 2007), is a voice building tool used with the Festival (Taylor, Black and Caley, 1998) concatenative speech synthesis system. It is principally aimed at researchers and as such, is not trivial to use for someone without specialist phonetic and computational knowledge. A high quality synthetic voice can be produced with around 1200 sentences or 80 minutes of continuous speech with a full coverage of the sounds of a language (Clark, Richmond and King, 2004). With less data there are fewer units available for concatenation which can make the output more inconsistent and sometimes unintelligible. Concatenative synthesis can produce very high quality natural-sounding speech but requires a large amount of recording to provide a database from which to select units and recombine them to produce speech. Once a database for a particular voice has been recorded it is not simple to modify as it will involve recording an entire database for any prosodic modification such as different emotions in speech or for speaker characteristics for personalization.

An approach specifically designed for people with progressive speech loss is ModelTalker (Yarrington, Pennington, Gray and Bunnell, 2005), a voice building service which can be used on any home computer to build a concatenative synthesis voice. The data collection tool, ModelTalker Voice Recorder (MTVR), requires approximately 1800 utterances to be recorded to build a good quality voice. MTVR prompts the individual to produce an utterance, screening it for consistency of pitch, loudness and pronunciation, aiming to collect only good quality consistent usable data. It does not require any specialist computer or linguistic knowledge by the user as the voice is recorded and uploaded via the internet to the developers who build the voice and send it back to the user.

Concatenative synthesis can produce very high quality synthesis that sounds very natural. It requires a lot of data to be recorded and can produce inconsistent output if the right coverage and amount of data is not recorded. Concatenative synthesis requires the recorded data to be intelligible as the data recorded is used directly as the voice output. This feature combined with the amount of data required makes these techniques more problematic for those individuals whose voices have started to deteriorate.

Parametric Synthesis

Parametric or formant synthesis has dominated VOCAs for many years because of its highly consistent and intelligible output and its relatively small memory footprint. Although lacking in naturalness in comparison to concatenative synthesis, certain features of the voice, particularly prosodic features, are more easily manipulable. This technique is based on the separate modelling of the excitation source and filter components of speech (Fant, 1960). The articulations of speech are modelled by a filter representing the resonant frequencies of the vocal tract at a point in time.

The flexibility of a parametric synthesizer lends itself to easier manipulation of the signal but the access to the appropriate parameters and the mapping between the parameters and particular characteristics of an individual is not trivial. This means that complete personalization for parametric synthesis is theoretically possible but practically complex, time-consuming and not possible without expert knowledge, if done at all. Further unsuitability for this purpose is due to the difficulties of extracting reliable parametric information once deterioration has begun.

Procedure Requirements

To allow people to be able to use an approximation of the characteristics of their own voice to personalize a speech synthesizer, there is a distinction to be made between building a personalized voice for an individual who is aware that they will lose their still functioning voice and building a voice for a person whose speech has already started to deteriorate or has a pre-existing speech impairment.

Building a synthetic voice for a particular individual will require some input data from them irrespective of their speech ability. Providing the required amount and quality of data to build a good concatenative synthesis voice is time-consuming and laborious for the speaker, which can be unsuitable for an individual with a severe speech impairment. They may often experience fatigue when speaking which will become audible and result in inconsistencies in the recordings. Recording utterances in small quantities over a period of time is one way of dealing with this issue but as the disorder continues to progress, the voice will continue to alter and production will become more difficult.

For a person whose speech has begun to deteriorate, there will have to be a way of capturing characteristics of the speaker while removing the effects of the dysarthria. Ideally, the voice would be captured before it has begun to deteriorate but it is clear that building a voice with the minimum amount of data possible is a requirement for this task.

For a person with a progressive condition, it is difficult not only to collect the data from a practical point of view but there are also emotional factors involved. In committing to this process, the person will be admitting that at some point they will lose their ability to speak. Therefore, this is a process that must be carefully timed to avoid unnecessary distress. The best time to collect recordings will be shortly after diagnosis when it is unlikely that their speech has begun to be affected, however this may not necessarily coincide with the individual's emotional readiness to deal with this prospect (Murphy, 2004).

The voice building process needs to involve minimal data input from the individual and should provide a way to use the speaker characteristics of a voice that has begun to deteriorate and compensate for the effects of dysarthria on the voice to produce an intelligible, natural-sounding output that sounds like the person using it.

An alternative approach to both concatenative and parametric synthesis known as model-based synthesis could provide the necessary requirements for personalization of synthetic speech. In addition it may be possible to realize a personalized synthetic voice using much less data than is required for concatentative approaches. Model-based synthesis statistically models the speech used to create the synthetic voice and has been shown to produce high quality output in the Blizzard challenge voice-building evaluations for a database of unimpaired speech (Zen, Toda, Nakamura and Tokuda, 2007). It requires a manageable amount of input data from the individual to adapt speaker-independent models which have been pre-trained on a large corpus. It has potential for compensating for speech with impairments by using adaptation techniques developed for speech recognition.

HMM-Based Speech Synthesis

Introduction

The HMM-based Speech Synthesis System (or HTS – 'H Triple S') (Zen, Nose, Yamagishi, Sako and Tokuda, 2007a, Tokuda et al., 2008) is a toolkit for building speech synthesizers using *Hidden Markov Models* (HMMs) (Rabiner, 1989) for speech synthesis. It uses HMMs to both model the speech production process probabilistically and generate new speech output. The procedure consists of three parts: training, adaptation and synthesis. The overall structure of HTS is detailed in figure 1. The following sections provide information on how speech is represented in HTS, an introduction to HMMs and details of the procedures involved to build synthetic voices.

Feature Vectors

Speech production is a continuous process. To model the acoustics, the speech has to be parameterized. Speech samples are taken at regular time intervals and represented by *feature vectors*: a set of numbers characterizing the spectral and excitation parameters at that time segment. The feature vectors are extracted from the corpus of speech every 5 milliseconds (ms) using STRAIGHT vocoding (Kawahara, Masuda-Katsuse and de Cheveigné, 1999).

In speech recognition, the feature vectors provide a compact representation of those acoustics of speech which are important for sound discrimination to accurately identify the output. This is usually restricted to a representation of the spectral acoustics without fundamental frequency (F0) information. In English, altering the F0 of a sound does not influence its phonemic representation. Speech synthesis, however, is not

Figure 1. Structure of the HTS 2.1 system

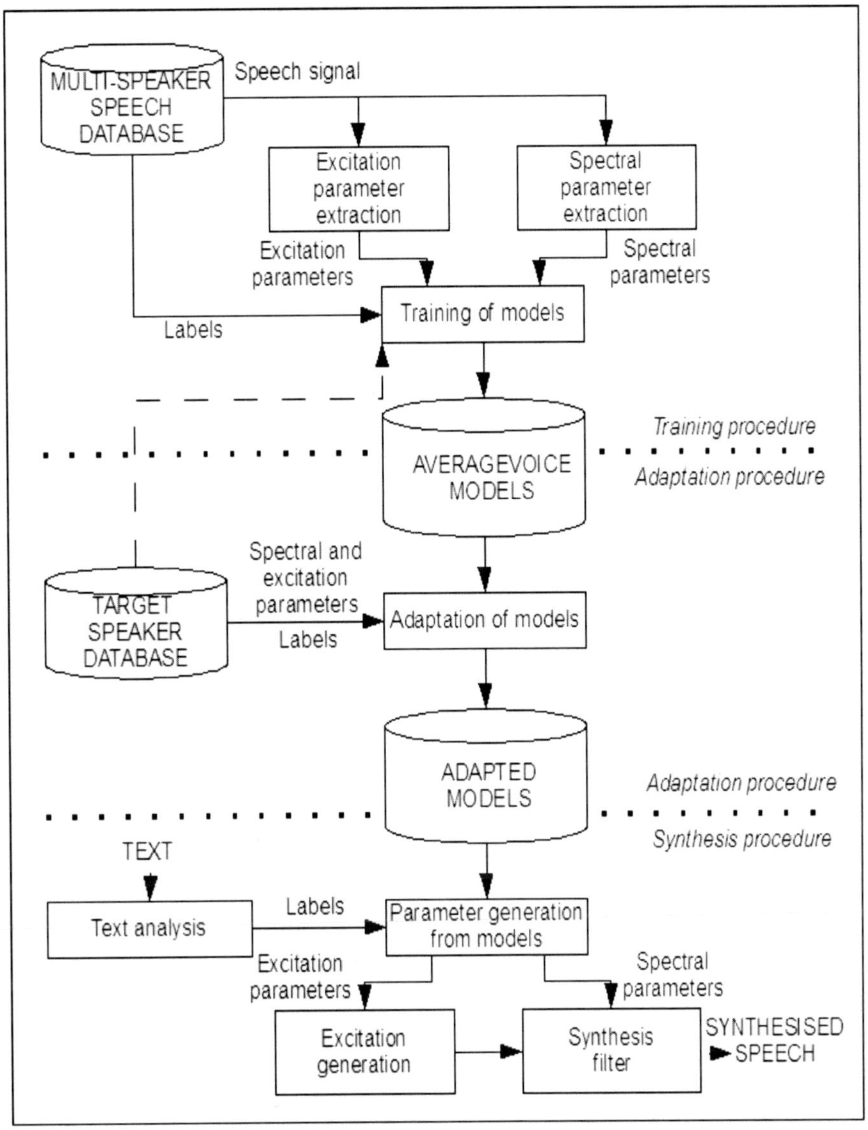

a classification task; the aim is to reproduce the speech signal as accurately as possible to produce a natural-sounding speech output. This requires much more information to be extracted into the feature vectors to be modelled. The feature vectors represent three different components or streams of the signal: spectral features in the form of mel-cepstral coefficients (including energy), which represent the shape of the vocal tract; log F0, which represents the pitch of the utterance and band aperiodicity, which helps to better model the excitation source. Aperiodicity provides a weighting for the aperiodic components in periodic frames across 5 frequency bands: 0-1, 1-2, 2-4, 4-6 and 6-8 kiloHertz (kHz).

Hidden Markov Models

HMMs can be used to probabilistically model sequences of feature vectors representing the acoustics of the speech signal. HMMs are generative models: an HMM for a word, represents the

Figure 2. Hidden Markov model (HMM). Emitting states are represented by circles and transitions are represented by arrows. There is a transition probability (a) associated with every transition and a Gaussian output probability (b) associated with every state.

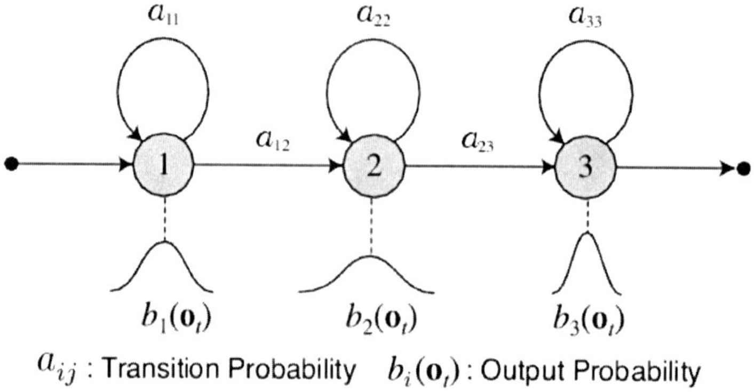

acoustics that are likely to be produced when that word is spoken. HMMs are extensively used in automatic speech recognition, where the question is 'what model, or sequence of models, is most likely to have produced the observed acoustics?'. HMMs are not only able to successfully characterize sequences of feature vectors, but they are also able to generate feature vectors dependent on the probabilistic modelling, from which speech waveforms can be synthesized.

An HMM consists of two parts: a model of the temporal sequence and a model of the observed data. The temporal sequence is modelled with a network of states and transitions between these states with associated probabilities. Figure 2 shows a diagrammatic representation of an HMM. The circles represent states containing the state output distribution probabilities (labelled b) and arrows represent transitions with associated transition probabilities. The transition probabilities (labelled a) model the number of time frames that the process will remain in a state and the possible next state to transition to in the sequence. Associated with each state is a statistical model of the observed data, usually a Gaussian (normally distributed) statistical representation of the acoustics of a particular section of speech. The number of states will define how many distinct sections of a feature vector sequence are modelled by that HMM. There should be enough states in an HMM to capture enough detail to model the sequence accurately while still accounting for natural variation in the acoustics.

HMM transition probabilities do not provide an accurate model for duration. The Markov property on which an HMM is based states that the description of the state that the process is in at a point in time fully captures all the information required that could influence the future of the process. However, if we want to model state occupancy by a normal distribution, the transition probability will depend on how long we have been in the state. To combat this problem, HTS estimates a normally distributed state duration probability density for each phoneme model during training and this is explicitly attached to the model for both training and synthesis. This alters some of the mathematical properties of the model and results in a *Hidden Semi-Markov Model* (HSMM) (Zen, Tokuda, Masuko, Kobayashi and Kitamura, 2007c) as shown in figure 3. The transition probabilities are replaced by a number of time frames to stay in that state, derived from the duration probability. The training corpus is then used to estimate the probability density function contained in the states to model the likelihood of that state generating that feature vector and the parameters of the duration model.

Figure 3. Hidden semi-Markov model (HSMM). Explicit duration probabilities (p) replace transition probabilities and define the number of time frames spent with the associated Gaussian output probability (b).

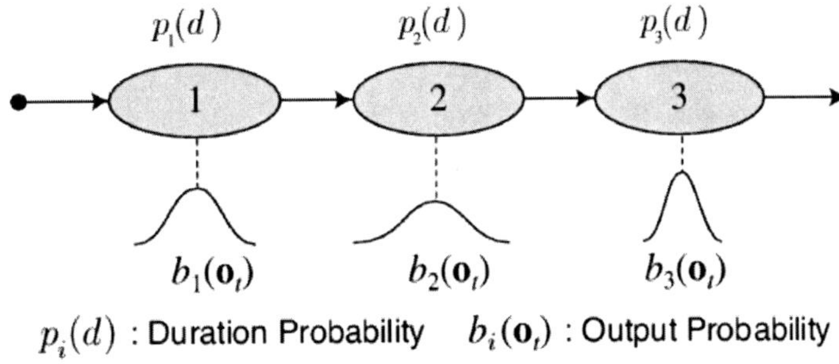

In order to model speech with HMMs, assumptions have to be made to simplify the probability calculations. The conditional independence assumption states that there is no dependency between the feature vector observations. This does not represent effectively the behaviour of the articulators whose configuration at one time frame is highly dependent on their configuration at the previous and following time frames. To approximate this correlation, other features are introduced into the feature vector which measure the change of the static observations, called deltas and delta-deltas, which capture the changes in the deltas. These features are introduced for spectral information, log F0 and aperiodicity.

An HSMM can be trained on a corpus of speech data to produce statistical models of the acoustics. Novel speech utterances are then formed by concatenating the appropriate models and generating a sequence of feature vectors from the model sequence from which a speech waveform can be synthesized. Unlike parametric synthesis, this data-driven technique does not demand human intervention for tuning any synthesis parameters; the variation is captured in the corpus of data on which the models are trained. Using HSMMs also creates the opportunity to use speaker adaptation techniques developed for speech recognition to personalize the voice of such a system from existing models built with several speakers' data, with a much smaller amount of data from the participant.

Training

For training, the data must be suitably labelled to align the feature vectors to the appropriate model. This is done by expanding an orthographic transcription of the spoken data into a set of context-dependent phoneme labels. The acoustic structure of a sound will vary depending on its surrounding context due to the continuous movement of the articulators in the production of speech. For speech recognition, the unit modelled by the HMM is usually a triphone: a phoneme-sized unit which takes into account the previous and following phoneme. Speech recognition aims to discriminate between sounds to classify them correctly using the minimal information required to do so. Speech synthesis aims to reproduce the speech waveform as accurately as possible, retaining features that contribute to the naturalness of speech. For a speech synthesis task, the contextual effects must be included as they contribute to the generation of phonetic and prosodic elements of the output speech.

In HTS, each model contains five emitting states and represents a context-dependent phoneme. Using this number of states for a phoneme-sized unit allows a high level of detail of the acoustics to be captured by the models, while still allowing for the natural variation present in speech. The contextual factors used in HTS are more detailed than in triphone modelling: they provide phonetic and prosodic information about the previous and following two phonemes at the phoneme, syllable, word, phrase and utterance levels. They use information about stress, position and part of speech of the unit.

Training a model for every context-dependent phoneme observed in the data will mean that to cover all possible contexts, an impractically large amount of data will have to be recorded by an individual. With such a specific model definition, each HSMM will be trained on very little data and will be unable to fully capture the acoustic variation present in speech. The problem of sparse data can be approached by sharing the parameters of the state output distribution between other acoustically similar states, clustering the data and training the models together. This is performed using phonetic decision trees which define clusters of acoustically similar data in a hierarchical structure, finding the structure of phonetic contexts which best split the data. Different factors will affect the acoustic distance between vectors for duration, spectral information, F0 and aperiodicity and so HTS uses separate decision trees for each. This means that there are separate models for the generation of each of these features, which will be combined at synthesis time.

Even with this approach, building a model based on the speech of one individual: a speaker-dependent model, will require a large amount data to fully capture the characteristics of that person's speech. The Blizzard challenge evaluation rated the speaker-dependent 2005 HTS system highest in a mean opinion score evaluation for naturalness and had the lowest word error rate representing high intelligibility (Bennett, 2005; Zen et al., 2007b). This voice was built with 80 minutes of speech from one person, which is equivalent to approximately 1200 sentences.

For individuals in this task who will have difficulties associated with their speech, it may be inappropriate and impractical to collect this amount of data. HTS uses adaptation techniques as introduced for speech recognition to deal with this problem of sparse data, adapting existing models towards those that would represent the target speaker but using a much smaller amount of data.

Adaptation

For adaptation, a large amount of data taken from several speakers is first used to build speaker-independent models. This process provides a robust model of the general characteristics of speech and the relationship between those characteristics. Having a full picture of speech provides a more informed starting point for adaptation, guaranteeing some shared characteristics between this *average voice* and the participant speaker. It will lead to fewer errors in estimating observations that can occur due to lack of data from the participant speaker. Adaptation data is provided by the target speaker and the parameters of the speaker-independent models are adapted to improve the fit to this data. In principle, the adaptation process aligns the correct sequence of existing models to the adaptation data and then re-estimates their parameters so that it is more likely that the models would generate the data (Yamagishi, Kobayashi, Nakano, Ogata, Isogai, 2009). This technique can be used for synthesis and using 100 sentences or approximately 6-7 minutes of speech data has been found to surpass the speaker-dependent technique for quality and similarity to speaker using voices trained on between 30 and 60 minutes of speech (Yamagishi and Kobayashi, 2007; Yamagishi, Zen, Toda and Tokuda, 2007).

HTS is robust to errors in the adaptation data as its statistical modelling can treat the occurrences as outliers. However, if the models are trained consistently on incorrect data the models will recreate that error in the output. To limit any inaccuracies in the data production an alignment is done as part of the adaptation process for each utterance between the data and the existing models corresponding to the label sequence. If there is an insufficient match between them, the utterance is rejected from the adaptation procedure.

Figure 4. The structure of HTS means that there can be a substitution of stream output probabilities between the average voice model and participant speaker model to compensate for deterioration in the participant's speech.

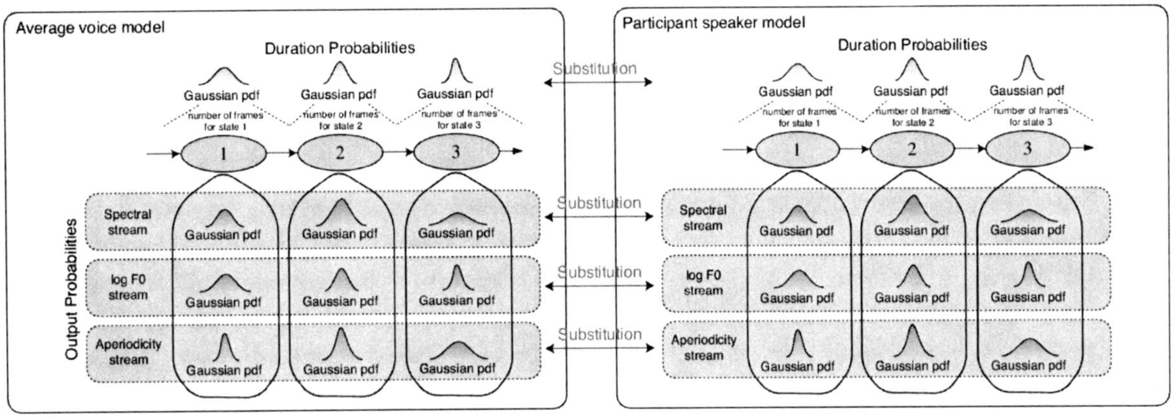

Dysarthria is a condition defined by inaccuracies in production containing disruption of the articulations, variability of speech rate, increased pauses and insertion of involuntary speech and non-speech segments into the output (Duffy, 2005). These inaccuracies, specifically insertions, can result in the rejection of the entire utterance from the adaptation data even if the utterance contains some usable data. The need to take minimal recordings from dysarthric individuals has been emphasized and so steps towards maximizing the use of the data should be taken. This can be done by extracting usable elements of data from within the utterances that would otherwise be rejected.

Any further inaccuracies in articulation that will not be rejected by the first iteration of the data should also be removed so that the speech modelled is based on well-articulated intelligible speech sections that match the label assigned to it. Telegraphic speech could be problematic as if not explicitly labelled as silence, a pause will be modelled as part of the adjoining model. Labelling the data for HTS produces a rich phonetic and prosodic representation which depends on the segment being part of a word. Rather than relabeling the speech, which could be difficult due to the presence of non-speech sounds in the data or other insertions which cannot be assigned to appropriate labels, the speech is extracted from the recordings and associated with labels taken from the original text. This links the speech with the planning in the brain of what was intended to be said as shown through the presence of coarticulation: the way in which articulations are affected by the surrounding context. Evidence of anticipatory movement of the articulators in the data, although disrupted by the effects of dysarthria on the movement of the articulators, means that the well-articulated segments of speech extracted from the data can be reasonably represented by the phonetic and prosodic information in the original labels.

The structure of HTS means that the models created during the training and adaptation processes generate the sequence of feature vectors for each stream separately: duration, log F0, aperiodicity and spectral coefficients. This structure allows some reconstruction of the voice by substituting models or information from the average voice to compensate for any disorder that occurs in the participant speaker's data. This is illustrated in figure 4. This procedure relies on the alignment between the states and the data being similar for both average voice and target speaker, which emphasizes the need to remove pauses from telegraphic speech.

Synthesis

For speech recognition, HMMs generate the most likely observations from the state sequence as determined by the state output distribution to compare to a set of feature vectors extracted from speech to be recognized. HTS makes use of the generative nature of these models and can directly synthesize a waveform from this generated feature vector sequence.

The first stage of synthesis is to convert the orthographic text to be synthesized into a context-dependent label sequence as used in training. An utterance HSMM is then created by traversing through the decision trees, using the label to answer phonetic contextual questions defined in training. Once a leaf node at the end of a branch in the tree is reached, that state output distribution is selected. This is done for each feature: spectral information, log F0 and aperiodicity. The decision tree for duration defines the number of time frames assigned to each state. A five emitting state model is built for each context-dependent phoneme with three associated distributions per state representing each stream. The utterance HSMM is built by concatenating together all the models.

Speech is generated by traversing through the model left to right using the state durations defined in the previous step. A state is reached at every time frame and an observation is generated. The excitation sequence is generated, firstly defining whether a state is voiced or voiceless. For voiced frames, an F0 value is assigned along with its corresponding aperiodicity weighting across the different frequency bands. The spectral feature sequence is generated using the parameter generation algorithm (Fukada, Tokuda, Kobayashi and Imai, 1992) and then with the excitation sequence, input into a mel log spectrum approximation (MLSA) filter to synthesize the speech.

Without using the dynamic features of speech, the deltas and delta-deltas, the models would output a sequence of the most likely feature vectors as defined by the state output distribution: the means of the distributions. By respecting the dynamic features in the parameter generation algorithm, it is ensured that the sequence of vectors produces a smoothly changing output.

Due to the statistical nature of this technique, output synthesis can be perceived as slightly muffled due to the spectral details being averaged out with high priority placed on producing a smooth output trace for each feature. In an attempt to improve the speech output and reduce this oversmoothing, a global variance measure for the spectral features, log F0 and aperiodicity is estimated from the adaptation data. This value is considered in the parameter generation algorithm ensuring that the parameters generated more accurately represent the full range of the data. Introducing this feature has been found to improve the output of the synthesis in listening tests (Toda and Tokuda, 2007; Yamagishi et al., 2009).

The ability of HTS to provide a personalized voice output that is highly intelligible with naturalness comparable to other synthesis systems using a minimal amount of data fulfils the requirements of a synthesis technique for this task. HTS is a proven technique for unimpaired speech data. It shows promise for the successful reconstruction of voices for individuals with dysarthria through selection of data and substitution of impaired features by corresponding information taken from the average voice model. Limitations of the HTS toolkit means that currently the synthesized output is not able to be produced at real-time speed, which could hinder the communication process, but as technology improves, this limitation is likely to reduce.

Using HTS with Dysarthric Speech

Isolated articulation errors occurring in the speech data will be averaged out due the statistical nature of this technique. Where these errors occur consistently, however, the error will be modelled and consequently appear in the output speech. Using the measurements of the dynamic properties of

Figure 5. Detailing the allowable substitution features to build up an output speaker model taking components from both average speaker and participant speaker models.

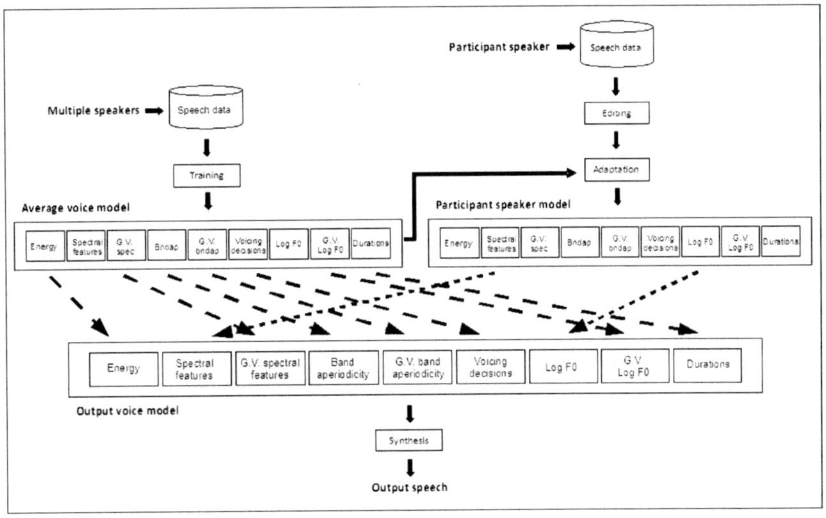

speech, deltas and delta-deltas will also help to remove any disruptions in the synthesis production aiming to produce a smooth output trajectory for each feature in the feature vector.

Selecting only intelligible sections of data to be used for adaptation will mean that only those sections will contribute to the re-estimation of the model parameters, limiting the reproduction of the impairments present in the speech.

Further alterations to the technique can be made to allow HMM synthesis to produce an appropriate output for dysarthric speech input. The following sections explain in more detail what components of the disordered speech can be replaced by that of the average voice and how they can compensate for those disordered characteristics found in dysarthric speech.

Any combination of the components can be substituted dependent on the particular pathology of the individual with dysarthria and their own preferences for the output. A representation of allowable substitutions and the structure of HTS for this task is shown in figure 5.

Data Selection

Editing the data will remove audible disruptions to the fluency of production in terms of repetitions, false starts, inappropriate silences or other speech and non-speech insertions. Where there is a long period of voicing onset, this can be removed from an otherwise usable section of speech. Any speech with unintelligible sections due to articulatory factors such as imprecise consonants or distorted vowels can also be removed. The data can be selected manually for those sections which are intelligible following a protocol to maintain consistency.

Spectral Information: Energy, Spectral Features, Global Variance for Spectral Information

The spectral part of the feature vectors contains information about the overall energy of the speech in each frame. Effects related to loudness variation in each frame of dysarthric speech, in the utterance as a whole or voice stress can be smoothed out by substituting the energy component from the average voice model into that of the participant speaker model. This will smooth out the output if there is much variation in the energy in the original speech and will produce a more appropriate speaker energy if the speaker's voice has either reduced or elevated energy levels.

The remaining mel-cepstral coefficients contain much of the speaker-specific information in the feature vector, representing the shape of the vocal tract of the individual. The selection of data to use only those sections which are intelligible allows the speaker's own spectral models to be retained for synthesis and produce an intelligible output.

The global variance measure for spectral information characterizes how much variation occurs in the data for each coefficient in the spectral part of the feature vector including energy. It aims to maximize the coverage of the variability as captured in the adaptation data. For those speakers with imprecise and therefore more variable articulation, this value will be higher. Replacing the global variance for spectral information with that corresponding to the average voice constrains the synthesis output and produces a more defined output.

Excitation Parameters: Log F0, Voicing Decisions, Aperiodicity, Global Variance for Log F0 and Aperiodicity

The F0 of a speaker contributes to the conveyance of speaker identity to the listener, therefore where the overall F0 of the speaker has not been altered by the condition, this information should be retained in the F0 models.

Phonatory irregularity such as problems with voicing initiation and control can take advantage of the robust model of speech by isolating the voicing decisions and substituting in that information from the average voice model.

Reduced control of the larynx and weakened vocal folds may also produce a change in voice quality. A person with dysarthria may have breathy or hoarse speech, where excessive breath through the glottis produces unwanted turbulent noise in the signal at high frequencies. The aperiodicity models input voiceless characteristics into voiced sounds to produce a more natural output. Substitution of the aperiodicity models from the average voice could produce a less breathy or hoarse output that is still natural sounding.

Where the dysarthric speaker has a monopitch or flat prosodic quality to their speech, the global variance of the F0 can be altered to make the pitch more variable and natural-sounding. This feature can be altered manually to suit the preferences of the individual.

Duration Information: State Duration Probability Densities, Overall Duration Control

For dysarthric speakers, the duration of segments is hugely variable and often disordered, contributing to difficulties in comprehension of the speech. This problem is mostly dealt with by the editing process but this will not remove the variability that occurs when the speech is of varying speeds but well-articulated. By substituting in the average voice model duration probability distributions, timing disruptions at both phoneme and utterance level can be modified and regulated. The overall rate of the speech can be further altered during synthesis to suit the preferences of and appropriateness for the individual.

Ideally an average voice with the same regional accent would be used to impose the durations for the dysarthric speaker's models as temporal aspects of the voice contributes to the accent, stress and rhythm of the speech, which is important to retain for vocal identity. An individual local donor speaker's durations would not offer that same level of robustness that can be found in the average voice model.

EVALUATION

The aim of the evaluation was to see if acceptable synthetic voices could be built for individuals with dysarthric speech. We tested the model-based synthesis techniques we have described above with two individuals with different speech pathologies. Example sound files accompany this evaluation section, which can be found at http://www.pitt.edu/~mullenni/cssbook.html.

With the evaluation we sought to answer three questions:

1. Can the individual recognize themselves in the voices built and which features contribute to this recognition?
2. Which features affect the quality of the voice output for the different participants?
3. Can features be altered to make the voices more appropriate for that participant?

We also discussed with the participants whether they liked the voices produced and if they would be happy for those voices to represent them in a VOCA.

Method

Participants

Participant 1 was male and 80 years old at the time of recording, two years post cerebrovascular accident (CVA), with moderate flaccid dysarthria. In his speech, overall energy varied, with imprecise and slow movement of the articulators resulting in a slow rate of production. The example sound file named "part1_original.wav" is a recording of his speech. Participant 2 was male, 69 years old at the time of recording and had been diagnosed with Parkinson's disease six years previously. He showed symptoms of mild hypokinetic dysarthria. His speech was quiet, with variable energy. There was little variation in pitch and a high perceived rate of articulation. The example sound file "part2_original.wav" is a recording of his speech.

Data Collection

Data was collected from the participants in a quiet room in the Department of Human Communication Sciences at the University of Sheffield using a Morantz PMD670 audio recorder with a Shure SM80 microphone.

The recorded speech material consisted of sentences taken from the Arctic dataset A (Kominek and Black, 2003). This set of utterances consists of 593 sentences taken from out-of-copyright books in English. The sentences are between 5-15 words in length to ensure ease of readability. The data set covers all diphones (a phone-sized unit consisting of half a phone plus half the following phone, used commonly in concatenative synthesis) found in US English. The participants completed the recordings in one sitting. Participant 1 recorded the first 200 sentences of the Arctic set A and participant 2 recorded the first 150.

Building Voices

The voices were built using HTS version 2.1 (internal) (Tokuda et al., 2008) using a 138-dimensional feature vector containing: 40 STRAIGHT mel-cepstra coefficients (including energy), deltas and delta-deltas; log F0 value, its delta and delta-delta; 5 band aperiodicity values, deltas and delta-deltas. The average voice used was provided with this version of HTS. It was built using full Arctic data sets (approximately 1150 sentences) as spoken by six male speakers: four US English speakers, one Canadian English speaker and one Scottish English speaker. An example of the average voice can be found in sound example file "avevoice.wav".

Voices were built with unedited data to compare the results with those built with data selected for intelligibility. For each participant, voices were built to combine together the model components from their own speech data and those taken from the average voice model to produce voices for the evaluation.

Evaluation Design

Stimuli

The stimuli presented to the participants were synthesized sentences and paragraphs taken from SCRIBE (Spoken Corpus Recordings in British English) (Huckvale, 2004). The SCRIBE paragraphs contain a high frequency of words which have features attributable to different regional accents of British English. It is important to retain these features to fully personalize a synthetic voice and is therefore an appropriate set of data for this task.

Procedure

The evaluation took place in a quiet room in the department of Human Communication Sciences at the University of Sheffield. The stimuli were presented to the participants individually using a laptop computer with external speakers.

The research was introduced as building voices for a computer to use to speak for that individual on days where their own voice was not clear. An example of the average voice was played and introduced as the starting point voice from which to change to an approximation of the participant's voice based on the data that they recorded previously. Original recordings of two non-disordered voices built with 500 sentences each were played, followed by the synthesized versions. This was to make the participants aware of the capabilities of this system. They were asked to rate the similarity of the synthesized version to the original recordings on a 1 (sounded like a different person) - 5 (sounded like the same person) scale. This attempted to gauge their reaction to the synthesized voices whilst getting them used to the task. It also provided an opportunity to attune their listening to synthesized speech.

1. Can the individual recognize themselves in the voices built and which features contribute to this recognition?

Comparisons were made between the average voice and versions of the average voice with features that display speaker characteristics replaced by those of the participant. The conditions were: average voice, average voice with participant log F0 features, average voice with participant spectral information and average voice with participant log F0 and spectral information. An original recording of the participant was played to remind the individual what their speech sounded like during the recordings and how it sounds when played out on a computer. They were asked to rate the difference between the original recording and the synthesis on a 1 (does not sound like me) - 5 (sounds like me) scale.

2. Which features affect the quality of the voice output for the different participants?

A choice was presented between the average voice with participant spectral and log F0 features and the same voice with one additional feature of the participant speaker's model substituted. The question asked was 'for each pair, which voice do you think sounds best?'. Conditions evaluated were using the participant's: durations, global variance for spectral features, energy and using the full set of unedited data. These conditions were chosen as they had a perceived effect on the output for one of the two participants. The participant was allowed to indicate that they perceived no difference between the two samples.

3. Can features be altered to make the voices more appropriate for that participant?

This question dealt with appropriateness for that participant and their preferences for the customizable features: rate of utterance and global variance for log F0. A pairwise comparison was made for three different sentences. For rate, the comparison was between the average voice durations and a slowed down version of the average voice durations. For global variance for log F0, the two options were that of the average voice or that of the participant. For each pair the question was asked 'can you tell a difference and if so, which one do you prefer?'.

Follow up questions were posed to clarify the responses given for the ratings and choices made.

Results

Participant 1's reaction to the non-disordered speech examples was that the synthesized versions sounded very like the original speakers whereas participant 2's rating was that the synthesis did not sound like the original speakers.

1. Can the individual recognize themselves in the voices built and which features contribute to this recognition?

After exposure to the stimuli, participant 1's rating of the average voice was 4 suggesting that his perception is that the average voice sounded similar to his own. The rating increased to 5 for all other conditions containing components of his model substituted into the output voice. Participant 2's ratings remained at 1 for each condition, stating that even when speaker information is substituted into the models, he did not recognize himself in the voice.

2. Which features affect the quality of the voice output for the different participants?

The results showed that both participants agreed that the use of average voice energy produced better output than when using their own energy information. Each participant noted different feature substitutions made a difference to their output voices. Using unedited data made no difference to participant 1 whereas participant 2 noticed a difference, preferring the unedited version. Using the participant's own durations did not make a difference between the two voices for participant 2 whereas participant 1 preferred his own durations. Using the participant's global variance for spectral features did not make a difference distinguishable by participant 1, but participant 2 preferred his own global variance for spectral features.

3. Can features be altered to make the voices more appropriate for that participant?

The results showed that differences are discernible and preferences made for both rate of utterance and global variance for log F0. Both participants noted differences between the two rates of production and showed a preference for the average voice durations rather than the slowed down versions. The results for global variance for log F0 showed that a difference was detectable between the two voices, with participant 1 preferring his own global variance for log F0 and participant 2 preferring that of the average voice.

For the rating of likeability of the voice, from 1 (do not like the voice) - 5 (like the voice), participant 1 rated his output as 5 and participant 2 rated his as 1.

Discussion

These results should be set within the context of the reactions to the first examples which were played to the participants. Participant 2's reaction to the non-disordered speech examples suggest that his ratings may be influenced by other factors than purely similarity between the stimuli. In previous listening tests with multiple participants (Creer, Cunningham, Green and Fatema, in press) one of these synthesized voices has shown a very high rating in similarity to the original speaker.

With sufficient data, it is possible to get voices with high similarity to an original recording. For participant 2, however, 150 sentences are not enough data to fully capture the likeness of his voice using that particular average voice model. The influence of the average voice becomes more apparent with less adaptation data and the American English dominated average voice prevented participant 2 from recognizing himself in the output voices. With a less intrusive average voice, that is closer in similarity to the voices being modelled, it is hypothesized that less data would be required to achieve such a likeness.

The different factors influencing the quality of the voice output were dependent on the individual and the effects of dysarthria on their speech. Where there were large perceptual differences, the voices containing factors that improved the output quality and intelligibility were perceived as best, except when it was perceived as more accurately representing the speech of that individual, seemingly confusing quality with similarity. For example, participant 1 preferred the voice where his own durations were used as he identified his own voice clearly in that example. Participant 2 also noted that although for one particular voice, the global variance for spectral information from the average voice made the output clearer, he preferred the voice with his own global variance for spectral information. This output produced a slightly muffled percept but this preference could be related to the perceived softness in the voice quality that it introduced which participant 2 noted was missing in other voice examples.

It was expected that for both speakers the preference would be for the edited data versions. Participant 2's preference for the unedited data version is difficult to interpret as there was a high level of similarity in output between stimuli for this condition.

The differences in output rate could be perceived by the speakers, although there is a limited extent to which the rate can be slowed until it starts to reduce intelligibility. The change of global variance for log F0 could also be perceived by the participants. Participant 2, who had a relatively narrow range of log F0 preferred to have a wider range than his own in the output. Participant 1's range was closer to the average voice and the preference showed it was more appropriate for him. These features can be customized to the extent where it would not impair the intelligibility of the output.

In relation to the pathologies of the speakers, both had variable energy in their speech and both preferred voices that normalized the energy output. Participant 2's monopitch output was reconstructed to have a preferred wider variability in pitch. Imprecise articulations were handled by using the average voice model durations and selecting data for adaptation. Examples of the speakers are attached. They were all built with edited data. The example sound files "part1_own_f0spec.wav" and "part2_own_f0spec.wav" are synthesized with the speakers' own log F0 and spectral features and all other features taken from the average voice. The example sound files "part1_own_energy.wav" and "part2_own_energy.wav" are synthesized with the speakers' own energy, log F0 and spectral features and all other features taken from the average voice. The example sound files "part1_own_gvlf0.wav" and "part2_own_gvlf0.wav" are synthesized with the speakers' own log F0, spectral features and global variance for log F0.

Between the two speakers, Participant 1's priority seemed to be clarity of output whereas Participant 2 did not want to be represented by a voice which he regarded as sounding nothing like his own and with which he had non-neutral associations. Participant 1 did not appear to associate the voices with anything other than himself and therefore was happy to be represented by them as long as the output was clear and intelligible.

FUTURE RESEARCH DIRECTIONS

Initial further evaluations are planned to determine whether these voices are recognizable and judged to be appropriate by others who are familiar with the participants and their pre-morbid speech. Further evaluation of the practicalities and implications of using a personalized voice in a communication aid should also be done to test the appropriateness of the voices for this application.

A technique for automating the data selection process is necessary to minimize the need for manual data selection. Selecting data manually can be very time-consuming and inconsistent as the selector becomes more attuned to the voice.

The results of this evaluation point to more success being achieved and better similarity judged for these British English speakers if average voices that were closer to the participant speakers' output were used. The average voice model should contain neutral associations which will not intrude on the participant's voice characteristics if there is insufficient data to fully adapt all the models. Ongoing work building HTS voices with British English data means that UK average voice models are now available along with multi-accented English speaking average voices, e.g. (Yamagishi, Zen, Wu, Toda and Tokuda, 2008).

These results hold for these speakers only. Further work in this area would fully test the reconstructive abilities of this technique for people with different pathologies and severity of dysarthria.

CONCLUSION

In an attempt to retain the purposes of speech: communication, maintenance and use of social interaction and displaying identity, an intelligible, natural-sounding voice which retains the individual's vocal identity can be constructed with the HTS toolkit. Using much less data than concatenative synthesis techniques require and less parameter manipulation than parametric synthesis techniques, the results of this evaluation suggest that this technique shows promise for building and reconstructing personalized synthetic voices for individuals with dysarthria once deterioration of their voice has begun.

ACKNOWLEDGMENT

STRAIGHT is used with permission from Hideki Kawahara. Sarah Creer's PhD. work was funded by the Engineering and Physical Sciences Research Council (EPSRC), UK.

REFERENCES

Allen, J. (2005). Designing desirability in an augmentative and alternative communication device. *Universal Access in the Information Society*, *4*, 135–145. doi:10.1007/s10209-005-0117-2

Angelo, D. H., Kokosa, S. M., & Jones, S. D. (1996). Family perspective on augmentative and alternative communication: families of adolescents and young adults. *Augmentative and Alternative Communication*, *12*(1), 13–20. doi:10.1080/07434619612331277438

Bennett, C. L. (2005). Large scale evaluation of corpus-based synthesizers: results and lessons from the Blizzard challenge 2005. In *Proceedings of the 9th European Conference on Speech Communication and Technology (Interspeech-2005/Eurospeech)* (pp. 105–108), Lisbon, Portugal.

Black, A. W., & Lenzo, K. A. (2007). *Building synthetic voices*. Retrieved February 2, 2007, from http://festvox.org/festvox/festvox_toc.html

Bloch, S., & Wilkinson, R. (2004). The understandability of AAC: a conversation analysis study of acquired dysarthria. *Augmentative and Alternative Communication*, *20*(4), 272–282. doi:10.1080/07434610400005614

Chambers, J. K. (1995). *Sociolinguistic theory.* Oxford: Blackwell.

Clark, R. A., Richmond, K., & King, S. (2004). Festival 2 – build your own general purpose unit selection speech synthesizer. In *Proceedings of the 5th International Speech Communication Association Speech Synthesis Workshop (SSW5)* (pp. 173–178), Pittsburgh, PA.

Coulston, R., Oviatt, S., & Darves, C. (2002). Amplitude convergence in children's conversational speech with animated personas. In *Proceedings of the 7th International Conference on Spoken Language Processing* (pp. 2689–2692), Boulder, CO.

Crabtree, M., Mirenda, P., & Beukelman, D. R. (1990). Age and gender preferences for synthetic and natural speech. *Augmentative and Alternative Communication*, *6*(4), 256–261. doi:10.1080/07434619012331275544

Creer, S. M., Cunningham, S. P., Green, P. D., & Fatema, K. (in press). Personalizing synthetic voices for people with progressive speech disorders: judging voice similarity. In *Proceedings of Interspeech2009.*

Darves, C., & Oviatt, S. (2002). Adaptation of users' spoken dialogue patterns in a conversational interface. In *Proceedings of the 7th International Conference on Spoken Language Processing* (pp. 561–564), Boulder, CO.

Duffy, J. (2005). *Motor speech disorders: substrates, differential diagnosis and management* (2nd ed.). St Louis, MO: Elsevier Mosby.

Fant, G. (Ed.). (1960). *Acoustic theory of speech production.* The Hague, Netherlands: Mouton.

Fukada, T., Tokuda, K., Kobayashi, T., & Imai, S. (1992). An adaptive algorithm for mel-cepstral analysis of speech. In *Proceedings of IEEE International Conference on Acoustics, Speech, and Signal Processing* (pp. 137–140), San Francisco, CA.

Gorenflo, D. W., & Gorenflo, C. W. (1991). The effects of information and augmentative communication technique on attitudes toward non-speaking individuals. *Journal of Speech and Hearing Research, 34*, 19–26.

Hetzroni, O. E., & Harris, O. L. (1996). Cultural aspects in the development of AAC users. *Augmentative and Alternative Communication, 12*(1), 52–58. doi:10.1080/07434619612331277488

Huckvale, M. (2004) *SCRIBE manual version 1.0.* Retrieved January 7, 2009, from http://www.phon.ucl.ac.uk/resource/scribe/scribe-manual.htm

Kawahara, H., Masuda-Katsuse, I., & de Cheveigné, A. (1999). Restructuring speech representations using a pitch-adaptive time-frequency smoothing and an instantaneous-frequency-based F0 extraction: possible role of a repetitive structure in sounds. *Speech Communication, 27*, 187–207. doi:10.1016/S0167-6393(98)00085-5

Kemp, B. (1999). Quality of life while ageing with a disability. *Assistive Technology, 11*, 158–163.

Kent, R., Weismer, G., Kent, J., & Rosenbek, J. (1989). Toward phonetic intelligibility testing in dysarthria. *The Journal of Speech and Hearing Disorders, 54*, 482–499.

Kominek, J., & Black, A. W. (2003). *CMU Arctic databases for speech synthesis.* Retrieved April 20, 2006, from http://festvox.org/cmu arctic/cmu arctic report.pdf

Light, J. (1988). Interaction involving individuals using augmentative and alternative communication systems: state of the art and future directions. *Augmentative and Alternative Communication, 4*(2), 66–82. doi:10.1080/07434618812331274657

Light, J., Page, R., Curran, J., & Pitkin, L. (2007). Children's ideas for the design of AAC assistive technologies for young children with complex communication needs. *Augmentative and Alternative Communication, 23*(4), 274–287. doi:10.1080/07434610701390475

Lilienfeld, M., & Alant, E. (2002). Attitudes of children toward an unfamiliar peer using an AAC device with and without voice output. *Augmentative and Alternative Communication, 18*(2), 91–101. doi:10.1080/07434610212331281191

Locke, J. L. (1998). Where did all the gossip go?: Casual conversation in the information age. *The Magazine of the American Speech-Language-Hearing Association, 40*(3), 26–31.

Miller, N., Noble, E., Jones, D., & Burn, D. (2006). Life with communication changes in Parkinson's disease. *Age and Ageing, 35*, 235–239. doi:10.1093/ageing/afj053

Moore, R., & Morris, A. (1992). Experiences collecting genuine spoken enquiries using WOZ techniques. In *Proceedings of DARPA Speech and Natural Language Workshop* (pp. 61–63), New York.

Moulines, E., & Charpentier, F. (1990). Pitch-synchronous waveform processing techniques for text-to-speech synthesis using diphones. *Speech Communication, 9*, 453–467. doi:10.1016/0167-6393(90)90021-Z

Murphy, J. (2004). 'I prefer contact this close': perceptions of AAC by people with motor neurone disease and their communication partners. *Augmentative and Alternative Communication, 20*(4), 259–271. doi:10.1080/07434610400005663

Nass, C., Moon, Y., & Green, N. (1997). Are machines gender neutral? Gender-stereotypic responses to computers with voices. *Journal of Applied Social Psychology, 27*, 864–876. doi:10.1111/j.1559-1816.1997.tb00275.x

O'Keefe, B. M., Brown, L., & Schuller, R. (1998). Identification and rankings of communication aid features by five groups. *Augmentative and Alternative Communication, 14*(1), 37–50. doi:10.1080/07434619812331278186

Parette, P., & Huer, M. B. (2002). Working with Asian American families whose children have augmentative and alternative communication needs. *Journal of Special Education Technology E-Journal, 17*(4). Retrieved January 4, 2009, from http://jset.unlv.edu/17.4T/parette/first.html

Rabiner, L. R. (1989). A tutorial on HMM and selected applications in speech recognition. *Proceedings of the IEEE, 77*(2), 257–286. doi:10.1109/5.18626

Smith, M. M. (2005). The dual challenges of aided communication and adolescence. *Augmentative and Alternative Communication, 21*(1), 76–79. doi:10.1080/10428190400006625

Stern, S. E. (2008). Computer synthesized speech and perceptions of the social influence of disabled users. *Journal of Language and Social Psychology, 27*(3), 254–265. doi:10.1177/0261927X08318035

Stern, S. E., Mullennix, J. W., Dyson, C.-L., & Wilson, S. J. (1999). The persuasiveness of synthetic speech versus human speech. *Human Factors, 41*, 588–595. doi:10.1518/001872099779656680

Stern, S. E., Mullennix, J. W., & Wilson, S. J. (2002). Effects of perceived disability on persuasiveness of computer synthesized speech. *The Journal of Applied Psychology, 87*, 411–417. doi:10.1037/0021-9010.87.2.411

Stern, S. E., Mullennix, J. W., & Yaroslavsky, I. (2006). Persuasion and social perception of human vs. synthetic voice across person as source and computer as source conditions. *International Journal of Human-Computer Studies, 64*, 43–52. doi:10.1016/j.ijhcs.2005.07.002

Street, R. L., & Giles, H. (1982). Speech accommodation theory: a social cognitive approach to language and speech. In M. Roloff, & C. R. Berger, (Eds.), *Social cognition and communication* (pp. 193–226). Beverly Hills, CA: Sage.

Taylor, P., Black, A. W., & Caley, R. (1998). The architecture of the Festival speech synthesis system. In *Proceedings of the 3rd ESCA Workshop in Speech Synthesis* (pp. 147–151), Jenolan Caves, Australia.

Toda, T., & Tokuda, K. (2007). A speech parameter generation algorithm considering global variance for HMM-based speech synthesis. *IEICE Transactions on Information and Systems . E (Norwalk, Conn.), 90-D*(5), 816–824.

Tokuda, K., Zen, H., Yamagishi, J., Masuko, T., Sako, S., Black, A., & Nose, T. (2008) *The HMM-based speech synthesis system (HTS) Version 2.1.* Retrieved June 27, 2008, from http://hts.sp.nitech.ac.jp/.

Wells, J. C. (1982). *Accents of English: an introduction.* Cambridge, UK: Cambridge Univ. Press.

Yamagishi, J., & Kobayashi, T. (2007). Average-voice-based speech synthesis using HSMM-based speaker adaptation and adaptive training. *IEICE Transactions on Information and Systems . E (Norwalk, Conn.), 90-D*(2), 533–543.

Yamagishi, J., Kobayashi, T., Nakano, Y., Ogata, K., & Isogai, J. (2009). Analysis of speaker adaptation algorithms for HMM-based speech synthesis and a constrained SMAPLR adaptation algorithm. *IEEE Transactions on Audio . Speech and Language Processing, 17*(1), 66–83. doi:10.1109/TASL.2008.2006647

Yamagishi, J., Nose, T., Zen, H., Ling, Z., Toda, T., & Tokuda, K. (2009). A robust speaker-adaptive HMM-based text-to-speech synthesis. *IEEE Transactions on Audio . Speech and Language Processing, 17*(6), 1208–1230. doi:10.1109/TASL.2009.2016394

Yamagishi, J., Zen, H., Toda, T., & Tokuda, K. (2007). Speaker-independent HMM-based speech synthesis system – HTS-2007 for the Blizzard challenge 2007. In *Proceedings of the Blizzard Challenge 2007* (paper 008), Bonn, Germany.

Yamagishi, J., Zen, H., Wu, Y.-J., Toda, T., & Tokuda, K. (2008). The HTS-2008 system: yet another evaluation of the speaker-adaptive HMM-based speech synthesis system in the 2008 Blizzard challenge. In *Proceedings of the Blizzard Challenge 2008*, Brisbane, Australia. Retrieved March 2, 2009, from http://festvox.org/blizzard/bc2008/hts_Blizzard2008.pdf.

Yarrington, D., Pennington, C., Gray, J., & Bunnell, H. T. (2005). A system for creating personalized synthetic voices. In [Baltimore.]. *Proceedings of ASSETS, 2005*, 196–197.

Zen, H., Nose, T., Yamagishi, J., Sako, S., & Tokuda, K. (2007a). The HMM-based speech synthesis system (HTS) version 2.0. In *Proceedings of the 6th International Speech Communication Association Speech Synthesis Workshop (SSW6)* (pp. 294–299), Bonn, Germany.

Zen, H., Toda, T., Nakamura, M., & Tokuda, K. (2007b). Details of the Nitech HMM-based speech synthesis system for the Blizzard challenge 2005. *IEICE Transactions on Information and Systems . E (Norwalk, Conn.), 90-D*(1), 325–333.

Zen, H., Tokuda, K., Masuko, T., Kobayashi, T., & Kitamura, T. (2007c). A hidden semi-Markov model-based speech synthesis system. *IEICE Transactions on Information and Systems . E (Norwalk, Conn.), 90-D*(5), 825–834.

SOUND FILES

URL for sound files: http://www.pitt.edu/~mullenni/cssbook.html.

KEY TERMS AND DEFINITIONS

Average Voice: A speaker-independent model of speech built from a large amount of data from multiple speakers. Participant adaptation data is used to adapt this model towards that of the participant.

Dysarthria: A group of motor speech disorders resulting from irregularities in the movement and control of the speech articulators.

Feature Vector: A parameterization of speech characterizing the spectral and excitation parameters at a segment of time.

Hidden Markov Model (HMM): A generative probabilistic model that represents the acoustics that are likely to be produced with an associated label.

Hidden Semi-Markov Model: An HMM that has a state duration probability density explicitly attached.

Participant Speaker: Individual speaker whose speech data is provided to adapt the speaker-independent models towards to provide speaker-dependent models and personalization of the output synthesis.

Voice Banking: A process of recording data for future use as voice prosthesis either directly playing back the recordings or using the data to build a full synthetic voice.

Voice Output Communication Aid: A communication device using digitized or synthesized speech output.

Chapter 7
Speech Technologies for Augmented Communication

Gérard Bailly
CNRS/Universities of Grenoble, France

Pierre Badin
CNRS/Universities of Grenoble, France

Denis Beautemps
CNRS/Universities of Grenoble, France

Frédéric Elisei
CNRS/Universities of Grenoble, France

ABSTRACT

The authors introduce here an emerging technological and scientific field. Augmented speech communication (ASC) aims at supplementing human-human communication with enhanced or additional modalities. ASC improves human-human communication by exploiting a priori knowledge on multimodal coherence of speech signals, user/listener voice characteristics or more general linguistic and phonological structure on the spoken language or vocabulary being exchanged. The nature of this a priori knowledge, the quantitative models that implement it and their capabilities to enhance the available input signals influence the precision and robustness of the perceived signals. After a general overview of the possible input signals characterizing speech production activity and available technologies for mapping these various speech representations between each other, three ASC systems developed at GIPSA-Lab are described in detail. Preliminary results of the evaluation of these three systems will be given and commented. A discussion on scientific and technological challenges and limitations of ASC concludes the chapter.

INTRODUCTION

Speech is very likely the most natural communication mean for humans. However, there are various situations in which audio speech cannot be used because of disabilities or adverse environmental conditions. Resorting to alternative methods such as *augmented speech* is a therefore an interesting approach. This chapter presents computer-mediated

DOI: 10.4018/978-1-61520-725-1.ch007

Figure 1. Computer-mediated communication consists in driving an artificial agent from signals captured on the source speaker. The embodiment of the agent may be quite diverse: from pure audio through audio-visual rendering of speech by avatars to a more videorealistic animations by means of of virtual clones of the source speaker or anthropoid robots - here the animatronic talking head Anton developed at U. of Sheffield (Hofe & Moore, 2008). The control signals of these agents can encompass not only audible and visible consequences of articulation but also control posture, gaze, facial expressions or head/hand movements. Signals captured on the source speaker provide partial information on speech activity such as brain or muscular activity, articulatory movements, speech or even scripts produced by the source speaker. Such systems exploit a priori knowledge on the mapping between captured and synthesized signals labelled here as "virtual human" and "phonological representation": these resources that know about the coherence between observed and generated signals can be either statistical or procedural.

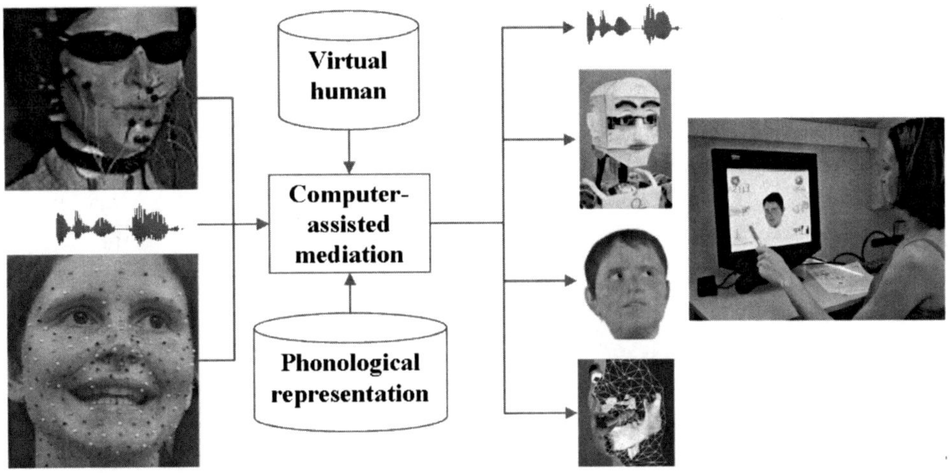

communication technologies that allow such an approach (see Figure 1). Speech of the emitter may in fact:

- not be captured by available hardware communication channels – camera, microphone
- be impoverished by the quality of the hardware or the communication channel
- be impoverished because of environmental conditions or because of motor impairments of the interlocutor

On the reception side, Augmented Speech Communication (ASC) may also compensate for perceptual deficits of the user by enhancing the captured signals or adding multimodal redundancy by synthesizing new perceptual channels or adding new features to existing channels. In order to improve human-human communication ASC can make use of *a priori* knowledge on multimodal coherence of speech signals, user/listener voice characteristics or more general linguistic and phonological structure on the spoken language or vocabulary being exchanged. The nature of this *a priori* knowledge, the quantitative models that implement it and their capabilities to enhance the available communication signals influence the precision and robustness of the communication.

The chapter will first present:

- the signals that can characterise the speech production activity i.e. from electromagnetic signals from brain activity, through articulatory movements, to their audiovisual traces

- devices that can capture these signals with various impact on articulation and constraints on usage
- available technologies that have been proposed for mapping these various speech representations between each other i.e. virtual human, direct statistical mapping or speech technologies using a phonetic pivot obtained by speech recognition techniques

Three ASC systems developed in the MPACIF Team at GIPSA-Lab will then be described in detail:

a. a system that converts non audible murmur into audiovisual speech for silent speech communication (Tran, Bailly, & Loevenbruck, submitted; Tran, Bailly, Loevenbruck, & Toda, 2008)
b. a system that converts silent cued speech (Cornett, 1967) into audiovisual speech and vice-versa. This system aims at computer-assisted audiovisual telephony for deaf users (Aboutabit, Beautemps, & Besacier, Accepted; Beautemps et al., 2007)
c. a system that computes and displays virtual tongue movements from audiovisual input for pronunciation training (Badin, Elisei, Bailly, & Tarabalka, 2008; Badin, Tarabalka, Elisei, & Bailly, 2008).

Preliminary results of the evaluation of these three systems will be given and commented. A discussion on both scientific and technological challenges and limitations will conclude the chapter.

CHARACTERIZING SPEECH PRODUCTION

The speech production chain sketched in Figure 2 consists of several signal transformations: the electrical activity of neural circuitry drives the contraction of several dozen of muscles that further shape the geometry of the vocal tract. The air flow generated by the pressure induced by the respiratory muscles interacts with the vocal tract walls in relation with the biomechanical properties of the speech articulators and generates various acoustic sources, such as pseudo-period signals at the glottis or noise signals at constrictions. These acoustic sources excite the vocal tract resonators and are finally radiated as speech sound through the mouth, the nose and skin. Speech production can be thus characterized by:

- **Neural activity:** Several brain areas are activated in motor control of speech. Nota and Honda (Nota & Honda, 2004) found for example that the bilateral motor cortex and the inferior cerebellum hemisphere were activated after the subtraction for breathing, non speech vocalization, and hearing. They asked subjects to plan speech in four different conditions: A) normal speech (spoken aloud), B) mouthed speech (mouthing silently with normal breathing), C) unarticulated speech (voicing "ah..." without articulation), and D) internal speech. Activations were also found in the superior temporal gyrus and inferior parietal lobule of the left hemisphere. Activations are also found in Broca's area, the supplementary motor area (SMA), or the insula, especially in case of difficult or unusual speech production task. Note also that most areas dedicated to speech perception are also activated during speech production and vice versa (Wilson, Saygin, Sereno, & Iacoboni, 2004).
- **Muscular activities:** Speech production involves the activation of the respiratory muscles (inhalation and exhalation), of muscles controlling the mandible, the lips, the soft palate, the pharynx and the larynx. Note also that the control of speech articulation involves the displacement of

Figure 2. The speech production chain. The intended message is decoded by the listener on the basis of audible and visible traces of speech articulation combined with a priori knowledge on the speaker, the language spoken and the message content given the history of the dialog and the situation.

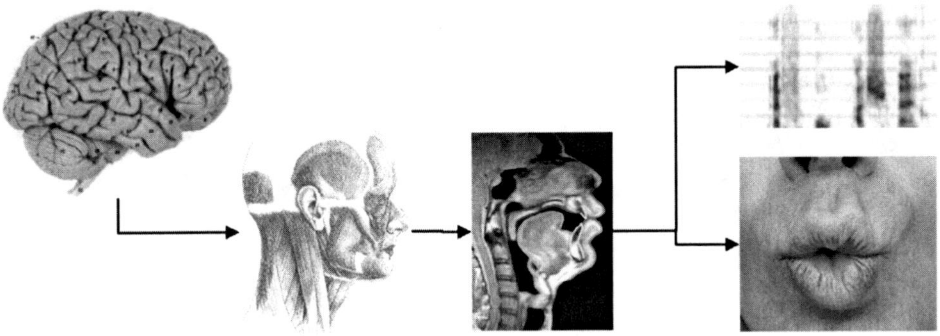

intermediate structures such as the hyoid bone. Speech production is thus accompanied by active and passive (resistive) action of both agonist and antagonist muscles.

- **Vocal tract geometry:** Contractions of muscles displace the above-mentioned speech articulators that shape the vocal tract. The dynamic range of this change of geometry depends on the interaction between the air flow and the articulatory movement: vocal folds typically oscillate in the range [50-400Hz], lips tongue tip or uvula oscillate at [20-30Hz] in trills, whereas the slowest articulator, the jaw, cycles at [5-6 Hz].
- **Audible signals:** Changes of vocal tract geometry are made audible as they change the acoustic resonances of the vocal tract and thus shape the spectrum of the speech signal that is finally radiated. The phonological structure of world's languages is strongly conditioned by the maximal acoustic dispersion of spectral characteristics of sounds (Schwartz, Boë, & Abry, 2007; Schwartz, Boë, Vallée, & Abry, 1997)
- **Visible signals:** Changes of vocal tract geometry are not all visible but movements of the jaw, the lips, parts of the movement of the larynx and the tongue are available to the interlocutor in face-to-face conversation. The benefit of audiovisual integration for speech detection, binding and comprehension has been clearly evaluated since many years (Summerfield, MacLeod, McGrath, & Brooke, 1989).

CAPTURING SPEECH

Various devices (see Figure 3) can capture dynamic representations of the current state of the speech production system. The aim of this section is to sketch the spectrum of available technology that can be used to record useful signals characterizing articulation and phonation.

The capture of sound vibration is usually performed by distant or head-mounted microphone. An alternative has been proposed to capture sound vibration:

- **The stethoscopic microphone:** Developed by Nakajima (Nakajima, Kashioka, Shikano, & Campbell, 2003) the stethoscopic microphone receives sound vibration through body tissue. This device is attached to the skin of the user, for instance behind the ear. The spectral bandwidth is reduced to 0-3 kHz.

Figure 3. Capturing signatures of speech-production. Left-to-right: ultrasound imaging (from Hueber, Chollet, Denby, Dreyfus, & Stone, 2007), electromagnetoarticulography (EMA), electromyography (EMG).

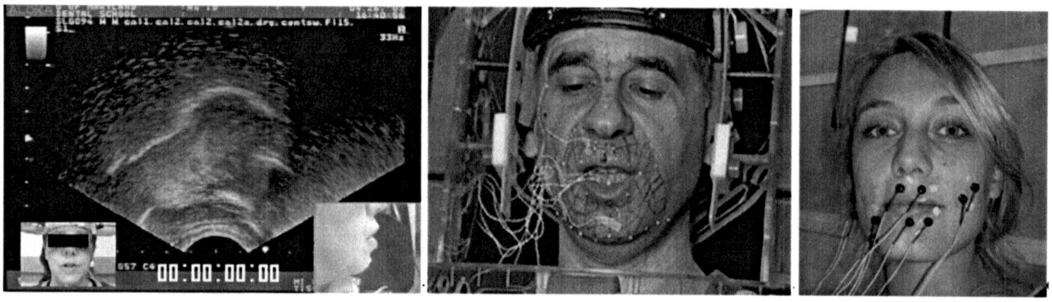

The observation of visible speech is typically done using two kinds of devices:

- **Surface deformation:** 3D range data scanners deliver very precise surface geometry together with texture information (e.g. structured light, time of flight or laser-based scanner technology). Further processing is required to compensate for head movement and to parameterize this surface with a constant number of parameters.
- **Movement of fleshpoints:** Motion capture devices (photogrammetric methods with optical flow calculation or active/passive markers) deliver movement of fleshpoints. They directly parameterize the surface with a constant number of parameters.

The observation of the internal organs does not really differ from the observation of facial movements. Three kinds of characteristics are typically monitored: density maps, positions of measurement points ("fleshpoints") and biological signals. Articulatory instrumentation includes:

- Magnetic Resonance Imaging (MRI), computerised tomography (CT), cineradiography as well as Ultra Sound Imaging (Whalen et al., 2005) provide information on the density of particular atoms or molecules within a specific volume. Some systems exploit directly the density maps as direct input. A further processing stage often retrieves surface information: if a simple threshold is often sufficient to identify the geometry of vocal tract walls in MRI or CT scan images, the determination of the tongue surface in X-ray images or ultrasound images is far more complicated. The ideal simultaneous resolution in time and space needed to observe speech movements is not available yet: the relaxation time of free hydrogen nuclei in MRI does not allow temporal sampling frequencies of more than 10-20 images per second, while noise increases drastically when acquisition rate of X-ray or ultrasound imaging are increased. Note that a further processing stage is required to determine the individual outline of the various organs in the vocal tract.
- ElectroMagnetic Articulography (EMA), ElectroPalatoGraphy (EPG) or X-ray MicroBeam (XRMB) (Kiritani, 1986) provide movement or contact information for a few measurement points attached to a speech organ. Note that EMA coils and thin wires going out of the mouth as well as the EPG artificial palate may interfere with speech movements (Recasens, 2002)
- Surface or needle ElectroMyoGraphy (EMG), ElectroGlottoGraphy (EGG) or

photoglotography and the various invasive systems for measuring oral or nasal airflows deliver signals that can be directly exploited for characterizing speech activity. They are however very noisy and must be cleaned via both signal processing and *a priori* knowledge.

Finally neuroprosthetics and brain-to-computer interfaces (BCI) exploit devices sensitive to the electromagnetic waves created by the neurons. Invasive (brain implants), partially-invasive (Electrocorticography or ECoG) and non-invasive (electroencephalography or EEG) devices that deliver signals related to speech planning as well as loud, silent or even simulated articulation.

MAPPING SIGNALS

ASC systems aim at restoring or even augmenting the signals characterizing articulation based on the signals that have been captured by some of the devices mentioned above. Most of these signals are noisy and deliver incomplete information on the articulation process. The many-to-one/one-to-many mapping between these signals is underspecified and both *a priori* knowledge and regularization techniques should be used to recover the necessary information on the articulation. *A priori* knowledge can be extracted from multiple sources:

- speech maps (Abry, Badin, & Scully, 1994) that are trained off-line and memorize the possible links between these signals that represent the coherence of the speech production process. Such a system builds a kind of speech homunculus that combines all kinaesthetic and sensory-motor information collected during speech production
- the phonetic and phonological structure of the language being spoken
- … as well as higher-level information on the linguistic content of the message.

Various technological tools (Guenther, Ghosh, & Tourville, 2006; Kröger, Birkholz, Kannampuzha, & Neuschaefer-Rube, 2006; Ouni & Laprie, 2005) have been proposed to model this *a priori* knowledge. We present here two solutions: Gaussian Mixture modelling (GMM; see Toda et al. (Toda, Ohtani, & Shikano, 2006) for its application to voice conversion) and Hidden Markov modelling (HMM, see Rabiner, 1989 for its application to speech recognition) that have been using in the applications of ASC presented below.

Direct Statistical Mapping

Speech mapping consists in building a model of the sensory-motor links based on a collection of parallel recordings of multiple characteristic signals. Though in some instances signals can actually be recorded simultaneously (see for example the combination between EMA and US in Aron, Berger, & Kerrien, 2008), the same speech items are usually recorded in different experimental setups; resulting signals must be then post-aligned, often using the acoustic signal as common reference. Voice conversion techniques (Toda, Black, & Tokuda, 2004; Toda & Shikano, 2005) can then be used to capture statistically significant correlations between pairs of input-output signals.

Characterizing Input Signals

Input feature vectors X_t are constructed by appending feature vectors from several frames around the current frame t. Data reduction techniques (principal component analysis in Toda & Shikano, 2005; or linear Discriminant analysis in Tran, Bailly, Loevenbruck, & Jutten, 2008) are often used to limit the number of model parameters to determine when the training material is too limited.

Characterizing Output Signals

Output feature vectors $Y_t = [y_t, \Delta y_t]$ consist of static and dynamic features at frame t.

A GMM (Toda, Black, & Tokuda, 2005) is then trained for representing the joint probability density $p(X_t, Y_t|\Theta)$, where Θ denotes a set of GMM parameters. The generation of the time sequence of the target static feature vector y from that of the source feature $X = [X_1, X_2 \ldots X_T]$ is performed so that a likelihood $L = p(Y/X, \Theta)$ is maximized. Note that the likelihood is represented as a function of y: the vector $Y = [Y_1, Y_2 \ldots Y_T]$ is represented as Wy, where W denotes a conversion matrix from the static feature sequence to the static and dynamic feature sequence, respectively y and Δy (Tokuda, Yoshimura, Masuko, Kobayashi, & Kitamura, 2000). Toda et al (Toda et al., 2005) have proposed an improved ML-based conversion method considering global variance (GV) of converted feature vectors that adds another term in the optimized likelihood.

The direct statistical mapping does not require any information on the phonetic content of the training data. Alignment of input and output feature vectors – if necessary – can be performed using an iterative procedure that combines Dynamic Time Warping with conversion so that prediction error diminishes as alignment and conversion improve.

The main advantage of direct statistical mapping resides in its ability to implicitly capture fine speaker-specific characteristics.

Mapping via Phoneme Recognition

In direct statistical mapping, the temporal structure of speech is implicitly modelled by considering (a) a sliding time window over the input frames and (b) both static and dynamic output features are combined to produce smooth and continuous parameter trajectories. Another way to account for the special temporal structure of speech is to consider that speech encodes phonological structures: in such an approach, a pivot phonetic representation that links all measurable signals is introduced.

The mapping process proceeds in two steps: a phonetic decoding using speech recognition techniques and an output trajectory formation using speech synthesis techniques. Both steps may use different mapping techniques between signals and phonemes such as classical HMM-based speech recognition combined with corpus-based synthesis.

But the recent success of HMM-based synthesis (Yamagishi, Zen, Wu, Toda, & Tokuda, 2008) opens the route to more integrated statistical approaches to "phonetic-aware" mapping systems.

The main advantage of phonetic-based mapping resides in its ability to explicitly introduce linguistic information as additional constraints in the underdetermined mapping problem. Both in the recognition and synthesis process, linguistic or even information structure may be exploited to enrich the constructed phonological structure and restore information that could not be predicted on the sole basis of input signals e.g. melodic patterns from silent articulation as required for silent communication interfaces (Hueber et al., 2007).

APPLICATIONS

Applications of ASC systems are numerous. Three main areas can be found in the literature: communication enhancement, aids to communication for speech impaired people, and language training.

Communication Enhancement

ASC systems, when addressing communication enhancement, aim either at fusing multimodal input in order to enhance input signals or at adding extra multimodal signals for the interlocutor so as to compensate for noisy channel or noisy perceptual conditions due to the environment. Si-

Figure 4. NAM-to-speech conversion (from Tran, Bailly, Loevenbruck, & Toda, 2009). (a) 3D facial articulation tracked using an active appearance model; the position of the NAM device is indicated by an arrow; (b) non audible murmur as captured by the NAM microphone is characterized by a strong low frequency noise and a band-limited signal; (c) a target sample of the same utterance pronounced loudly in a head-set microphone; (d) the loud signal generated using GMM-based mapping from input signals (a) and (b).

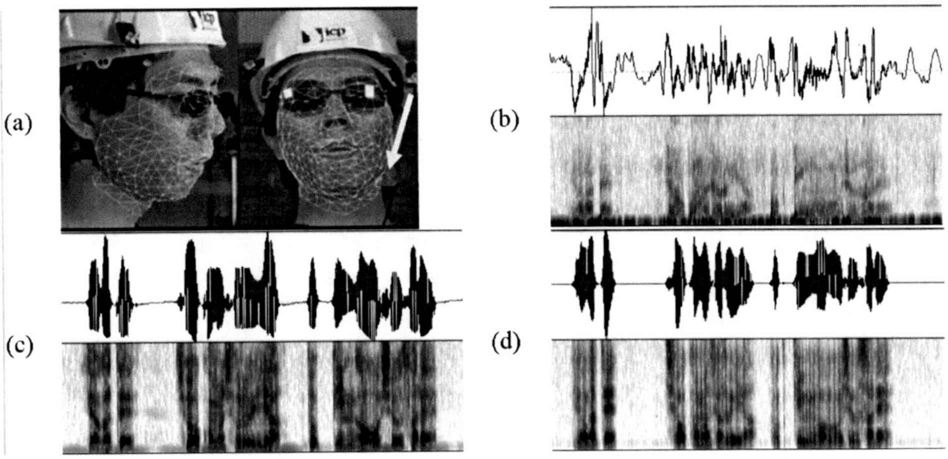

lent speech interfaces (SSI) fall into this category: SSI should enable speech communication to take place without emitting an audible acoustic signal. By acquiring sensor data from the human speech production process, an SSI computes audible – and potentially visible – signals. Both mapping approaches have been explored:

- Bu et al (Bu, Tsuji, Arita, & Ohga, 2005) generate speech signals from EMG signals recorded during silent speech articulation via an intermediate recognition of 5 vowels and the nasal sound /n/ by a hybrid ANN-HMM speech recognition system. The linguistic model has the hard job of restoring missing consonants based on phonotactic constraints of Japanese phonology. Similarly Hueber et al (Hueber et al., 2007) combine HMM-based speech recognition with corpus-based speech synthesis to generate an audible speech signal from silent articulatory gestures captured by US imaging and video.
- Conversely Toda et al (Toda & Shikano, 2005) use direct statistical mapping for converting non audible murmur captured by a stethoscopic microphone to audible speech signal.

We have recently shown that direct statistical mapping outperforms phonetic-aware HMM-based mapping and that multimodal input improves significantly the prediction (Tran, Bailly, Loevenbruck, & Jutten, 2008). A perceptual identification task performed on a very difficult vocabulary of Japanese VCV stimuli (see Figure 4) shows that listeners can retrieve from converted speech more than 70% of the phonetic contrasts whereas amplified input NAM is unintelligible.

Aids to Communication for Speech Impaired People

ASC systems, when addressing communication impairment, aim to compensate for motor or perceptual deficits of one or both interlocutors. BCI can for example be exploited to offer people suffering from myopathy the ability to communicate with other people. Nakamura et al (Nakamura, Toda, Saruwatari, & Shikano, 2006) have used voice conversion of body-transmitted artificial speech to predict the structure of speech recorded before laryngectomy from speech produced after the surgery. This computer-assisted recovery of speech (Verma & Kumar, 2003) can also be performed by adapting voice fonts (Verma & Kumar, 2003) to the speaker's characteristics.

In our group, Beautemps et al (Beautemps et al., 2007) are working on a system that will enable deaf people using cued speech (CS) to have visiophonic conversations with normal hearing interlocutors. CS recognition (Aboutabit, Beautemps, Clarke, & Besacier, 2007) and synthesis (Gibert, Bailly, Beautemps, Elisei, & Brun, 2005) systems have been developed to allow conversion between speech movements and hand and lips movements. The CS-to-speech system either drives the movement of a virtual hand superposed on the video of the normal hearing speaker that produces audio speech (Bailly, Fang, Elisei, & Beautemps, 2008) or controls the movements of the face, head and hand of a virtual talking head. CS synthesis may restore more than 95% of the phonetic contrasts that could not be solved on the basis of lip reading alone (Gibert, Bailly, & Elisei, 2006).

Language Training

Some ASC systems can also be used as tools for helping learners of a second language to master the articulation of foreign sounds. ASC systems thus perform acoustic-to-articulatory inversion: they compute the articulatory sequence that has most likely produced the sound sequence uttered by the learner. This articulation can be then displayed by means of a talking head in an augmented reality manner (see Figure 6), and compared to the required articulation so that proper corrective strategies are elicited. Several projects of virtual tutors have been launched (Engwall & Bälter, 2007; Massaro, 2006).

We have shown that despite the fact that such displays of internal articulation appear very unusual to them, listeners / viewers possess, to a certain extent, native tongue reading capabilities without intensive training (some subjects gain up to 40% recognition rate when watching the tongue display in absence of sound) (Pierre Badin et al., 2008). Such technologies may thus help people in pronunciation training.

Figure 5. Cued speech processing. Left, impressive recognition scores (Aboutabit et al., 2007) are obtained by fusing lip and hand movements. Motion capture is simplified here by make-up. Right, text-to-cued speech synthesis (Gibert et al., 2005) is performed by concatenating elementary gestural units gathered by motion capture on a human speech cuer.

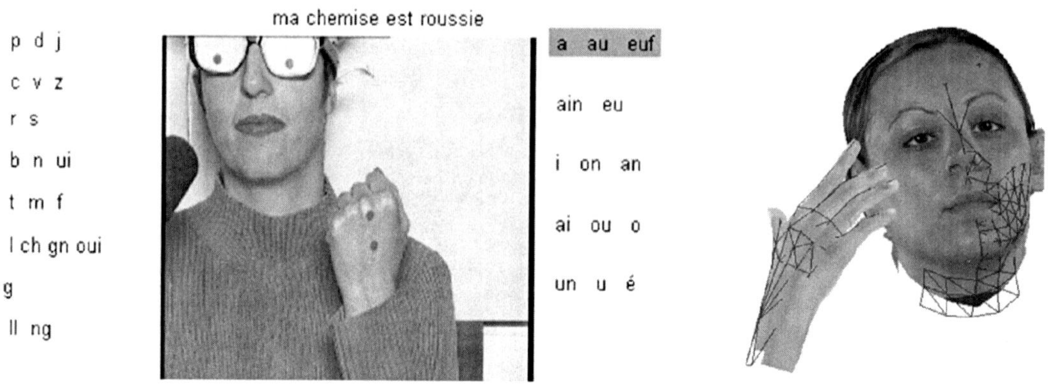

Figure 6. Artificial tongue displays that can be used as feedback for pronunciation training (Pierre Badin et al., 2008)

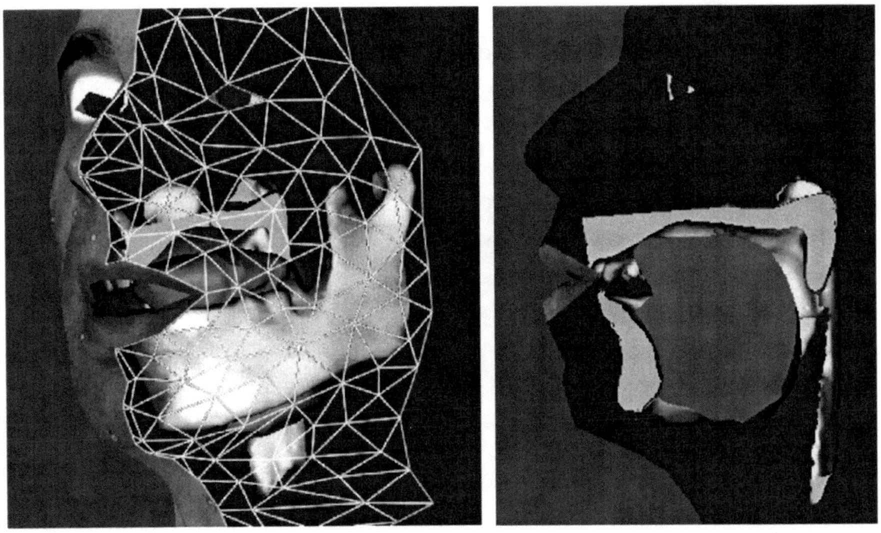

CONCLUSION

Augmented speech communication is a very challenging research theme that requires better understanding and modelling of the speech production and perception processes. ASC systems require *a priori* knowledge to be injected in the underdetermined inversion process so as to restore the coherence of multimodal signals that deliver incomplete information on the speech articulation or that are corrupted by noise.

A number of open issues need to be dealt with before this technology can be deployed in everyday life applications:

- The problem of speaker normalization is a hot topic: Pairs of input/output training data are only available for a limited number of subjects that have accepted to be monitored with quite invasive recording devices. To be practically acceptable, ASC systems should be able to adapt to a specific user quickly using a limited quantity of input/output data;
- Similar to speech recognition systems, ASC systems rely a lot on top-down information that constraints the mapping or inverse mapping problem. ASC should be able to benefit from language-specific constraints to gain robustness;
- Real-time issues are also very important. Guéguin et al (Guéguin, Le Bouquin-Jeannès, Gautier-Turbin, Faucon, & Barriac, 2008) have shown that full-duplex conversation is possible as long as one-way transmission delays are below 400ms. ASC systems should thus exploit limited contextual information to estimate output features. This imposes notably important constraints on speech recognition techniques;

Such technologies that connect two human brains benefit from cortical plasticity: people can learn to cope with imperfect mappings and noisy signals. Technologies that combine multimodal input and output are likely to enable computer-mediated conversation with minimum cognitive load. Evaluation issues are critical: people can cope with very crude communication channels but at the expense of the recruitment of intensive cognitive resources that may forbid any parallel activity.

ACKNOWLEDGMENT

Some of the PhD students of the team have largely contributed to settle this research in the laboratory: Nourredine Aboutabit and Viet-Ahn Tran are warmly thanked. We also thank our colleagues Panikos Héracleous, Hélène Loevenbruck and Christian Jutten for discussion and common work. Tomoki Toda from NAIST/Japan was very helpful. This experimental work could not have been conducted without the technical support from Christophe Savariaux and Coriandre Vilain. Part of this work has been supported by the PPF "Interactions Multimodales", PHC Sakura CASSIS, ANR Telma and Artis.

REFERENCES

Aboutabit, N., Beautemps, D., Clarke, J., & Besacier, L. (2007). A HMM recognition of consonant-vowel syllables from lip contours: the cued speech case. Paper presented at the Interspeech, Antwerp, Belgium.

Aboutabit, N. A., Beautemps, D., & Besacier, L. (Accepted). Lips and hand modeling for recognition of the cued speech gestures: The French vowel case. *Speech Communication*.

Abry, C., Badin, P., & Scully, C. (1994). Sound-to-gesture inversion in speech: the Speech Maps approach. In K. Varghese & S. Pfleger & J. P. Lefèvre (Eds.), Advanced speech applications (pp. 182-196). Berlin: Springer Verlag.

Aron, M., Berger, M.-O., & Kerrien, E. (2008). Multimodal fusion of electromagnetic, ultrasound and MRI data for building an articulatory model. Paper presented at the International Seminar on Speech Production, Strasbourg, France.

Badin, P., Elisei, F., Bailly, G., & Tarabalka, Y. (2008). An audiovisual talking head for augmented speech generation: Models and animations based on a real speaker's articulatory data. Paper presented at the Conference on Articulated Motion and Deformable Objects, Mallorca, Spain.

Badin, P., Tarabalka, Y., Elisei, F., & Bailly, G. (2008). Can you "read tongue movements"? Paper presented at the Interspeech, Brisbane, Australia.

Bailly, G., Fang, Y., Elisei, F., & Beautemps, D. (2008). Retargeting cued speech hand gestures for different talking heads and speakers. Paper presented at the Auditory-Visual Speech Processing Workshop (AVSP), Tangalooma, Australia.

Beautemps, D., Girin, L., Aboutabit, N., Bailly, G., Besacier, L., Breton, G., et al. (2007). TELMA: telephony for the hearing-impaired people. From models to user tests. Toulouse, France.

Bu, N., Tsuji, T., Arita, J., & Ohga, M. (2005). Phoneme classification for speech synthesiser using differential EMG signals between muscles. Paper presented at the IEEE Conference on Engineering in Medicine and Biology, Shanghai, China

Cornett, R. O. (1967). Cued speech. *American Annals of the Deaf, 112*, 3–13.

Engwall, O., & Bälter, O. (2007). Pronunciation feedback from real and virtual language teachers. *Journal of Computer Assisted Language Learning, 20*(3), 235–262. doi:10.1080/09588220701489507

Gibert, G., Bailly, G., Beautemps, D., Elisei, F., & Brun, R. (2005). Analysis and synthesis of the 3D movements of the head, face and hand of a speaker using cued speech. *The Journal of the Acoustical Society of America, 118*(2), 1144–1153. doi:10.1121/1.1944587

Gibert, G., Bailly, G., & Elisei, F. (2006). Evaluating a virtual speech cuer. Paper presented at the InterSpeech, Pittsburgh, PE.

Guéguin, M., Le Bouquin-Jeannès, R., Gautier-Turbin, V., Faucon, G., & Barriac, V. (2008). On the evaluation of the conversational speech quality in telecommunications. EURASIP Journal on Advances in Signal Processing, Article ID 185248, 185215 pages.

Guenther, F. H., Ghosh, S. S., & Tourville, J. A. (2006). Neural modeling and imaging of the cortical interactions underlying syllable production. *Brain and Language*, *96*(3), 280–301. doi:10.1016/j.bandl.2005.06.001

Hofe, R., & Moore, R. K. (2008). AnTon: an animatronic model of a human tongue and vocal tract. Paper presented at the Interspeech, Brisbane, Australia.

Hueber, T., Chollet, G., Denby, B., Dreyfus, G., & Stone, M. (2007). Continuous-speech phone recognition from ultrasound and optical images of the tongue and lips. Paper presented at the Interspeech, Antwerp, Belgium.

Kiritani, S. (1986). X-ray microbeam method for measurement of articulatory dynamics: techniques and results. *Speech Communication*, *5*(2), 119–140. doi:10.1016/0167-6393(86)90003-8

Kröger, B. J., Birkholz, P., Kannampuzha, J., & Neuschaefer-Rube, C. (2006). Modeling sensory-to-motor mappings using neural nets and a 3D articulatory speech synthesizer. Paper presented at the Interspeech, Pittsburgh, PE.

Massaro, D. W. (2006). A computer-animated tutor for language learning: Research and applications. In P. E. Spencer & M. Marshark (Eds.), Advances in the spoken language development of deaf and hard-of-hearing children (pp. 212-243). New York, NY: Oxford University Press.

Nakajima, Y., Kashioka, H., Shikano, K., & Campbell, N. (2003). Non-audible murmur recognition Input Interface using stethoscopic microphone attached to the skin. Paper presented at the International Conference on Acoustics, Speech and Signal Processing.

Nakamura, K., Toda, T., Saruwatari, H., & Shikano, K. (2006). Speaking aid system for total laryngectomees using voice conversion of body transmitted artificial speech. Paper presented at the InterSpeech, Pittsburgh, PE.

Nota, Y., & Honda, K. (2004). Brain regions involved in motor control of speech. *Acoustical Science and Technology*, *25*(4), 286–289. doi:10.1250/ast.25.286

Ouni, S., & Laprie, Y. (2005). Modeling the articulatory space using a hypercube codebook for acoustic-to-articulatory inversion. *The Journal of the Acoustical Society of America*, *118*(1), 444–460. doi:10.1121/1.1921448

Rabiner, L. R. (1989). A tutorial on hidden Markov models and selected applications in speech recognition. *IEEE Transactions on Audio, Speech, and Language Processing*, *77*, 257–286.

Recasens, D. (2002). An EMA study of VCV coarticulatory direction. *The Journal of the Acoustical Society of America*, *111*(6), 2828–2840. doi:10.1121/1.1479146

Schwartz, J. L., Boë, L. J., & Abry, C. (2007). Linking the Dispersion-Focalization Theory (DFT) and the Maximum Utilization of the Available Distinctive Features (MUAF) principle in a Perception-for-Action-Control Theory (PACT). In M. J. Solé & P. Beddor & M. Ohala (Eds.), Experimental approaches to phonology (pp. 104-124): Oxford University Press.

Schwartz, J.-L., Boë, L.-J., Vallée, N., & Abry, C. (1997). The Dispersion -Focalization Theory of vowel systems. *Journal of Phonetics*, *25*, 255–286. doi:10.1006/jpho.1997.0043

Summerfield, A., MacLeod, A., McGrath, M., & Brooke, M. (1989). Lips, teeth, and the benefits of lipreading. In A. W. Young & H. D. Ellis (Eds.), Handbook of research on face processing (pp. 223-233). Amsterdam: Elsevier Science Publishers.

Toda, T., Black, A. W., & Tokuda, K. (2004). Mapping from articulatory movements to vocal tract spectrum with Gaussian mixture model for articulatory speech synthesis. Paper presented at the International Speech Synthesis Workshop, Pittsburgh, PA.

Toda, T., Black, A. W., & Tokuda, K. (2005). Spectral conversion based on maximum likelihood estimation considering global variance of converted parameter. Paper presented at the International Conference on Acoustics, Speech and Signal Processing (ICASSP), Philadelphia, PE.

Toda, T., Ohtani, Y., & Shikano, K. (2006). Eigenvoice conversion based on gaussian mixture model. Paper presented at the InterSpeech, Pittsburgh, PE.

Toda, T., & Shikano, K. (2005). NAM-to-Speech Conversion with Gaussian Mixture Models. Paper presented at the InterSpeech, Lisbon - Portugal.

Tokuda, K., Yoshimura, T., Masuko, T., Kobayashi, T., & Kitamura, T. (2000). Speech parameter generation algorithms for HMM-based speech synthesis. Paper presented at the IEEE International Conference on Acoustics, Speech, and Signal Processing, Istanbul, Turkey.

Tran, V.-A., Bailly, G., & Loevenbruck, H. (submitted). Improvement to a NAM-captured whisper-to-speech system. Speech Communication - special issue on Silent Speech Interfaces.

Tran, V.-A., Bailly, G., Loevenbruck, H., & Jutten, C. (2008). Improvement to a NAM captured whisper-to-speech system. Paper presented at the Interspeech, Brisbane, Australia.

Tran, V.-A., Bailly, G., Loevenbruck, H., & Toda, T. (2008). Predicting F0 and voicing from NAM-captured whispered speech. Paper presented at the Speech Prosody, Campinas - Brazil.

Tran, V.-A., Bailly, G., Loevenbruck, H., & Toda, T. (2009). Multimodal HMM-based NAM-to-speech conversion. Paper presented at the Interspeech, Brighton.

Verma, A., & Kumar, A. (2003). Modeling speaking rate for voice fonts. Paper presented at the Eurospeech, Geneva, Switzerland.

Whalen, D. H., Iskarous, K., Tiede, M. T., Ostry, D., Lehnert-LeHoullier, H., & Hailey, D. (2005). The Haskins optically-corrected ultrasound system (HOCUS). *Journal of Speech, Language, and Hearing Research: JSLHR*, *48*, 543–553. doi:10.1044/1092-4388(2005/037)

Wilson, S. M., Saygin, A. P., Sereno, M. I., & Iacoboni, M. (2004). Listening to speech activates motor areas involved in speech production. *Nature Neuroscience*, *7*, 701–702. doi:10.1038/nn1263

Yamagishi, J., Zen, H., Wu, Y.-J., Toda, T., & Tokuda, K. (2008). The HTS-2008 system: Yet another evaluation of the speaker-adaptive HMM-based speech synthesis system. Paper presented at the Proc. Blizzard Challenge, Brisbane, Australia.

Section 3
Specific Applications

Chapter 8
CSS and Children:
Research Results and Future Directions

Kathryn D. R. Drager
The Pennsylvania State University, USA

Joe Reichle
University of Minnesota, USA

ABSTRACT

Currently, many computer-based augmentative and alternative communication (AAC) systems use speech output, either synthesized or digitized speech. The goal of this chapter is to provide a review of the research to date on computerized synthesized speech (CSS) with children. Information on the intelligibility and comprehension of CSS for children is presented, and the variables that may affect these, including context, speech rate, age of the child, the language(s) spoken by the listener, experience with CSS, and background noise. Each of these factors and the research support with child participants are discussed. The intelligibility of digitized speech is also discussed. Additionally, this chapter will address the attitudes and preferences of children regarding CSS, as well as hypotheses about the role that CSS may play for children with significant communication disabilities that require AAC. Finally, future research priorities are presented.

INTRODUCTION

Children encounter computerized synthesized speech (CSS) in a variety of places. Synthesized and digitized speech is found in educational software and computer games, as well as in augmentative and alternative communication (AAC) systems. Computerized speech in each of these applications should be as intelligible as possible to maximize educational opportunities and, for a child with significant communication disabilities, the potential for peer interaction.

Approximately 8-12 individuals per 1,000 experience speech and language impairments severe enough to significantly limit effective communication with others (Beukelman & Ansel, 1995). Many of these individuals use gestural- or graphic-based AAC systems. Approximately 12% of children receiving special education services require AAC (Binger & Light, 2006). For many of these children,

DOI: 10.4018/978-1-61520-725-1.ch008

computerized AAC systems with speech output are available to support their communication, using digitized, synthesized, or a combination of digitized and synthesized speech.

Digitized speech is recorded human voice stored as sampled segments of sound waves (Schlosser, 2003). Synthesized speech is computer generated according to a set of rules in an algorithm. Different synthesizers have used different types of coding to produce speech; some are based on the human voice. There is a wealth of research on the intelligibility and listener comprehension of synthesized speech for adults under ideal listening conditions. However we know relatively little about the usefulness of synthesized or digitized speech when young children serve as listeners. For the purposes of this chapter, the term computerized synthesized speech (CSS) will encompass both synthesized and digitized speech.

Intelligible speech output has several advantages for children who require AAC. First, intelligible CSS may allow children who require AAC an opportunity to experience more naturalized interaction with peers. Speech output may be a more comfortable method of communicative exchanges for peers, who are accustomed to communicating with one another via speech. CSS may assist in providing children who require AAC with opportunities to develop critical social skills and relationships that otherwise would not be available. Second, there is some evidence that CSS may enhance learning of AAC symbols (Schlosser, Belfiore, Nigam, Blischak, & Hetzroni, 1995). Third, CSS may increase comprehension of spoken language for children learning to use AAC using naturalistic language instruction (Sevcik & Romski, 2002). Fourth, the use of CSS allows for increased independence in communication with a wide range of communication partners, such as other children who are not literate or who are visually impaired, as well as in groups or over the telephone. In addition to these reasons, there are numerous applications for speech output in educational software and other computer games. To fully realize these advantages, it is necessary to examine the intelligibility and listener comprehension of CSS and the factors that influence these outcomes. It is also necessary to determine the effects of using CSS on attitudes of listeners, as well as the preferences of children regarding these voices. Lastly, it is also important to consider the role that speech output plays for children who rely on CSS for communication.

BACKGROUND

A processing constraint model has driven the majority of research examining the intelligibility and listener comprehension of CSS with adults. Theoretically, humans have a finite capacity for attention (Moray, 1967), with the brain allocating these resources across tasks. Tasks that require a large amount of processing resources will be completed at the expense of other tasks. Natural speech is characterized by redundant acoustic cues (Klatt, 1987). The information from the natural speech signal is rich, and little attention needs to be allocated by the listener for speech perception. In contrast, synthesized speech contains very few of these redundant cues, requiring increased processing resources for perception (Duffy & Pisoni, 1992). Fewer resources remain for comprehension and other higher order processing, and few remain for any other demands in communication interactions. Children, however, are working within the constraints of a more limited working memory capacity than adults (Case, 1985; Dempster, 1981). The limited capacity will impact the attentional resources available for deciphering synthesized speech. Thus, it may not be possible to generalize the results of research on speech output with adults as listeners.

INTELLIGIBIILITY OF SYNTHESIZED SPEECH

Intelligibility is the adequacy of the acoustic signal to transmit sounds (Dowden, 1997; Yorkston, Strand, & Kennedy, 1996). Intelligibility is often measured by having listeners repeat or transcribe stimuli, or by identifying stimuli within a closed-set. Repeating meaningful words and sentences likely also involves some comprehension of the material, although intelligibility measures cannot provide an estimate of the level of comprehension for the listener. Synthesized speech has been shown to be consistently lower in intelligibility compared to natural speech for adults (e.g., Hoover, Reichle, & Van Tasell, & Cole, 1987; Mirenda & Beukelman, 1987, 1990; Mitchell & Atkins, 1989).

Greene and Pisoni (1982) used a picture identification task to investigate the ability of second grade children (ages 7-9) to identify words presented either with natural speech or with a text-to-speech synthesizer. The results showed that the intelligibility of words presented in synthesized speech was significantly lower than for words presented in natural speech. During a second experiment in the same study, Green and Pisoni used a digit span task with 34 fourth graders (ages 9-11). In this task, the children repeated progressively longer digit sequences, between two and eight digits long, in both natural and synthetic speech. The fourth grade children showed higher levels of performance with natural speech than with synthesized speech. For both tasks, picture identification and digit span recall, the authors reported that the children made more errors than adults who had participated in the same tasks during previous experiments in the researchers' laboratory. Greene (1983) repeated this series of experiments with younger children (ages 5-6) and again with fourth graders. The results for the picture identification task with Kindergarten children were consistent with those for the earlier experiment. In contrast, the second group of fourth grade children showed no difference in performance in digit span recall with natural or synthesized speech.

The main conclusions of these early studies were: a) children were able to process CSS, b) the children experienced decreased intelligibility of CSS compared to natural speech, and c) the intelligibility of CSS for children was lower than for adults. Signal-independent variables will likely influence the intelligibility of synthesized speech in many ways. These variables may be related to the stimuli, such as context and speech rate. Or they may be related to aspects of the listener, such as age of the child, the native language(s) of the listener, and the experience of the listener with synthesized speech, or practice effects. Lastly, environmental variables may also affect the intelligibility of CSS, such as background noise.

Factors that Influence Speech Intelligibility

Context

Contextual information, which may take a variety of forms, has been consistently demonstrated to facilitate intelligibility of CSS for adults. Research has investigated the influence of longer messages (e.g., sentences) versus single words (Mirenda & Beukelman, 1987, 1990). Sentences appear to be more intelligible unless the listeners are presented with a closed response set (Koul & Hanners, 1997; Logan, Greene, & Pisoni, 1989). Additionally, stories are more intelligible than isolated sentences (Drager & Reichle, 2001b). These longer messages (sentences and paragraphs) generally contain more linguistic context than single words. Another form of context, predictability and meaningfulness of the spoken message, also increases the intelligibility of CSS for adults (Hoover, et al., 1987; Oshrin & Siders, 1987; Slowiaczek & Nusbaum, 1985). Lastly, contextual information in the form of a keyword (specifying the topic of a sentence) improves intelligibility of CSS with adult listeners (Marics & Williges, 1988).

Three studies have investigated the effect of context with children as listeners (Drager, Clark-Serpentine, Johnson, & Roeser, 2006; Mirenda & Beukelman, 1987, 1990). Mirenda and Beukelman (1987) compared the intelligibility of single words and sentences for three speech synthesizers (seven separate voices) and natural speech. Two listener groups were comprised of children: one younger (6-8 years old) and one slightly older (10-12 years old). The third group was adults (26-40 years old). While the intelligibility of single words for all synthesizers was significantly lower than the intelligibility of single words in natural speech, the sentence intelligibility of three synthesized voices (DECtalk™ male, female, and child) was statistically equivalent to the intelligibility of natural speech sentences for children and adults. At least for DECtalk™, the contextual information available in synthesized sentences may help to facilitate intelligibility.

In a follow-up study, Mirenda and Beukelman (1990) used the same procedures to investigate an additional five synthesizers (seven voices), again across three age groups. The study included seven each of: second grade children (7-8 years old), older elementary children (11-12 years old), and adults (22-50 years old). For both groups of children, the speech produced by the speech synthesizers were significantly less intelligible than natural speech in both word and sentence conditions. One synthesizer resulted in intelligibility that was statistically equivalent to natural speech for sentences for adults (Smoothtalker 3.0 male). In both Mirenda and Beukelman studies (1987, 1990), the intelligibility of sentences was consistently higher than for words, for all age groups. However, the reported results of this investigation did not resolve whether the difference was statistically significant, as single words and sentences were separate dependent variables, and analyses were not conducted to determine intelligibility differences.

Drager, Clark-Serpentine, et al. (2006) examined context as a variable with typically developing 3-5 year old children. The children listened to three types of speech output: DECtalk™ (Kit the Kid), MacinTalk™ (Junior), and digitized speech (sampled at 11 kHz). There were two contextual variables: single words and sentences, and the presence or absence of a topic cue (e.g. bedtime). Word and sentence intelligibility for 4- and 5-year-old children was significantly higher than intelligibility for 3-year-old children. However, there was a three-way interaction for the variables of message length (words versus sentences), context (topic cues), and speech type. When words or sentences were presented within the context of a topic cue, there were no significant differences between any of the three speech types. When words were presented without a topic cue, the intelligibility of both digitized speech and MacinTalk™ were significantly higher than the intelligibility of DECtalk™. When sentences were presented without a topic cue, the intelligibility of digitized speech was significantly higher than both of the two synthesizers. It appears that context interacted in complex ways to influence intelligibility.

Although sentences are more intelligible than single words for children ages 3 to 12 (Drager, Clark-Serpentine, et al., 2006; Mirenda & Beukelman, 1987, 1990), there are no simple conclusions. In two of the studies, statistical analyses were not conducted to compare these two stimulus types (Mirenda & Beukelman, 1987, 1990). In the third study, two types of context interacted with the variable of speech type (Drager, Clark-Serpentine, et al., 2006). Future research is necessary to determine the effects of different contexts on the intelligibility of CSS for children. If facilitative, it will be important to provide contextual cues as much as possible when children are required to understand CSS. This may be accomplished by several means that include using phrases or sentences where appropriate, providing topic cues, or repeating important messages.

Speech Rate

There is little research available on the effect of speech rate on the intelligibility of CSS. For adults, the intelligibility of a lower quality speech synthesizer (Echo II) was significantly higher when pauses between words were increased slightly (Venkatagiri, 1991). However, increasing pause duration even further did not result in significant intelligibility increases. Though not an intelligibility measure, Higginbotham, Drazek, Kowarsky, Scally, and Segal (1994) found that adults were able to summarize texts more accurately when speech was presented at slow rates (i.e., 10 sec between each word, which was equivalent to 5.5 words per min) than at normal speeds (140 words per min). In contrast, Drager, Anderson, DeBarros, Hayes, Liebman, and Panek (2007) found that pauses between words did not significantly improve intelligibility for adults listening in background noise. However, the pauses were not systematically inserted. Instead the sentences were presented as they were being formulated using iconic encoding which resulted in pauses of varying lengths between words.

Only one study has investigated the effect of rate on intelligibility of CSS for children. Segers and Verhoeven (2005) examined Kindergartners' skill in discriminating between two synthesized words presented at different rates. The participants included children who were diagnosed with Specific Language Impairment (SLI) (average age 69.6 months), and children who were considered to have normal language (average age 69.5 months). A slowed speech rate was accomplished in two ways: first, by lengthening the word by 200%, and second, by lengthening the transition of the second formant from 45 to 90 ms (affecting the vowel). The children with SLI had lower scores overall than the children with normal language. Additionally, both groups showed higher intelligibility when the speech rates were slowed, regardless of the rate reduction type that was used. The largest advantage was seen for children who were considered to have "poor" speech discrimination at the normal speech rate (8 participants with SLI and 3 participants with normal language). Because this study used a speech discrimination task, rather than an intelligibility measure per se (with a restricted set [two words]), it is impossible to draw any firm conclusions about speech rate and intelligibility of CSS for children.

Listener Variables that Influence Intelligibility

Age

Overall, the intelligibility of synthesized speech for children appears to be lower than for adults (Greene, 1983; Greene & Pisoni, 1982), at least with one synthesizer. However, there is very little evidence available that the age of the child listener (younger children versus older children) has a significant impact on the intelligibility of synthesized speech. Mirenda and Beukelman (1987, 1990) found that, overall the younger children (6-8 year olds between both studies) had lower intelligibility scores than the older children (10-12 year olds between both studies), and the intelligibility for both groups of children was lower than it was for adults. However, these differences either were not statistically significant using a conservative analysis (1987), or were qualified by an interaction with another variable (1990). There was a relatively small number of participants in each group in these studies (five and seven respectively), which may have restricted the power of the analyses.

In contrast, as noted earlier, Drager, Clark-Serpentine, et al. (2006) found that the intelligibility of DECtalk™, MacinTalk™, and digitized speech was significantly lower for the 3-year-old children than for the 4- and 5-year-old children (but not between the 4-year-olds and the 5-year-olds). The development from age 3 to age 4 is accompanied by tremendous changes in language. At this point in development comprehension begins to shift from being primarily context-dependent to an emergence of reliance on syntactic information (Miller & Paul, 1995). At the same time, the average receptive vocabulary size increases from approximately 500 words to 3000 words (Miller & Paul, 1995). The increased mastery of language comprehension, in addition to increases in working memory capacity, should allow children's perception and understanding of synthesized speech to improve over this period of development.

Listener's Native Language

The listener's native language is one factor that influences the intelligibility of CSS with adults. Adult listeners who are non-native speakers of the language being presented experience lower intelligibility of synthesized speech compared to native speakers (Mack, Tierney, & Boyle, 1990; Reynolds, Bond, & Fucci, 1996). Axmear, Reichle, Alamsaputra, Kohnert, Drager, and Sellnow (2005) investigated this variable with 20 children between the ages of 4-6. Half of the children were monolingual English speakers, and the other half were bilingual. For both groups, natural speech was significantly more intelligible than sentences presented in CSS. Overall, intelligibility for the monolingual children was significantly higher than intelligibility for the bilingual children. Additionally, the bilingual children experienced a greater decline in performance relative to natural speech than the children in the monolingual group. The investigation was conducted in the children's homes or church, and background noise was not tightly controlled. However, despite this limitation, there remains some initial evidence that the language of the listeners is a factor that will affect intelligibility for children, as well as adults. Axmear et al. caution that interventionists may assume a lack of compliance among bilingual listeners, when in fact the children may have difficulty understanding CSS. Because there are also very few studies that have investigated this variable in adults the evidence is preliminary.

Experience with Synthesized Speech

Synthesized speech intelligibility appears to improve with increased exposure (e.g., Schwab, Nusbaum, & Pisoni, 1985), and practice effects may be most apparent in early exposure (Venkatagiri, 1994). Several studies have investigated the effects of children's practice on synthesized speech intelligibility. Rounsefell, Zucker, and Roberts (1993) investigated the effects of practice with adolescents (ages 15-19) in a secondary classroom setting. They found that adolescents who were repeatedly exposed to synthesized speech showed a significant improvement in intelligibility compared to adolescents who received no training (control group). McNaughton, Fallon, Tod, Weiner, and Neisworth (1994) investigated the effects of practice with elementary children (ages 6-10) and adults (ages 19-44). Both groups showed increased intelligibility of single words over sessions.

Koul and Clapsaddle (2006) investigated the effects of practice with individuals with mild-to-moderate intellectual disabilities (ages 22-55) and a group of typically developing children (ages 4-8 years). The investigators used a closed-set picture identification task (the participants were asked to point to the line drawing that best represented the word or sentence provided, from a field of four). Both groups demonstrated evidence of learning across sessions. Additionally, both groups identified significantly more words than sentences. This appears to be in contrast to the earlier reported findings on the effects of linguistic context. However, it is not possible to compare performance on a picture identification task with performance on a repetition task.

The practice effect identified for synthesized speech is thought to be due to a "perceptual tuning" on the part of the listeners (Venkatagiri, 1994). Theoretically, through practice, listeners are learning specific detailed acoustic-phonetic information about the structural properties of CSS. The listener learns to make better use of the few acoustic cues that are available in the signal, leading to increases in intelligibility. With younger children, however, it is possible that the additional information available due to perceptual tuning will be insufficient to overcome working memory capacity constraints. Two studies have investigated the effects of practice on very young children, ages 2-4.

Drager et al. (2008) investigated the performance of typically developing 3- and 4-year-old children over four sessions. Ten children participated in each of four groups at each age level (80 children total). The four groups included: practicing with single words, practicing with sentences, practicing with short stories, and no practice (control). Overall, intelligibility was significantly higher for the 4-year-old children than for the 3-year-old children. For both single words and sentences, all groups except the control group (which showed no change from the first to the last sessions) showed evidence of learning. Significant improvements in intelligibility were seen by the third session for single words, and by the second session for sentences, compared to the first session. Young children appeared to benefit from practice with either words or sentences. However, the children who practiced with stories had the lowest intelligibility scores with both single words and sentences. It is possible that stories, with several sentences but one unifying theme, provide a smaller sample of speech (phonemes and word boundaries).

Koul and Hester (2006) examined the effect of practice with even younger children. This investigation involved individuals with severe intellectual disabilities (ages 13-54) and typically developing children (ages 2.5-3). As in the Koul and Clapsaddle (2006) study, the dependent measure was based on a picture identification task. In this study, there was no significant difference in intelligibility across sessions for either group. Overall, the typically developing children were more accurate identifying pictures than the group with intellectual disabilities. There are several potential explanations for a lack of learning found in this study, compared to the previous research reviewed. One explanation is that a picture identification task was not as sensitive to changes in intelligibility as repetition task might have been. A second explanation is that the participants did not receive enough practice (16 words in each of three sessions compared to 60 words in each of four sessions for the Drager et al. 2008 study). Finally, although 3-year-old children appeared to be influenced by practice effects in the Drager et al. study, the children in the Koul and Hester (2006) study were slightly younger (mean age 3.12 years). There may be a critical difference in working memory capacity for 2-year-old children than 3-year-old children.

Relative to some of the other variables that may influence the intelligibility of synthesized speech, practice effects have received a fair amount of attention in the literature. The majority of studies reviewed showed a significant increase in intelligibility of synthesized speech for children from age 3 to adolescence. Two of these studies also included a control group which decreased potential threats to internal validity (Drager et al., 2008; Rounsefell et al., 1993).

Environmental Variables that Influence Intelligibility

Background Noise

Much of the research on synthesized speech intelligibility has been conducted in ideal conditions (i.e. sound-treated rooms). However, intelligibility of CSS may be influenced by natural conditions, which often have background noise. Background noise of +10 dB signal to noise ratio (SNR) resulted in significantly reduced intelligibility for adult listeners (Fucci, Reynolds, Bettagere, & Gonzales, 1995), and this effect appears to be more pronounced for CSS than for natural speech (Koul & Allen, 1993).

Few studies have examined background noise as an independent variable with children as listeners. At least three studies were conducted in natural environments, which would include the presence of background noise (Axmear et al., 2005; Drager, Clark-Serpentine, et al., 2006; Drager et al., 2008). However, it is impossible from these studies to make any determinations about the relationship of background noise and intelligibility of synthesized speech for children. In each of the studies, care was taken by the researchers to ensure an environment that was as quiet as possible (e.g., separate rooms away from the classroom). The intelligibility outcomes that resulted might actually be lower had the measures been taken in the natural environment.

Because of a lack of studies that have investigated the effect of background noise on the intelligibility of CSS for children, it is impossible to draw any conclusions. It might be hypothesized that background noise would present a challenge for child listeners, given the lack of redundant acoustic cues in synthesized speech. If background noise interferes with the reception of the signal, there are fewer other cues available to assist with perception.

LISTENER COMPREHENSION OF SYNTHESIZED SPEECH

While many studies have focused on synthesized speech intelligibility (particularly for adults), few studies have focused on listeners' comprehension of CSS. Comprehension has been described as the adequacy of the speech signal to impart meaning in a functional context (Dowden, 1997; Yorkston et al., 1996). Theoretically, intelligibility requires more resources for CSS than for natural speech, resulting in a reduction of resources for higher-level comprehension processes. However, for adults, comprehension of synthesized discourse passages is not significantly lower than comprehension of natural speech (e.g., Schwab, Nusbaum, & Pisoni, 1985; Jenkins & Franklin, 1982).

Only one study investigated children's comprehension of synthesized speech. Massey (1988) used the Token Test for Children to present children with a series of tasks to complete (e.g., find the small white circle). One group was diagnosed with a language impairment (8-10 years old), while the other group had normal language skills (matched for age and sex to the children with language impairment). Consistent with the adult literature, the children with normal language showed no difference in comprehension between the natural speech commands and the synthesized commands. The children with language impairments, however, did significantly better when following commands given in natural speech than synthesized speech. These children's comprehension was already compromised compared to the children with normal language, even with natural speech. Therefore it appears that comprehension of CSS may be more negatively affected for individuals who already have comprehension impairments.

The processing costs imposed by comprehending synthesized speech may only become apparent with more sensitive dependent measures such as response latency (Duffy & Pisoni, 1992). Increased latencies to CSS would reflect more processing time required for comprehension (Pisoni, Manous, & Dedina, 1987; Ralston, Pisoni, Lively, Greene, & Mullennix, 1991). One task that has been used to assess response times is a sentence verification task, in which participants are required to judge whether a presented sentence is true or false.

Three studies have used a sentence verification task with children (Koul & Hanners, 1997; Reynolds & Fucci, 1998; Reynolds & Jefferson, 1999). Reynolds and Jefferson (1999) compared children from two age groups (6-7 and 9-11 year olds). Response latencies for both groups were measured only for sentences that were verified accurately and repeated correctly by the participants. These latencies were significantly longer for synthesized sentences than for natural speech sentences. The children also responded more quickly to true sentences than to false sentences.

Overall, responses for the older children were significantly faster than the younger children.

Reynolds and Fucci (1998) used a similar design to investigate comprehension of CSS for two groups of children: children with SLI (ages 6-11) and children with normal language skills (matched with the children with SLI by age and sex). Both groups of children responded more quickly to natural speech sentences than synthesized sentences, and more quickly to sentences that were true than sentences that were false. Children with normal language demonstrated significantly shorter response latencies than did the children with SLI.

Finally, Koul and Hanners (1997) implemented a sentence verification task with children to compare listeners' comprehension of different synthesizers. The treatment group included individuals with mild-to-moderate intellectual disabilities (ages 14-48). A control group consisted of 10 typically developing children (ages 3-13) who were matched with the treatment group on mental age. Participants with intellectual disabilities had lower mean accuracy scores than the typically developing children. Both groups made consistently made more accurate judgments and shorter latencies of responding for the higher quality synthesizer than for the lower quality synthesizer. This suggests that the quality of the synthesizer might influence comprehension.

The limited research that is available on children's comprehension of synthesized speech suggests similar patterns to those seen with adults. Comprehension, as measured by the ability of children to understand the meaning of a message, does not seem to be negatively affected by synthesized speech for children with normal language skills. However, children's comprehension of synthesized speech does appear to be associated with processing costs when measured by response latencies. In adults, several variables have been identified that affect comprehension of synthesized speech, including the rate of speech, the output method for presenting speech, and divided attention (Drager & Reichle, 2001a; Higginbotham et al., 1994; Higginbotham, Scally, Lundy, & Kowarsky, 1995). However, these variables have not been investigated in children.

INTELLIGIBILITY OF DIGITIZED SPEECH

Digitized speech is the conversion of speech into numbers, which are then converted back into speech output (Drager, Clark-Serpentine, et al., 2006). Typically, digitized speech varies in terms of sampling rate, or the number of samples per second. Higher sampling rates equate into more information that is available in the signal, at the cost of more memory necessary to encode the speech (Venkatagiri, 1996), and thus, more expensive equipment. While digitized speech is accompanied by limitations, such as the need to predetermine each message and a finite amount of memory available, it has often been associated with high intelligibility, presumed to be close to or as intelligible as natural speech (Mirenda & Beukelman, 1987). This is likely true for digitized speech that has been sampled at very high rates. In fact, in most studies that have compared the intelligibility of synthesized speech and natural speech, the "natural speech" is in fact digitized speech sampled at CD-ROM quality (44.1 kHz). However, the digitized speech generated by most AAC devices used by young children samples speech at significantly lower sampling rates, from 5-11 kHz.

Drager, Clark-Serpentine, et al. (2006) compared the intelligibility of digitized speech to two synthesizers for children ages 3-5. As noted earlier, intelligibility of all of the speech types was influenced by all the variables of interest: age, context (topic cue), and message length. For sentences presented without a topic cue, digitized speech was significantly more intelligible than the two speech synthesizers, DECtalk™ and MacinTalk™. When words were presented without a topic cue, the intelligibility of digitized speech was significantly higher than one synthesizer, but equivalent to the second. This suggests that the relationship is not a straightforward one. In some situations, digitized speech is not significantly more intelligible than synthesized speech for young children. For example, the intelligibility of digitized single words was 73% on average, a level that will not be functional for natural communication.

In a second study, Drager, Ende, Harper, Iapalucci, and Rentschler (2004) compared the performance of typically developing 3-5 year olds with digitized speech differing in sampling rate. The sampling rates included 44.1 kHz (called natural speech), 11 kHz, and <6 kHz. Overall, the intelligibility of natural speech was significantly higher than the intelligibility of both of the digitized speech samples, suggesting that digitized speech is not equivalent to natural speech. Additionally, overall, the intelligibility of the higher quality digitized speech was significantly higher than that of the lower quality digitized speech. These results were qualified by a significant three-way interaction of message (words versus sentences), age (3-, 4-, and 5-year-olds), and speech type. For single words, the pattern of results was the same as the overall results: natural speech was significantly more intelligible than both qualities of digitized speech and the high quality digitized speech was significantly more intelligible than the lower quality digitized speech. However, for sentences, the high quality digitized speech was equivalent to natural speech for the 3- and 5-year-olds (but not the 4-year-olds). The high quality digitized sentences were significantly more intelligible than the lower quality digitized sentences for all ages.

The premise that digitized speech is equivalent to natural speech may only be true for sentences, where linguistic context assists with intelligibility. However, sampling rate has a large impact on intelligibility of digitized speech. Additionally, there will be many situations where it would be desirable to use single words. In these situations it may be necessary to increase intelligibility (e.g., use accompanying visual cues, provide contextual cues, and establish potential practice effects).

CHILDREN'S ATTITUDES TOWARD AND PREFERENCES FOR CSS

Considering the intelligibility and comprehension of CSS isolates only one aspect of interaction, without accounting for other variables. There may also be a significant impact of CSS on children's attitudes toward other children using CSS for communication. Children may also show specific preferences regarding synthesized voices. For adults, a speaker using his own voice was perceived as more trustworthy than a speaker using CSS (Stern, Mullennix, Dyson, & Wilson, 1999). However, when told that the speaker using CSS had a disability, adults responded to CSS almost as positively as natural speech (Stern, Mullennix, & Wilson, 2002). It is important to understand the perceptions of children as well.

Two studies have investigated the attitudes of children toward CSS where the speech output was the independent variable (Bridges Freeman, 1990; Lilienfeld & Alant, 2002). In the first, Bridges Freeman (1990) asked fourth grade children to complete an attitude scale and quality rating for natural speech (child's voice) and three synthesizers. The children's attitude scores for all the voices were high and not significantly different from attitude scores for natural speech. However, they did show a clear preference for natural speech and for DECtalk over other synthesizers. The children's attitudes were related to their preferences, with a significant, but low, correlation. Lilienfeld and Alant (2002) investigated the effect of speech output on the attitudes of children, ages 11-13. The children watched videotaped examples of an unfamiliar peer with cerebral palsy, with and without speech output. These investigators found a significant main effect for voice. That is, the children's attitudes were significantly higher for the voice group than for the non-voice group.

Results suggested that children may have more tolerance for CSS than adults, although they do appear to prefer natural speech. The use of CSS is preferable to no speech output at all. Given the limited available empirical information, additional research is necessary to adequately determine the influence of CSS on children's attitudes.

Mirenda, Beukelman, and colleagues addressed the preferences for three different age groups regarding CSS. Mirenda, Eicher, and Beukelman (1989) investigated the preferences of children 6-8 years old, 10-12 years old, and 15-17 years old, and adults 24-45 years old regarding 11 voices (seven synthesizers and four natural speakers). The listeners were asked to judge the voices for six potential users of the voice: a male adult, a female adult, a male child, a female child, a computer, and themselves. The groups rated the synthesized voices as less acceptable for humans than natural speech, but acceptability for synthesized voices increased when the voice was being chosen for computers. Additionally, the youngest children chose a less intelligible synthesized voice (Votrax) as an acceptable choice for computers, while adults chose a natural speaker for computers. There was also a gender-influenced difference when the listeners were asked to rate voices for themselves. Boys 6-8 years old rated the male adult and male child voices as acceptable for themselves, while 10-12 year old boys preferred the male child, but rated the male adult as unacceptable. All ages of females rated the female adult and female child as acceptable for themselves, and rated these significantly higher than any other voices. Crabtree, Mirenda, and Beukelman (1990) provided a follow-up study, extending the earlier study to additional synthesizers. For the most part, the results were consistent with the Mirenda et al. (1989) study, except that all males rated both male adult and male child voices as acceptable for themselves. Clearly, individuals of all ages display apparent preferences for synthesized voices, particularly when asked to consider a choice of voice for themselves.

THE ROLE OF SPEECH OUTPUT FOR CHILDREN

For many individuals, their voice may serve as an extension of their personality. Consequently, it might not be surprising that people demonstrate preferences. However, this raises the question of the role that CSS serves for children with disabilities who rely on AAC with speech output. Some adults who use AAC have very specific preferences regarding choice of voice, with some females choosing the male voice because they feel it is easier to understand. Others have expressed that the speech output is simply a tool to deliver messages, and does not represent their "voice", which sounds very different to them inside their heads. There is no research available to inform these issues, with either adults or children.

Speech output may serve several roles for children who use AAC. One may be that the CSS serves truly as the "voice" for the child. In fact, it may be the only public voice that communication partners will be able to hear and/or understand. Lee, Liao, and Ryu (2007) found that fifth grade children apply gender-based rules to gender-identified synthesized speech. When the gender of the voice matched the stereotypical gender-bias of the content (e.g., a female voice talking about princesses or a male voice talking about dinosaurs), the children responded with more positive evaluations. These results suggest that listeners consider the speech output as the voice of the individual using it.

Another role that CSS may play is as a vehicle for communication, much like an e-mail or a letter read aloud by another person. It transmits a message, but does not imply that the voice that is heard is the voice of the sender. Lastly, the voice may serve as an input mechanism for the child, particularly a young child who is learning the AAC system. This last role is clearly not the primary consideration for most facilitators who program AAC systems. Parents from many cultures make modifications to their speech when talking to children (Ochs & Scheiffelin, 2008). However, speech output used with children does not vary prosody or intonation according to these modifications.

It is impossible to determine which role(s) that CSS serves for children who require AAC. There is evidence that children who use AAC are aware of the speech output. Sigafoos, Didden, and O'Reilly (2003) taught three children with autism (ages 3, 4, and 13) to request using a single switch with digitized speech output. Once the children had acquired the requesting behavior, they alternated the speech output condition on and off. The children had similar rates of use of the switch whether the speech output was turned on or not, suggesting that the requesting behavior was maintained by access to preferred objects, and not the speech output. However, the children did show some evidence of being aware of the digitized speech, depressing the switch repeatedly during the speech off condition and showing puzzlement. In another study, Schlosser et al. (2007) taught five children with autism to request with and without speech output. Although the children engaged in frequent requesting in both conditions, two of the children requested more often with speech output. One child requested more often without speech output, and there was no difference for the remaining two children. The impact of speech output and the role it plays may be different for different individuals.

FUTURE RESEARCH DIRECTIONS AND CONCLUSION

Despite over 15 years of study, the research on CSS with children is in the early stages. Based on the studies reviewed, it is clear that children are able to process and understand synthesized speech. However, relative to the intelligibility and comprehension for adults, children may have greater difficulty with synthesized speech. Future research is required to adequately define this relationship, and the variables that may contribute to improving or decreasing the perception and understanding of synthesized speech. Maximizing intelligibility and comprehension may be a one important step in facilitating learning of AAC systems by children with significant communication disabilities, potentially enhancing their comprehension of spoken language, and improving relationships among children who require AAC and their peers. There is some evidence that the many of the variables that influence intelligibility for adults also influence intelligibility for children. But little is known about each of these variables. Additionally, there is limited information on the intelligibility of digitized speech under various conditions, although many AAC technologies in use with young children use digitized speech output. Specifically, future research should investigate the variables of context, speech rate, age, native language of the child, experience of the child with CSS, and background noise on the intelligibility and listener comprehension of synthesized and digitized speech.

Given the increasing incidence of students in public schools that are English-language learners (Kindler, 2002), it will be critical to further investigate the intelligibility of CSS for children who are non-native speakers of English. With this group of children, speech synthesis software increasingly comes into play in educational software that young learners access. The literature addressing this population as consumers of synthesized speech applications is quite limited. Available evidence suggests that it is possible that at least some synthesized speech applications are less intelligible for English as a second language students than for monolingual students. If this finding is replicated there may be significant implications for utilizing educational software applications to supplement instruction for this population.

In school settings, there is no information on the effect that background noise has on the intelligibility of CSS. Children may be in background noise levels of 55-65 dBA in elementary classrooms (Nelson, Soli, & Seitz, 2002). The bulk of the available synthesized intelligibility and comprehension literature with children has been conducted in sound controlled environments under relatively optimal listening conditions. Those investigations that have utilized less optimal listening environments have not attempted to tightly control noise as an independent variable. In examining the effect of signal to noise ratios on speech intelligibility, it will likely be important to also treat the specific speech synthesis stimulus as an independent variable in that it is quite possible that different products or voice types within products will react differentially to noise. One interesting consideration is whether the facilitating effects of practice would be sufficient to overcome the debilitating effects of background noise for children.

As with adults, there are few studies that have specifically investigated the comprehension of synthesized speech with children. Like intelligibility studies, the studies that are available suggest that children's comprehension of synthesized speech is affected in much the same way as adults' comprehension. Typically developing children are able to comprehend synthesized speech as well as natural speech (Massey, 1988), but performance deficits become apparent when more subtle dependent measures are investigated, such as response latency. It is unclear whether these longer response times, which the researchers hypothesize reflect longer processing times, significantly affect performance in natural situations.

Improvements in CSS may also lead to improved attitudes of listeners and the other perceptions of listeners. Listener perception of synthesized speech applications is likely to be particularly important for several reasons. First, a more intelligible the synthesized speech application may place less communicative burden on the listener. Among younger children this is critically important since they are less apt to invite communicative repair. Secondly, for AAC users, having to engage in communicative repair can further slow communicative exchanges in an already very slow communicative modality (compared to natural speech output). Third, speech output applications on speech generating devices may act as a logical overture to recruit social approaches from peers. Among very young communicators, it would be useful to examine the relationship between the match between voice and the actual speaker for age and gender and the probability of a peer's approach.

Further, available literature addressed in this chapter suggests that characteristics of augmentative communication systems are apt to directly influence a listener's perception of an AAC user's intellectual level. This, in turn, has implications for the listener's selection of age appropriate topics. Perceived intellectual level of a communicative partner is also apt to influence semantic, morphological, and grammatical aspects of communicative output addressed to the user of a speech generating device. Although not extensively explored to date, these variables may have significant implications for language intervention strategies in natural environments that depend on modeling and feedback from communicative partners.

We believe that repeated exposure and practice effects with synthesized and digitized speech applications for children represents an under investigated but very important area for further scrutiny. Limited evidence discussed in this chapter suggests that under some conditions there is a practice effect (particularly for less competent communicators). Even more limited evidence suggests that this practice effect can occur as a result of being exposed to novel words rather than the same repeated words. Further demonstrations of the extent to which improvement as a result of general exposure to synthesized speech occurs as well as the amount of exposure to yield an educationally significant effect would be of significant assistance to educators.

Finally, there is some evidence limited evidence that voice output (even when of limited intelligibility) can have a facilitating effect on natural speech production (Romski & Sevcik, 1996). There is also very preliminary evidence that pairing speech output with graphic symbol presentations may facilitate comprehension of spoken language (Harris & Reichle, 2004; Drager, Postal, Carrolus, Castellano, Gagliano, & Glynn, 2006). With very young children and with children who experience significant developmental disabilities, further examination of this facilitating effect that synthesized and digitized speech applications may have represents a critically important area for future research. If parents can be reassured that implementing a speech generating device will not compromise speech development and comprehension of naturally produced spoken language, speech-language pathologists will have a much easier case to make in promoting the more preventative implementation of speech generating devices with young children who are "at significant risk" for natural speech production and/or comprehension of natural speech.

This chapter has attempted to present the current state of knowledge about the intelligibility and comprehension of CSS for children, as well as attitudes, preferences, and the roles that speech output plays. To fully realize the potential advantages of CSS for children, such as the opportunity for children who require AAC to experience more naturalized interaction with peers and to develop critical social skills and relationships, it is necessary to fully understand the nature of CSS with children. CSS will need to be highly intelligible, comprehensible, and natural. Perhaps one of the most surprising areas requiring attention is the need to further explore the intelligibility of human recorded speech. The limited available literature suggests that it may be far less intelligible than previously assumed. Synthesized and digitized speech applications in augmentative and alternative communication have made substantial advances in the past 20 years. We have moved from speech applications in single words that were functionally unintelligible (Votrax and Echo speech synthesis) to applications just beginning to be incorporated in speech generating devices that are increasingly difficult to distinguish from live speech. We are hopeful that the next 20 years will render discussions of practical applications of speech synthesis intelligibility unnecessary.

ACKNOWLEDGMENT

Portions of this chapter were based on an article: Drager, K.D.R., & Reichle, J. (2009). Synthesized speech output and children: A systematic review. *Manuscript submitted for publication.*

REFERENCES

Axmear, E., Reichle, J., Alamsaputra, M., Kohnert, K., Drager, K., & Sellnow, K. (2005). Synthesized speech intelligibility in sentences: A comparison of monolingual English speaking and bilingual children. *Language, Speech, and Hearing Services in Schools, 36*, 244–250. doi:10.1044/0161-1461(2005/024)

Beukelman, D., & Ansel, B. (1995). Research priorities in augmentative and alternative communication. *Augmentative and Alternative Communication, 11*, 131–134. doi:10.1080/07434619512331277229

Binger, C., & Light, J. (2006). Demographics of preschoolers who require augmentative and alternative communication. *Language, Speech, and Hearing Services in Schools, 37*, 200–208. doi:10.1044/0161-1461(2006/022)

Bridges Freeman, S. (1990). Children's attitudes toward synthesized speech varying in quality. (Doctoral dissertation, Michigan State University, 1990). *Dissertation Abstracts International, 52*(06), 3020B. (UMI No. 9117814)

Case, R. (1985). *Intellectual development: Birth to adulthood.* Toronto, ON: Academic Press, Inc.

Crabtree, M., Mirenda, P., & Beukelman, D. R. (1990). Age and gender preferences for synthetic and natural speech. *Augmentative and Alternative Communication, 6*, 256–261. doi:10.1080/07434619012331275544

Dempster, F. N. (1981). Memory span: Sources of individual and developmental differences. *Psychological Bulletin, 89*, 63–100. doi:10.1037/0033-2909.89.1.63

Dowden, P. (1997). Augmentative and alternative communication decision making for children with severely unintelligible speech. *Augmentative and Alternative Communication, 13*, 48–59. doi:10.1080/07434619712331277838

Drager, K., Ende, E., Harper, E., Iapalucci, M., & Rentschler, K. (2004). *Digitized Speech Output for Young Children Who Require AAC.* Poster presented at the annual convention of the American Speech-Language-Hearing Association, Philadelphia, PA.

Drager, K., Finke, E., Gordon, M., Holland, K., Lacey, L., Nellis, J., et al. (2008, August). *Effects of Practice on the Intelligibility of Synthesized Speech for Young Children.* Poster presented at the biennial conference of the International Society for Augmentative and Alternative Communication, Montréal, Québec, Canada.

Drager, K. D. R., Anderson, J. L., DeBarros, J., Hayes, E., Liebman, J., & Panek, E. (2007). Speech synthesis in background noise: Effects of message formulation and visual information on the intelligibility of American English DECTalk®. *Augmentative and Alternative Communication, 23*, 177–186. doi:10.1080/07434610601159368

Drager, K. D. R., Clark-Serpentine, E. A., Johnson, K. E., & Roeser, J. L. (2006). Accuracy of repetition of digitized and synthesized speech for young children in background noise. *American Journal of Speech-Language Pathology, 15*, 155–164. doi:10.1044/1058-0360(2006/015)

Drager, K. D. R., Postal, V. J., Carrolus, L., Castellano, M., Gagliano, C., & Glynn, J. (2006). The effect of aided language modeling on symbol comprehension and production in two preschoolers with autism. *American Journal of Speech-Language Pathology, 15*, 112–125. doi:10.1044/1058-0360(2006/012)

Drager, K. D. R., & Reichle, J. E. (2001a). Effects of age and divided attention on listeners' comprehension of synthesized speech. *Augmentative and Alternative Communication, 17*, 109–119.

Drager, K. D. R., & Reichle, J. E. (2001b). Effects of discourse context on the intelligibility of synthesized speech for young adult and older adult listeners: Applications for AAC. *Journal of Speech, Language, and Hearing Research: JSLHR, 44*(5), 1052–1057. doi:10.1044/1092-4388(2001/083)

Duffy, S. A., & Pisoni, D. B. (1992). Comprehension of synthetic speech produced by rule: A review and theoretical interpretation. *Language and Speech, 35*, 351–389.

Fucci, D., Reynolds, M. E., Bettagere, R., & Gonzales, M. D. (1995). Synthetic speech intelligibility under several experimental conditions. *Augmentative and Alternative Communication, 11*, 113–117. doi:10.1080/07434619512331277209

Greene, B. G. (1983). Perception of synthetic speech by children. In *Research on Speech Perception Progress Report No. 9.* Bloomington, IN: Speech Research Laboratory, Indiana University.

Greene, B. G., & Pisoni, D. B. (1982). Perception of synthetic speech by children: A first report. In *Research on Speech Perception Progress Report No. 8.* Bloomington, IN: Speech Research Laboratory, Indiana University.

Harris, M. D., & Reichle, J. (2004). The impact of aided language stimulation on symbol comprehension and production in children with moderate cognitive disabilities. *Am. Journ. of Speech-Language Pathology, 13*, 155–167. doi:10.1044/1058-0360(2004/016)

Higginbotham, D. J., Drazek, A. L., Kowarsky, K., Scally, C., & Segal, E. (1994). Discourse comprehension of synthetic speech delivered at normal and slow presentation rates. *Augmentative and Alternative Communication, 10*, 191–202. doi:10.1080/07434619412331276900

Higginbotham, D. J., Scally, C. A., Lundy, D. C., & Kowarsky, K. (1995). Discourse comprehension of synthetic speech across three augmentative and alternative communication (AAC) output methods. *Journal of Speech, Language, and Hearing Research: JSLHR, 38*, 889–901.

Hoover, J., Reichle, J., VanTasell, D., & Cole, D. (1987). The intelligibility of synthesized speech: Echo II versus Votrax. *Journal of Speech and Hearing Research, 30*, 425–431.

Jenkins, J. J., & Franklin, L. D. (1982). Recall of passages of synthetic speech. *Bulletin of the Psychonomic Society, 20*(4), 203–206.

Kindler, A. (2002). *Survey of the states' limited English proficient students and available educational programs and services, summary report.* Washington, DC: National Clearinghouse for English Language Acquisition & Language Instruction Educational Programs.

Klatt, D. H. (1987). Review of text-to-speech conversion for English. *The Journal of the Acoustical Society of America, 82*, 737–793. doi:10.1121/1.395275

Koul, R., & Clapsaddle, K. C. (2006). Effects of repeated listening experiences on the perception of synthetic speech by individuals with mild-to-moderate disabilities. *Augmentative and Alternative Communication, 22*, 112–122. doi:10.1080/07434610500389116

Koul, R., & Hanners, J. (1997). Word identification and sentence verification of two synthetic speech systems by individuals with mental retardation. *Augmentative and Alternative Communication, 13*, 99–107. doi:10.1080/07434619712331277898

Koul, R., & Hester, K. (2006). Effects of listening experiences on the recognition of synthetic speech by individuals with severe intellectual disabilities. *Journal of Speech, Language, and Hearing Research: JSLHR, 49*, 47–57.

Koul, R. K., & Allen, G. D. (1993). Segmental intelligibility and speech interference thresholds of high-quality synthetic speech in presence of noise. *Journal of Speech and Hearing Research, 36*, 790–798.

Lee, K. M., Liao, K., & Ryu, S. (2007). Children's responses to computer-synthesized speech in educational media: Gender consistency and gender similarity effects. *Human Communication Research, 33*, 310–329. doi:10.1111/j.1468-2958.2007.00301.x

Lilienfeld, M., & Alant, E. (2002). Attitudes of children toward an unfamiliar peer using an AAC device with and without voice output. *Augmentative and Alternative Communication, 18*, 91–101. doi:10.1080/07434610212331281191

Logan, J. S., Greene, B. G., & Pisoni, D. B. (1989). Segmental intelligibility of synthetic speech produced by rule. *The Journal of the Acoustical Society of America, 86*, 566–581. doi:10.1121/1.398236

Mack, M., Tierney, J., & Boyle, M.E.T. (1990). The intelligibility of natural and LPC-coded words and sentences of native and non-native speakers of English. *Massachusetts Institute of Technology Lincoln Laboratory Technical Report, 869.*

Marics, M. A., & Williges, B. H. (1988). The intelligibility of synthesized speech in data inquiry systems. *Human Factors, 30*, 719–732.

Massey, H. (1988). Language-impaired children's comprehension of synthetic speech. *Language, Speech, and Hearing Services in Schools, 19*, 401–409.

McNaughton, D., Fallon, K., Tod, J., Weiner, F., & Neisworth, J. (1994). Effect of repeated listening experiences on the intelligibility of synthesized speech. *Augmentative and Alternative Communication, 10*, 161–168. doi:10.1080/07434619412331276870

Miller, J. F., & Paul, R. (1995). *The clinical assessment of language comprehension.* Baltimore: Brookes.

Mirenda, P., & Beukelman, D. R. (1987). A comparison of speech synthesis intelligibility with listeners from three age groups. *Augmentative and Alternative Communication, 3*, 120–128. doi:10.1080/07434618712331274399

Mirenda, P., & Beukelman, D. R. (1990). A comparison of intelligibility among natural speech and seven speech synthesizers with listeners from three age groups. *Augmentative and Alternative Communication, 6*, 61–68. doi:10.1080/07434619012331275324

Mirenda, P., Eicher, D., & Beukelman, D. R. (1989). Synthetic and natural speech preferences of male and female listeners in four age groups. *Journal of Speech and Hearing Research, 32*, 175–183.

Mitchell, P. R., & Atkins, C. P. (1988). A comparison of the single word intelligibility of two voice output communication aids. *Augmentative and Alternative Communication, 4*, 84–88.

Moray, N. (1967). Where is capacity limited? A survey and a model. *Acta Psychologica, 27*, 84–92. doi:10.1016/0001-6918(67)90048-0

Nelson, P., Soli, S., & Seitz, A. (2002). *Acoustical barriers to learning.* Melville, NY: Technical Committee on Speech Communication of the Acoustical Society of America.

Ochs, E., & Schieffelin, B. (2008). Language socialization: An historical overview. In P. A. Duff & N. H. Hornburger (Eds.), *Encyclopedia of language and education (2nd edition), 8*, 3-15.

Oshrin, S. E., & Siders, J. A. (1987). The effect of word predictability on the intelligibility of computer synthesized speech. *Journal of Computer-Based Instruction, 14*, 89–90.

Pisoni, D. B., Manous, L. M., & Dedina, M. J. (1987). Comprehension of natural and synthetic speech: II. Effects of predictability on the verification of sentences controlled for intelligibility. *Computer Speech & Language, 2*, 303–320. doi:10.1016/0885-2308(87)90014-3

Ralston, J. V., Pisoni, D. B., Lively, S. E., Greene, B. G., & Mullennix, J. W. (1991). Comprehension of synthetic speech produced by rule: Word monitoring and sentence-by-sentence listening times. *Human Factors, 33*, 471–491.

Reynolds, M., & Jefferson, L. (1999). Natural and synthetic speech comprehension: Comparison of children from two age groups. *Augmentative and Alternative Communication, 15*, 174–182. doi:10.1080/07434619912331278705

Reynolds, M. E., & Fucci, D. (1998). Synthetic speech comprehension: A comparison of children with normal and impaired language skills. *Journal of Speech, Language, and Hearing Research: JSLHR, 41*, 458–466.

Reynolds, M. E. D., Bond, Z. S., & Fucci, D. (1996). Synthetic speech intelligibility: Comparison of native and non-native speakers of English. *Augmentative and Alternative Communication, 12*(1), 32. doi:10.1080/07434619612331277458

Romski, M. A., & Sevcik, R. A. (1996). *Breaking the speech barrier: Language development through augmented means.* Baltimore: Paul H. Brookes Publishing.

Rounsefell, S., Zucker, S. H., & Roberts, T. G. (1993). Effects of listener training on intelligibility of augmentative and alternative speech in the secondary classroom. *Education and Training in Mental Retardation, 28*, 296–308.

Schlosser, R., Belfiore, P., Nigam, R., Bilischak, D., & Hetzroni, O. (1995). The effects of speech output technology in the learning of graphic symbols. *Journal of Applied Behavior Analysis*, *28*, 537–549. doi:10.1901/jaba.1995.28-537

Schlosser, R. W. (2003). Roles of speech output in augmentative and alternative communication: Narrative review. *Augmentative and Alternative Communication*, *19*, 5–27. doi:10.1080/0743461032000056450

Schlosser, R. W., Sigafoos, J., Luiselli, J. K., Angermeier, K., Harasymowyz, U., Schooley, K., & Belfiore, P. J. (2007). Effects of synthetic speech output on requesting and natural speech production in children with autism: A preliminary study. *Research in Autism Spectrum Disorders*, *1*, 139–163. doi:10.1016/j.rasd.2006.10.001

Schwab, E. C., Nusbaum, H. C., & Pisoni, D. B. (1985). Some effects of training on the perception of synthetic speech. *Human Factors*, *27*, 395–408.

Segers, E., & Verhoeven, L. (2005). Effects of lengthening the speech signal on auditory word discrimination in kindergartners with SLI. *Journal of Communication Disorders*, *38*, 499–514. doi:10.1016/j.jcomdis.2005.04.003

Sevcik, R. A., & Romski, M. A. (2002). The role of language comprehension in establishing early augmented conversations. In J. Reichle, D. Beukelman, & J. Light (Eds.), *Exemplary practices for beginning communicators: Implications for AAC* (pp. 453-474). Baltimore: Paul H. Brookes Publishing Co., Inc.

Sigafoos, J., Didden, R., & O'Reilly, M. (2003). Effects of speech output on maintenance of requesting and frequency of vocalizations in three children with developmental disabilities. *Augmentative and Alternative Communication*, *19*, 37–47. doi:10.1080/0743461032000056487

Slowiaczek, L. M., & Nusbaum, H. C. (1985). Effects of speech rate and pitch contour on the perception of synthetic speech. *Human Factors*, *27*, 701–712.

Stern, S. E., Mullennix, J. W., Dyson, C., & Wilson, S. J. (1999). The persuasiveness of synthetic speech versus human speech. *Human Factors*, *41*, 588–595. doi:10.1518/001872099779656680

Stern, S. E., Mullennix, J. W., & Wilson, S. J. (2002). Effects of perceived disability on persuasiveness of computer-synthesized speech. *The Journal of Applied Psychology*, *87*, 411–417. doi:10.1037/0021-9010.87.2.411

Venkatagiri, H. S. (1991). Effects of rate and pitch variations on the intelligibility of synthesized speech. *Augmentative and Alternative Communication*, *7*(4), 284. doi:10.1080/07434619112331276023

Venkatagiri, H. S. (1994). Effect of sentence length and exposure on the intelligibility of synthesized speech. *Augmentative and Alternative Communication*, *10*, 96–104. doi:10.1080/07434619412331276800

Venkatagiri, H. S. (1996). The quality of digitized and synthesized speech: What clinicians should know. *American Journal of Speech-Language Pathology*, *5*, 31–42.

Yorkston, K. M., Strand, E. A., & Kennedy, M. R. T. (1996). Comprehensibility of dysarthric speech: Implications for assessment and treatment planning. *American Journal of Speech-Language Pathology*, *5*, 55–66.

Chapter 9
Systematic Review of Speech Generating Devices for Aphasia

Rajinder Koul
Texas Tech University, USA

Diana Petroi
Texas Tech University, USA

Ralf Schlosser
Northeastern University, USA

ABSTRACT

The purpose of this chapter is to integrate and synthesize, using a meta-analytic approach, the research literature on the effectiveness of augmentative and alternative communication (AAC) intervention using speech generating devices (SGDs) for people with aphasia. Many individuals with little or no functional speech as a result of severe aphasia rely on non-speech communication systems to augment or replace natural speech. These systems include SGDs and software programs that produce synthetic speech upon activation. Based on this quantitative review, the following conclusions are evident. The first is that the existing state of knowledge on whether AAC interventions using SGDs work for people with aphasia is seriously affected not only because of the lack of data but also because most of the available data are compromised because of serious internal validity concerns. Keeping in mind this first conclusion as a context, the second conclusion is that AAC intervention options that utilize SGDs seem to be effective in changing the dependent variables in the experimental contexts. However, the variability among dependent measures across studies and of results within and across studies precludes meta-analytic techniques. Thus, any statements as to the effectiveness of AAC interventions using SGDs for persons with aphasia cannot be made yet.

INTRODUCTION

Aphasia is a language impairment resulting from damage to areas of the brain that are responsible for comprehension and formulation of language. Many persons with aphasia demonstrate severe speech and language deficits, and their ability to use natural language is permanently and severely impaired (Koul & Corwin, 2003). Such individuals may benefit from augmentative and alternative

DOI: 10.4018/978-1-61520-725-1.ch009

communication (AAC) methods. These include aids, techniques, strategies, and symbols for either augmenting speech and/or providing an alternative means of communication (Lloyd, Fuller, & Arvidson, 1997). AAC aids such as speech generating devices (SGDs), graphic symbols, and/or text-based software programs that turn computers into speech output communication devices have become increasingly available to persons with aphasia as a result of rapid advancements in computer technology (Beukelman & Mirenda, 2005; Garrett & Kimelman, 2000; Koul & Corwin, 2003; Koul, Corwin, & Hayes, 2005; Koul & Harding, 1998; Koul & Schlosser, 2004; Rostron, Ward, & Plant, 1996; Schlosser, 2003; Schlosser, Blischak, & Koul, 2003). Studies involving AAC intervention using either SGDs or graphic symbol software programs indicate that persons with chronic severe Broca's aphasia and global aphasia are able to access, identify, and combine graphic symbols to produce sentences and phrases in experimental contexts (Koul, Corwin, & Hayes, 2005; Koul, Corwin, Nigam, & Oetzel, 2008; Koul & Harding; McCall, Shelton, Weinrich, & Cox, 2000; Weinrich, Boser, McCall, & Bishop, 2001; Weinrich, Shelton, McCall, & Cox, 1997). However, their ability to use these alternative forms of communication outside structured treatment contexts has been limited. Persons with chronic severe Broca's aphasia have difficulty expressing themselves through speech. Their expressive speech is non-fluent and is comprised of few unintelligible words produced with significant effort. However, their comprehension is relatively intact. In contrast, persons with global aphasia demonstrate severe impairments across expressive speech, comprehension, reading and writing.

With the advent of evidence-based practice in AAC, it has become critical to evaluate the evidence before us. Schlosser and Raghavendra (2004) define evidence-based practice in AAC as "the integration of best and current research evidence with clinical/educational expertise and relevant stakeholders perspectives, in order to facilitate decisions about assessment and intervention that are deemed effective and efficient for a given direct stakeholder." (p.3). In times of dwindling resources and increased accountability, funding agencies for assistive devices and services increasingly require documentation that interventions actually work. Similarly, many consumers are seeking evidence from professionals that communication interventions using assistive technology such as SGDs really work before they are willing to consider using that technology. Are sufficient data to that end available? Although several individual intervention studies using SGDs with persons with aphasia have been published over the last three decades, it is difficult to draw definite conclusions based on single studies. It is critical that this body of studies be synthesized in a systematic manner (Cooper & Hedges, 1994; Schlosser, Wendt, & Sigafoos, 2007). Only then can we draw more definitive conclusions concerning the efficacy of AAC interventions using SGDs. Thus, the primary purpose of this chapter is to conduct a systematic review of the extant research literature on the effectiveness of AAC interventions for people with severe aphasia. AAC intervention approaches for the purposes of this review include use of the SGDs and software programs that produce synthetic and/or digitized speech output upon selection of a symbol or a written text.

METHODS

Inclusion Criteria

To be included, studies had to meet the following criteria:

1. The intervention and/or measured outcomes of the studies related to the implementation of AAC using SGDs and/or graphic symbol or text-based software programs that turn

computers into speech output communication devices. The speech output may be in digitized and/or synthetic form.

2. The dependent variables of the studies related to outcomes in which some type of change in behavior was observed secondary to AAC intervention using SGDs. These included but were not limited to identification of graphic symbols, production of words and/or sentences using symbols, and functional communication using SGDs.
3. The participants were diagnosed with aphasia, with etiologies for aphasia primarily including but not limited to stroke and traumatic brain injury.
4. Statistical data from group designs allowed for effect sizes (Cooper & Hedges, 1994) to be calculated, and data from single-subject experimental designs allowed for percentage of non-overlapping data (PND) (Scruggs, Mastropieri, & Casto, 1987) to be determined.
5. Pre-experimental designs, such as AB designs or pre-test post-test group designs without control group were excluded.
6. Studies ruled out internal validity concerns by using appropriate single-subject or group experimental designs.
7. Studies were published in English between 1980 and 2008. This time frame was selected to allow for the inclusion of early through up-to-date publications related to AAC intervention for aphasia.
8. Studies were published as articles in peer-reviewed journals and were accessible through the following search methods.

Search Methods

A systematic review methodology was utilized to limit bias in locating, appraising and synthesizing all relevant AAC intervention studies that used SGDs. This involved a comprehensive search for treatment studies. Electronic data-base searches were conducted using the Cumulative Index for Allied Health Literature (CINAHL), PubMed, and the Educational Resources Information Center (ERIC) as well as bibliographic database searches (e.g., Academy of Neurologic Communication Disorders and Sciences (ANCDS). In addition, we implemented hand searches of selected journals such as Augmentative and Alternative Communication and Aphasiology. Finally, ancestry searches involved examining reference lists of previously published studies related to AAC intervention and aphasia. Database searches involved locating articles using specific search terms (e.g., AAC and aphasia) and/or searching for articles specifically related to aphasia intervention and/or AAC intervention. Some journals (e.g.,) were also selectively hand searched for potentially relevant articles. Ancestry searches involved examining reference lists of previously published studies related to AAC intervention and aphasia. Each of the search methods utilized consisted of reviewing titles, abstracts, and/or full-text articles to determine the relevancy of each study.

The first and second authors independently decided on study inclusion. Once relevant studies were found, inclusion criteria were applied to determine which articles met the data extraction.

Data Extraction

The coding procedures used in this analysis were adapted from Schlosser and Wendt (2006). Tables 1 and 2 present the coding manual and form that were prepared to facilitate systematic data extraction related to specific categories. Each study was also appraised for methodological quality on ten dimensions (see Tables 1 and 2).

Data Extraction for Single-Subject Experimental Designs

PND, as discussed by Scruggs et al. (1987), was calculated for single-subject experimental designs. PND is an indicator of "effect size" that involves

Table 1. Coding procedures and categories for single-subject experimental designs

Article	
Design/Type	Single-subject
Purpose	
Type of research	Efficacy or effectiveness
Participant(s)	Entered study: Completed study:
Independent variable	
Dependent variable(s)	
Treatment integrity	1 – Reported 2 – Not reported
Treatment integrity: % of sessions	1 – N/A 2 – Enter % 3 – Not reported
Assessment of methodological quality Yes / No Yes / No Yes / No Yes / No Yes / No Yes / No Yes / No Yes / No Yes / No Yes / No	**Appraising single-subject experimental designs:** 1. Participants and participant selection were described with sufficient detail to allow other researchers to select similar participants in future studies. 2. Critical features of the physical setting were described with sufficient precision to allow for replication. 3. The dependent variables were sufficiently operationalized. 4. The dependent variables were measured repeatedly using sufficient assessment occasions to allow for identification of performance patterns prior to intervention and comparison of performance patterns across conditions/phases (level, trend, variability). 5. Inter-observer agreement (IOA) met minimal standards (i.e., IOA = 80%; Kappa = 60%). 6. Baseline data were sufficiently compared with data gathered during the intervention phase under the same conditions as baseline. 7. Baseline data were sufficiently consistent before intervention was introduced to allow prediction of future performance. 8. Experimental control was demonstrated via three demonstrations of the experimental effect (predicted change in the dependent variable varies with the manipulation of the independent variable) at different points in time (a) within a single participant (within-subject replication) or (b) across different participants (between-subject replication). 9. The independent variable was defined with replication precision. 10. Treatment integrity was at an appropriate level given the complexity of the treatment, independently verified, and based on relevant procedural steps.
Participant ID:	
Participant characteristics	Age: Gender: Race/ethnicity Education: Lesion site: Cause: Time post-onset:
Characteristics of aphasia	Type/severity: Acute/chronic:
Speech before treatment	1 – Little or no functional speech 2 – Some speech, but not intelligible 3 – Some speech, but echolalic 4 – Speech as primary mode
Length of treatment	1 – Unable to determine based on reported data 2 – Intervention was conducted for __ months, __ weeks, __ sessions
Density of treatment schedule	1 – Unable to determine based on reported data 2 – Intervention was conducted for __ daily (e.g., number of sessions)
Calculation of PND-Intervention &/or PND-Generalization	

Table 2. Coding procedures and categories for group designs

Article	
Design/Type	
Purpose	
Type of research	Efficacy or effectiveness
Participant(s)	Entered study: Completed study:
Independent variable	
Dependent variable(s)	
Treatment integrity	1 – Reported 2 – Not reported
Treatment integrity: % of sessions	1 – N/A 2 – Enter % 3 – Not reported
Assessment of methodological quality Yes / No Yes / No Yes / No Yes / No Yes / No Yes / No Yes / No Yes / No Yes / No Yes / No	**Appraising group designs:** 1. Participants were randomly allocated to interventions (in a crossover study, the participants were randomly allocated to an order in which treatments were received). 2. Allocation was concealed. 3. The intervention groups were similar at baseline regarding the most important prognostic indicators. 4. There was blinding of all participants. 5. There was blinding of all therapists who administered therapy. 6. There was blinding of all assessors who measured at least one key outcome. 7. Measures of at least one key outcome were obtained from more than 85% of participants originally allocated to groups. 8. All participants for whom outcome measures were available received the treatment or control condition as allocated, or if this was not the case, data for at least one key outcome was analyzed by "intention to treat." 9. The results of between-intervention group statistical comparisons were reported for at least one key outcome. 10. The study provided both point measures and measures of variability for at least one key outcome.
Participant ID:	
Participant characteristics	Age: Gender: Race/ethnicity Education: Lesion site: Cause: Time post-onset:
Characteristics of aphasia	Type/severity: Acute/chronic:
Speech before treatment	1 – Little or no functional speech 2 – Some speech, but not intelligible 3 – Some speech, but echolalic 4 – Speech as primary mode
Length of treatment	1 – Unable to determine based on reported data 2 – Intervention was conducted for __ months, __ weeks, __ sessions
Density of treatment schedule	1 – Unable to determine based on reported data 2 – Intervention was conducted for __ daily (e.g., number of sessions)
Calculation of effect size	1- Unable to determine based on reported data 2- Able to determine based on reported data

calculating the percentage of non-overlapping data points between baseline and intervention, baseline and generalization, and/or baseline and maintenance. In a multiple baseline design across subjects, for example, a single PND was calculated for each participant, the PNDs were then added, and a mean was obtained by dividing the summed PNDs across participants by the number of tiers (see Schlosser, Lee, & Wendt, 2008, for a review of PND applications). Data for PND calculations were obtained from graphic displays. Single-subject experimental studies that did not provide graphs were not included because PND data could not be extracted. PNDs were interpreted according to criteria presented by Scruggs et al.: greater than 90 = highly effective, 90 - 70 = fairly effective, 70 - 50 = questionable, and less than 50 = unreliable.

Data Extraction for Group Designs

Cohen's *d* was used to calculate effect sizes for group studies. Web-based calculators (Becker, 1999; Thalheimer & Cook, 2002) were used to determine Cohen's *d* for *F*-statistics and/or *t*-statistics. Based on Cohen's (1988, 1992) interpretation of the magnitude of the effect size, effect sizes of .20, .50, and .80 were considered as small, medium, and large effects, respectively.

The second author independently extracted all the data with the first author reviewing the data. Inter-observer agreement for the coding procedures was based on the first author coding at least 20% of the data from the studies included. Disagreements between the two authors were resolved upon discussion, which resulted in 100% agreement.

RESULTS

As there are no accepted methods available for integrating data from single-subject and group designs (Robey, 1998; Schlosser & Wendt, 2008), results are reported separately for these two different experimental designs.

Single-Subject Experimental Designs

Five single-subject experimental design studies involving a total of 23 participants met the inclusion criteria. Data are summarized in Table 3.

Participant Characteristics

The studies included a total of 23 participants with aphasia. The number of participants with aphasia across studies ranged from 1 to 9. Age of participants ranged from 27 to 86 years with mean age of 63.73 years. Eleven (48%) of the total participants were male, and 12 (52%) were female. For 22 of the participants, mean months post-onset of aphasia was 52.65 months (range = 8 to 106 months). However, for one participant, specific time post-onset of aphasia was not available. Speech and language characteristics prior to AAC intervention indicated that participants had primarily little or no functional speech.

Intervention

All five studies evaluated the effectiveness of AAC intervention either using SGDs or graphic symbol software programs that turned computers into speech output communication devices. Length of intervention varied across studies.

Design

All five studies used multiple baseline designs.

Measures

Categories of dependent variables that were measured included identification of graphic symbols, sentence production using graphic symbols, and learning to use SGDs in structured as well as functional treatment contexts.

Table 3. Summary of results for single-subject design studies

Study authors	Subject number	Time post onset	Severity/ type of aphasia	Dependent variable(s)	Research design	PND-Intervention	PND-Generalization
Koul & Harding (1998)	1	9 months	Severe aphasia	1. Identification of single symbols 2. Identification of two-symbol combinations	Multiple baseline design across behaviors replicated across subjects	Symbol identification: 100% Two-symbol combinations: 100%	N/A
	2	8 months	Severe aphasia			Symbol identification: 100% Two-symbol combinations: 100%	N/A
	3	48 months	Global			Symbol identification: 92.10% Two-symbol combinations: 100%	N/A
	4	48 months	Severe aphasia			Symbol identification: 87.5% Two-symbol combinations: 90.90%	N/A
	5	60 months	Global			Symbol identification: 100% Two-symbol combinations: 100%	N/A
Koul, Corwin, & Hayes (2005)	1	13 months	Severe Broca's	1. Producing sentences of varying grammatical complexity using graphic symbols	Multiple baseline across behaviors replicated across subjects	43.43%	13.33%
	2	81 months	Severe Broca's			58.58%	0%
	3	105 months	Severe Broca's			42.52%	22.22%
	4	96 months	Global			0%	0%
	5	56 months	Severe Broca's			15%	6.66%
	6	56 months	Severe Broca's			26.97%	13.33%
	7	>12 months	Global			15.5%	0%
	8	43 months	Severe Broca's			42.23%	0%
	9	81 months	Severe Broca's			13.56%	0%
Koul, Corwin, Nigam, & Oetzel (2008)	1	12 months	Severe Broca's	1. Producing sentences of varied grammatical complexity using graphic symbols	Multiple baseline across behaviors replicated across subjects	79.44%	N/A
	2	106 months	Severe Broca's			77.46%	N/A

Table continued next page

Table 3. continued

Study authors	Subject number	Time post onset	Severity/ type of aphasia	Dependent variable(s)	Research design	PND-Intervention	PND-Generalization
	3	35 months	Severe Broca's			77.15%	N/A
McKelvey, Dietz, Hux, Weissling, & Beukelman (2007)	1	96 months	Broca's	Use of Visual Scene Displays during conversation interactions: 1. Disability talk instances 2. Navigation/organization talk instances 3. Inappropriate question-answer exchanges	Multiple baseline across behaviors	Disability talk instances: 30% Navigation/ organization talk instances: 10% Inappropriate question-answer exchanges: 50%	N/A
Nicholas, Sinotte, & Helms-Estabrooks (2005)	1	90 months	Severe non-fluent	Use of *C-Speak Aphasia* during functional communication tasks: 1. Responding to questions 2. Describing pictures 3. Describing videos 4. Making phone calls 5. Writing	Multiple baseline across behaviors replicated across subjects	Autobiographical task: 100% Picture description: 100% Video description: unable to calculate Telephone calls: 100% Writing: unable to calculate	N/A
	2	19.2 months	Severe non-fluent			Autobiographical task: 50% Picture description: 75% Video description: unable to calculate Telephone calls: 75% Writing: unable to calculate	N/A
	3	27.6 months	Severe non-fluent			Autobiographical task: 55.55% Picture description: 77.77% Video description: unable to calculate Telephone calls: 0% Writing: unable to calculate	N/A
	4	18 months	Severe non-fluent			Autobiographical task: 100% Picture description: 60% Video description: unable to calculate Telephone calls: 100% Writing: unable to calculate	N/A
	5	50.4 months	Severe non-fluent			Autobiographical task: 16.66% Picture description: 100% Video description: 50% Telephone calls: 66.66% Writing: unable to calculate	N/A

Outcomes

PNDs were calculated for single-subject experimental designs. PNDs for dependent measures ranged from 0 to 100. As the studies varied in terms of specific independent and dependent measure employed, it was considered inappropriate to aggregate the outcomes across studies. Table 3 indicates that 15 (36.58%) out of 41 PND values for intervention are classified in the highly effective range (i.e., above 90), seven (17.07%) PND values are classifiable in the fairly effective range (70-90), seven (17.07%) PND values are classified in the questionable range (50-70), and 12 (29.26%) PND values are classified in the ineffective range (i.e., below 50). In one study (Nicholas, Sinotte, & Helms-Estabrooks, 2005), 9 of the 25 PND values for intervention could not be calculated based on the data provided; therefore, those values were not included in the 41 above mentioned values. Because generalization data were available for only one study, PND values for generalization were calculated only for that study (Koul et al., 2005). All PND values for generalization for that study fell in the ineffective range.

Group Designs

Two group studies involving 42 participants with aphasia met the inclusion criteria. The data are summarized in Table 4.

Participant Characteristics

The data provided on participant characteristics varied across studies. However, most of the participants had severe aphasia with limited verbal expression. Mean time post onset of aphasia ranged from equal to or greater than 6 months to 30 months.

Intervention

Both studies involved the use of SGDs as a primary component of AAC intervention.

Design

One study used a between group design and another study used a within subject design.

Measures

The dependent variables measured varied between studies. Beck and Fritz (1998) measured recall of abstract and concrete icons and recall of one, two, and three icon messages. Van de Sandt-Koenderman, Wiegers, and Hardy (2005) measured number of therapy sessions required for SGD training, as well as the effect of mean age and time post-onset on training outcome.

Outcomes

Effect sizes were calculated for all significant results for each study. Large effect sizes were revealed for the dependent variables in both the studies. However, for one of the two studies (van de Sandt-Koenderman et al., 2005), effect sizes could not be calculated for 2 of the 3 dependent measures.

Appraisal of Evidence for Single-Subject Experimental Designs and Group Designs

Single-subject experimental design studies reviewed above were appraised on their methodological quality using the framework proposed by Schlosser and Raghavendra (2003). Schlosser and Raghavendra described four basic types of research evidence: inconclusive evidence, suggestive evidence, preponderant evidence, and conclusive evidence. Inconclusive evidence indicates that the outcomes of the study are not plausible and

Table 4. Summary of results for group design studies

Study authors	Number of subjects[1]	Mean time post onset	Severity/Type of aphasia	Dependent variable(s)	Research design	Effect size (Cohen's *d*)
Beck & Fritz (1998)	$N = 20$ Aphasia group: $n = 10$ Control group: $n = 10$	≥ 6 months	Anterior lesions (high compre-hension): $n = 5$ Posterior lesions (low comprehend-sion): $n = 5$	1. Recalling abstract vs. concrete icon messages using IntroTalker SGD[2] 2. Recalling one, two, and three icon messages using IntroTalker SGD	Between group design	**Aphasia vs. control group (final probe):** Aphasia group: $n = 10$ Control group: $n = 10$ Aphasia vs. control: Cohen's $d = 1.27$ Abstract vs. concrete: Cohen's $d = 3.47$ Group vs. abstract/concrete: not significant Icon length: Cohen's *d*: 6.69 Group vs. icon length: Cohen's *d*: 1.1 Abstract/concrete vs. icon length: Cohen's *d*: 0.92 Group vs. abstract/concrete vs. icon: Cohen's *d*: 0.98 **High comprehension vs. low comprehension (final probe):** Aphasia group: $n = 10$ (used 5 and 5 for *n*'s for treatment and condition subjects, respectively) High vs. low: Cohen's *d*: 2.94 Abstract vs. concrete: Cohen's *d*: 3.82 Group vs. abstract/concrete: not significant Icon length: Cohen's *d*: 6.54 Group vs. icon length: not significant Abstract/concrete vs. icon length: Cohen's *d*: 2.37 Group vs. abstract/concrete vs. icon: Cohen's *d*: 2.39
van de Sandt-Koenderman, Wiegers, & Hardy (2005)	$N = 22$ (included subjects with LHD[3], RHD[4], subarachnoid hemorrhage, and traumatic brain injury)	30 months	Not specified – limited verbal expression but fairly good auditory comprehension	1. Number of therapy sessions required for PCAD[5] training, 2. Outcome of PCAD training 3. Mean age and time post-onset for successful and unsuccessful subjects	Within subject design	1. Number of therapy sessions needed for PCAD training: Cohen's *d*: unable to calculate Cohen's *d* based on data provided 2. Outcomes of PCAD training: unable to calculate Cohen's *d* based on data provided 3. Mean age and time post-onset for successful and unsuccessful clients: a. Mean age: Cohen's *d*: 1.30 b. Time post-onset: not significant

[1]Number of participants who completed each study
[2]SGD: Speech generating device
[3]LHD: Left hemisphere damage
[4]RHD: Right hemisphere damage
[5]PCAD: Portable communication assistant for people with dysphasia

clinical, and/or educational implications should not be considered because of serious threats to internal validity. Suggestive evidence indicates that the study has minor design flaws or an adequate design with insufficient inter-observer or treatment integrity. Preponderant evidence indicates that the study has either minor design flaws with sufficient inter-observer agreement or treatment integrity or a strong design with questionable inter-observer agreement or treatment integrity. Conclusive evidence suggests that the study has a strong design with sufficient inter-observer and treatment integrity. Thus, the Koul and Harding (1998); Koul et al. (2008); and McKelvey, Dietz, Hux, Weissling, and Beukelman (2007) studies were appraised as providing preponderant evidence based on the use of a strong design with acceptable inter-observer agreement but lack of treatment integrity. The Koul et al. (2005) study was considered to provide conclusive evidence based on the use of a strong research design as well as acceptable inter-observer agreement and treatment integrity. In contrast, the Nicholas et al. (2005) study was appraised as providing inconclusive evidence based on serious threats to internal validity as well as lack of inter-observer agreement and treatment integrity.

The group design study by van de Sandt-Koenderman et al., 2005 included for meta-analysis in this chapter suffers from serious internal validity concerns as this study did not include a control group or a control condition. In contrast, the Beck and Fritz (1998) study included a control group. However, the small number of subjects with aphasia in their study reduces the strength of the study.

DISCUSSION AND CONCLUSION

This chapter presented a systematic review of studies that evaluated the efficacy of AAC intervention using SGDs in individuals with severe aphasia. Results indicate that AAC intervention options using SGDs seem to be effective in changing the dependent variables under study. However the variability of results within and across single-subject design studies indicates that predictions about effectiveness of AAC interventions using SGDs for persons with aphasia cannot be made yet. Additionally, there were only two group design studies included in this review. The primary reasons for excluding most of the group design studies were the concerns related to internal validity. Further, many case studies that examined effectiveness of AAC intervention using SGDs were not included in this systematic review because case studies by their very nature can neither exclude threats to internal validity nor contribute to external validity.

DIRECTIONS FOR FUTURE RESEARCH

It becomes impossible to adequately support individuals with aphasia in maximizing their full inclusion, social integration, employment, and independent living without knowing which interventions work and which interventions work better than others. There is a serious paucity of data as to the efficacy of AAC interventions using SGDs in persons with aphasia. Thus, it is critical that future research focus on collecting efficacy data on AAC interventions using designs that eliminate concerns related to internal validity as well as generality.

REFERENCES

Beck, A. R., & Fritz, H. (1998). Can people who have aphasia learn iconic codes? *Augmentative and Alternative Communication*, *14*, 184–196. doi:10.1080/07434619812331278356

Becker, L. A. (1999). *Effect size calculators*. Retrieved on July 21, 2008, from http://web.uccs.edu/lbecker/Psy590/escalc3.htm

Beukelman, D. R., & Mirenda, P. (2005). *Augmentative and alternative communication: Supporting children and adults with complex communication needs.* (3rd ed.) Baltimore: Paul H. Brookes.

Cohen, J. (1988). *Statistical power analysis for the behavioral sciences* (2nd ed). Hillsdale, NJ: Lawrence Erlbaum Associates.

Cohen, J. (1992). A power primer. *Psychological Bulletin, 112*, 15–159.

Cooper, H. M., & Hedges, L. V. (Eds.). (1994). Research synthesis as a scientific enterprise. In *The handbook of research synthesis* (pp. 3-14). New York: Russell Sage Foundation.

Garrett, K. L & Kimelman M. D. Z. (2000) AAC and aphasia: Cognitive-linguistic considerations. In: Beukelman D. R, Yorkston K. M & Reichle J (Eds.) *Augmentative and alternative communication for adults with acquired neurologic disorders* (pp.339-374). Baltimore: Paul H. Brookes.

Koul, R., Corwin, M., & Hayes, S. (2005). Production of graphic symbol sentences by individuals with aphasia: Efficacy of a computer-based augmentative and communication intervention. *Brain and Language, 92*, 58–77. doi:10.1016/j.bandl.2004.05.008

Koul, R., Corwin, M., Nigam, R., & Oetzel, S. (2008). Training individuals with severe Broca's aphasia to produce sentences using graphic symbols: Implications for AAC intervention. *Journal of Assistive Technologies, 2*, 23–34.

Koul, R., & Harding, R. (1998). Identification and production of graphic symbols by individuals with aphasia: Efficacy of a software application. *Augmentative and Alternative Communication, 14*, 11–24. doi:10.1080/07434619812331278166

Koul, R., & Schlosser, R. W. (2004). Effects of synthesized speech output in the learning of graphic symbols of varied iconicity [Electronic version]. *Disability and Rehabilitation, 26*, 1278–1285. d oi:10.1080/09638280412331280299

Koul, R. K., & Corwin, M. (2003). Efficacy of AAC intervention in chronic severe aphasia. In R.W. Schlosser, H.H. Arvidson, & L.L. Lloyd, (Eds.), *The efficacy of augmentative and alternative communication: Toward evidence-based practice* (pp. 449-470). San Diego, CA: Academic Press.

Lloyd, L. L., Fuller, D. R., & Arvidson, H. H. (1997). *Augmentative and alternative communication: A handbook of principles and practices.* Needham Heights, MA: Allyn & Bacon.

McCall, D., Shelton, J. R., Weinrich, M., & Cox, D. (2000). The utility of computerized visual communication for improving natural language in chronic global aphasia: Implications for approaches to treatment in global aphasia. *Aphasiology, 14*, 795–826. doi:10.1080/026870300412214

McKelvey, M. L., Dietz, A. R., Hux, K., Weissling, K., & Beukelman, D. R. (2007). Performance of a person with chronic aphasia using personal and contextual pictures in a visual scene display prototype. *Journal of Medical Speech-Language Pathology, 15*, 305–317.

Nicholas, M., Sinotte, M. P., & Helms-Estabrooks, N. (2005). Using a computer to communicate: Effect of executive function impairments in people with severe aphasia. *Aphasiology, 19*, 1052–1065. doi:10.1080/02687030544000245

Robey, R. R. (1998). A meta-analysis of clinical outcomes in the treatment of aphasia. *Journal of Speech, Language, and Hearing Research: JSLHR, 41*, 172–187.

Rosenberg, W., & Donald, A. (1995). Evidence based medicine: An approach to clinical problem-solving. *BMJ (Clinical Research Ed.), 310*, 1122–1126.

Rostron, A., Ward, S., & Plant, R. (1996). Computerised augmentative communication devices for people with dysphasia: Design and evaluation. *European Journal of Disorders of Communication, 31*, 11–30. doi:10.3109/13682829609033149

Schlosser, R. W. (2003). Roles of speech output in augmentative and alternative communication: Narrative review [Electronic version]. *Augmentative and Alternative Communication, 19*, 5–27. doi:10.1080/0743461032000056450

Schlosser, R. W., Blischak, D. M., & Koul, R. K. (2003). Roles of speech output in AAC: An integrative review. In R.W. Schlosser, H.H. Arvidson, & L.L. Lloyd, (Eds.), *The efficacy of augmentative and alternative communication: Toward evidence-based practice* (pp. 471-531). San Diego, CA: Academic Press.

Schlosser, R. W., Lee, D. L., & Wendt, O. (2008). Application of the percentage of non-overlapping data in systematic reviews and meta-analyses: A systematic review of reporting characteristics. *Evidence-Based Communication Assessment and Intervention, 2*, 163–187. doi:10.1080/17489530802505412

Schlosser, R. W., & Raghavendra, P. (2003). Toward evidence-based practice in AAC. In R.W. Schlosser, H.H. Arvidson, & L.L. Lloyd, (Eds.), *The efficacy of augmentative and alternative communication: Toward evidence-based practice* (pp. 259-297). San Diego, CA: Academic Press.

Schlosser, R. W., & Raghavendra, P. (2004). Evidence-based practice in augmentative and alternative communication. *Augmentative and Alternative Communication, 20*, 1–21. doi:10.1080/07434610310001621083

Schlosser, R. W., & Wendt, O. (2006). *The effects of AAC intervention on speech production in autism: A coding manual and form.* Unpublished manuscript, Northeastern University, Boston.

Schlosser, R.W., & Wendt, O. (2008). Effects of augmentative and alternative communication intervention on speech production in children with autism: A systematic review. *American Journal of Speech-language Pathology: A Journal of Clinical practice, 17*, 212-230.

Schlosser, R. W., Wendt, O., & Sigafoos, J. (2007). Not all systematic reviews are created equal: considerations for appraisal. *Evidence-Based Communication Assessment and Intervention, 1*, 138–150. doi:10.1080/17489530701560831

Scruggs, T. E., Mastropieri, M. A., & Castro, G. (1987). The quantitative synthesis of single subject research methodology: Methodology and validation. *Remedial and Special Education, 8*, 24–33. doi:10.1177/074193258700800206

Thalheimer, W., & Cook, S. (2002, August). *How to calculate effect sizes from published research articles: A simplified methodology*. Retrieved on July 28, 2008, from http://work- learning.com/effect_sizes.htm

van de Sandt-Koenderman, M., Wiegers, J., & Hardy, P. (2005). A computerized communication aid for people with aphasia. *Disability and Rehabilitation, 27*, 529–533. doi:10.1080/09638280400018635

Weinrich, M., Boser, K. I., McCall, D., & Bishop, V. (2001). Training agrammatic subjects on passive sentences: Implications for syntactic deficit theories. *Brain and Language, 76*, 45–61. doi:10.1006/brln.2000.2421

Weinrich, M., Shelton, J. R., McCall, D., & Cox, D. M. (1997). Generalization from single sentence to multisentence production in severely aphasic patients. *Brain and Language, 58*, 327–352. doi:10.1006/brln.1997.1759

ENDNOTE

* References marked with an asterisk indicates studies included in the meta-analyses.

Chapter 10
Are Speech-Generating Devices Viable AAC Options for Adults with Intellectual Disabilities?

Dean Sutherland
University of Canterbury, New Zealand

Jeff Sigafoos
Victoria University of Wellington, New Zealand

Ralf W. Schlosser
Northeastern University, USA

Mark F. O'Reilly
The University of Texas at Austin, USA

Giulio E. Lancioni
University of Bari, Italy

ABSTRACT

Many adults with intellectual disabilities have severe communication impairments and are therefore potential candidates for the use of speech-generating technologies. However, there may be reluctance to prescribe speech-generating devices for adults with intellectual disabilities in the absence of evidence demonstrating that such persons are capable of learning and interested in using this technology. In this chapter, the authors provide an overview of intellectual disability and the use of speech-generating technologies for adults with intellectual disability. This overview is followed by a systematic review of intervention studies that have sought to teach the use of speech-generating technologies to adults with intellectual disability. An overview and review of this type may help to inform and advance evidence-based practice in the provision of communication intervention for adults with intellectual disability.

DOI: 10.4018/978-1-61520-725-1.ch010

INTRODUCTION

Imagine an adult who has failed to acquire the ability to speak and remains unable to communicate his/her most basic wants and needs; an adult unable to request a drink when thirsty or a snack when hungry; an adult unable to inform others when in pain or ill; an adult unable to enjoy the simple pleasure of conversing with loved ones. There are literally millions of such adults. They are to be found among those diagnosed with intellectual disability (Carr & O'Reilly, 2007; Sigafoos, O'Reilly, & Green, 2007). Would the resulting communicative handicaps experienced by these millions of people be reduced if they could be taught to use speech-generating devices (SGDs)?

For the purpose of this chapter, SGDs are defined as any switch-operated, electronic, or computer-based communication aid that produces either digitized (i.e., recorded) or synthesized speech output. Such devices are typically used to augment unintelligible speech or provide an alternative mode of communication in cases where natural speech has failed to develop sufficiently. When used for these purposes, SGDs represent a mode or system of augmentative and alternative communication (AAC). AAC and SGDs are more fully described in a subsequent section of this chapter.

In this chapter, we attempt to determine whether adults with intellectual disabilities can benefit from SGDs by systematically reviewing intervention studies that have sought to teach the use of SGD to these individuals. A review of this type may help to inform and advance evidence-based practice in the provision of communication intervention for adults with intellectual disability. Our chapter begins with overviews of intellectual disability and the use of AAC by adults with intellectual disability.

DEFINING AND DESCRIBING INTELLECTUAL DISABILITY

The term intellectual disability covers a range of more specific disorders and syndromes, all of which share several common diagnostic criteria (Carr & O'Reilly, 2007; Matson, 2007). The essential feature of intellectual disability (or mental retardation) is "significantly sub-average general intellectual functioning . . . accompanied by significant limitations in adaptive functioning . . ." (American Psychiatric Association, 2000, p. 41). The communication domain is one area of adaptive functioning that is often significantly limited in persons with intellectual disability (Sigafoos et al., 2007). Epidemiological and assessment studies consistently show that people with intellectual disabilities often present with major speech, language, and communication problems (Abbeduto, Evans, & Dolan, 2001). The nature and extent of their communication problems depends, in part, on the etiology and severity of intellectual disability (Duker, van Driel, & van Bercken, 2002; Sigafoos et al., 2007).

In terms of etiology, there is some research suggesting that certain intellectual disability syndromes are associated with distinct and possibly unique communication profiles. Duker et al. (2002), for example, compared the communication profiles of individuals with Down syndrome to individuals with Angelman syndrome. They found that individuals with Down syndrome tended to have greater deficits in the communication functions related to requesting and rejecting/protesting in comparison to echoic or imitative functions. The opposite was true of individuals with Angelman syndrome. These data highlight the importance of etiology in designing communication interventions for individuals with intellectual disability.

Intellectual disability is a heterogeneous condition. It is therefore possible that promising interventions for one etiological group, such as communication interventions involving the use of SGDs, may prove unsuitable for another etiological group. In addition to the skills that the individuals present with, consideration of person's the current and future environments and the communication partners they are expected to interact with in those environments may lead to the selection of an appropriate intervention. Thus consideration of participant characteristics, as noted by Bedrosian (2003), is important when reviewing studies on the use of speech-generating technologies in communication interventions for adults with intellectual disability.

In terms of severity, four degrees or levels of intellectual disability have been delineated: (a) mild, (b) moderate, (c) severe, and (d) profound (American Psychiatric Association, 2000). These four degrees of severity are based largely on IQ scores. Generally, individuals with IQ scores indicative of severe to profound intellectual disability (i.e., IQ less than 40) will have more pronounced and obvious speech and language problems than individuals with mild to moderate intellectual disability (i.e., IQ of 40-70).

Sigafoos et al. (2007) summarized the nature of the communication problems associated with mild/moderate versus severe/profound intellectual disability. Briefly, individuals with mild/moderate intellectual disability typically present with delayed speech acquisition, but most will eventually develop a sufficient amount of speech to meet their daily communication needs. Their acquired speech repertoires are, however, often characterized by (a) limited vocabulary, (b) shorter mean length of utterance, (c) articulation and intelligibility problems, and (d) poor language comprehension. For these individuals, AAC is not often used as an alternative to speech as most will acquire a fair amount of functional speech and language. Rather AAC might be indicated during the early years of development to temporarily compensate for delayed speech acquisition. In addition, AAC might be used to augment the person's unintelligible speech when necessary, such as when communicating in noisy environments or with unfamiliar people. AAC might also be used to provide a source of visual input to aid comprehension (Mirenda & Brown, 2009).

Individuals with severe/profound intellectual disabilities, in contrast, often fail to acquire sufficient speech and language to meet daily communication needs. Even with intensive speech training, many adults with severe/profound intellectual disability remain essentially mute. Given the severe nature of their communication impairments, AAC could be seen as necessary for providing such persons with a viable mode of communication. In the absence of successful efforts to teach AAC, many of these individuals rely on prelinguistic acts, such as vocalizations, facial expressions, and body movements (Sigafoos et al., 2000). However such prelinguistic acts are often so informal and idiosyncratic as to be indecipherable to most listeners (Carter & Iacono, 2002). In such cases, Sigafoos, Arthur-Kelly, and Butterfield (2006) argued that AAC interventions should aim to enhance the person's prelinguistic repertoire by developing more formal and sophisticated forms of non-speech communication, such as teaching the person to use a SGD.

DEFINING AND DESCRIBING AAC

AAC is a specialist area of research and clinical practice within the fields of speech-language pathology, special education, and rehabilitation (Beukelman & Mirenda, 2005). In clinical practice, AAC professionals focus on enhancing adaptive functioning via non-speech communication modes. Common non-speech communication modes include: (a) gestures and manual signs, (b) communication boards, and (c) SGDs with either digitized (i.e., recorded) or synthesized speech output. Intervention to teach non-speech communication is often indicated in cases of aphasia, autism, brain injury, cerebral palsy, deaf/blindness, intellectual disability, and stroke (Bedrosian, 2003; Beukelman & Mirenda, 2005; Mirenda & Iacono, 2009; Sigafoos et al., 2008).

Non-speech communication modes are typically classified as unaided or aided (Beukelman & Mirenda, 2005; Lloyd, Fuller, & Arvidson, 1997). Unaided AAC modes do not require any external material or equipment. Examples of unaided AAC are informal gestures and manual signs, which might be drawn from formal sign language systems such as American Sign Language. One potential advantage of unaided AAC is that the person does not require access to supplementary materials or equipment in order to communicate. However, a potential disadvantage of unaided AAC is that successful communicative exchanges require communicative partners who can interpret the person's gestures or signs. Rotholz, Berkowitz, and Burberry (1989) demonstrated that the use of manual signs in community settings was largely ineffective because most people in the community did not comprehend manual signs.

Aided AAC approaches require acting upon some materials or equipment, such as pointing to line drawings on a communication board, giving a photograph to a communicative partner, or touching a switch to activate a pre-recorded message. A potential disadvantage of aided AAC is that the person can only communicate when he/she is in possession of the materials or equipment. This potential disadvantage may be offset by the fact that unlike manual sign-based communication, aided AAC is often easier for a wider range of communicative partners to interpret, thus making such systems potentially more functional in inclusive settings (Rotholz et al., 1989).

Among the various aided AAC options, SGDs would appear to have certain additional and unique advantages (Schlosser & Blischak, 2001). Schepis, Reid, and Behrman (1996), for example, delineated several potential advantages of using SGDs over other AAC options in communication intervention programs for individuals with intellectual and developmental disabilities. Specifically, the speech output feature, whether this be digitized or synthesized speech, could be seen as providing a more natural and understandable communicative signal to listeners. In addition, speech output combines an attention-gaining function with the communicative act and this may increase the probability of listeners attending to the person's communicative attempts. This combination of attention-gaining with functional communication may be especially important for individuals with intellectual disabilities who often lack appropriate attention-gaining skills (Sobsey & Reichle, 1989). Furthermore, many of the existing and emerging speech output technologies can be programmed to generate digitized or synthesized speech output that is so precise (e.g., *"I would like a decaffeinated coffee with skim milk please."*) that misunderstandings are reduced. This too may be especially important for individuals with intellectual disabilities who often lack effective strategies to repair communicative breakdowns that arise when listeners do not understand their initial communicative attempts (Brady & Halle, 2002; Brady, McLean, McLean, & Johnston, 1995; Sigafoos et al., 2004).

USE OF SPEECH-GENERATING DEVICES IN AAC INTERVENTIONS FOR ADULTS WITH INTELLECTUAL DISABILITIES

Adults with intellectual disability are the focus of this chapter because they represent a seemingly less studied, but important and challenging clinical group for AAC professionals. Many such adults attended school at a time when AAC was less developed as a field of research and practice and were therefore less likely to have benefited from recent advances in AAC, such as the development of new speech-generating technologies and more effective intervention procedures for teaching AAC. Our clinical experiences suggest that many adults with intellectual disabilities continue to be excluded from effective communication interventions due, in part, to limited knowledge and competence in AAC among direct-care staff.

When AAC intervention is provided, our collective experiences suggest a general reluctance to consider the use of SGDs.

Schlosser and colleagues (Schlosser, 2003; Schlosser & Blischak, 2001) highlighted the potential value of speech output technology in AAC interventions, but also considered some of the possible reasons for the relatively limited use of SGDs in such interventions, especially for persons with intellectual disabilities. First, there may be a tendency to view speech output as less relevant for people with poor language comprehension skills. Second, there may be a perception that individuals with more severe disabilities will express only basic communicative functions (e.g., requesting preferred objects) and thus they will have little need for more sophisticated SGDs. In short, SGDs may be perceived as an over-optioned AAC system. But this perception might in turn create a self-fulfilling prophecy. Third, SGDs are generally more expensive than other AAC systems and the mere provision of a SGD is no guarantee that the person will be capable of learning to use, or interested in using, that device for communicating with others. Thus, there is the potential risk that the money spent on an expensive SGD could be money wasted if the person either cannot learn to use the device or lacks the interest and motivation to use the device. This concern may be more common in services for adults as there could be a perception that adults with intellectual disabilities are, by virtue of age-related cognitive decline and long histories of failure, less responsive to AAC intervention overall and perhaps less capable of learning to use sophisticated communication technologies.

Whether adults with intellectual disabilities are capable of learning and interested in using SGDs are empirical questions. Schlosser, Wendt, and Sigafoos (2007) argued that systematic reviews are one way to provide clinically-meaningful answers to these types of questions. A good systematic review that includes: (a) clear and specific research questions, (b) replicable search and appraisal procedures, and (c) a clear statement of the clinical bottom-line can be extremely useful in guiding clinical practice. What follows is our systematic review of intervention studies that have sought to teach the use of speech-generating technologies to adults with intellectual disability. The aim is to determine if there is in fact any evidence relevant to the questions of whether adults with intellectual disabilities are capable of learning, and interested in using, SGDs for functional communication. The specific objectives of this review are to describe the characteristics of these studies (e.g., participants, target behaviors, and intervention procedures), evaluate intervention outcomes, and appraise the certainty of the evidence for the existing corpus of intervention studies. A review of this type is primarily intended to guide and inform evidence-based practice with respect to the use of SGDs in AAC interventions for adults with intellectual disability. A secondary aim is to identify gaps in the existing database so as to stimulate future research efforts aimed at developing new and more effective applications of emerging speech-generating technologies for this population.

METHOD

Search Strategies

Systematic searches were conducted in five electronic databases: Cumulative Index of Nursing and Allied Health Literatures (CINAHL), Education Resources Information Center (ERIC), Medline, Linguistics and Language Behavior Abstracts (LLBA), and PsycINFO. Publication year was not restricted, but the search was limited to English-language journal articles. On all five databases, the terms Intellectual Disability (or Mental Retardation) and Augmentative Communication (or Speech-Generating Device or SGD or VOCA) were inserted as free-text search terms. Abstracts of the records returned from these electronic searches were reviewed to identify studies for review (see Inclusion and Exclusion Criteria). The reference lists for the included studies were also reviewed to identify additional articles for possible inclusion.

Inclusion and Exclusion Criterion

To be included in this review, the article had to be a research study that examined the effects of an intervention to teach the use of a SGD for expressive communication with at least one adult with intellectual disability. Any study in which at least one of the adult participants was described as having mental retardation or intellectual disability was considered, regardless of whether or not the participants had additional handicapping conditions (e.g., cerebral palsy, vision impairment). SGDs could include any device intended as an expressive communication aid that produced either digitized or synthesized speech output. An adult was defined as anyone aged 18 years or older. Communication intervention was defined as implementing one or more therapeutic/teaching procedures for the purpose of trying to increase or improve the person's communication skills using a SGD. Examples could include: teaching the person to use a SGD to make requests, recruit attention, initiate a conversation, or repair a communicative breakdown.

Studies were excluded from the review if they (a) focused only on children, (b) did not report original new data (e.g., review papers), (c) focused only on the assessment of communication skills, (d) reported only demographic characteristics and not the results of an intervention, or (e) focused only on teaching receptive language, such as pointing to pictures or symbols named by the teacher (cf. Schlosser, Belfiore, Nigam, Blischak, & Hetzroni, 1995).

Data Extraction

Each identified study was first assessed to determine if it met the pre-determined inclusion criteria. Each identified study that met the pre-determined inclusion criteria was then analyzed and summarized in terms of: (a) participants (age and severity of intellectual disability), (b) mode of communication (e.g., type of SGD used), (c) communication skill(s) taught to the participants, (d) intervention procedures, (e) results of the intervention, (f) length of follow-up if any, and (g) certainty of evidence. The certainty of evidence for each study was rated as either conclusive or inconclusive based on the definitions applied by Millar, Light, and Schlosser (2006).

Appraising the certainty of evidence (for included studies only) followed a two-stage process. First, only studies that included a recognized experimental design (e.g., multiple-baseline, ABAB) could be considered as having the potential to provide conclusive evidence. Thus any study that lacked a recognized experimental design was automatically classified as capable of providing only inconclusive evidence. This included narrative case studies, pre-post testing without a control group, and studies using A-B or intervention-only designs. Second, studies that made use of a recognized experimental design also had to meet four additional standards to be classified as providing conclusive evidence. First, the data had to provide a convincing demonstration of an intervention effect. This determination was based on visual inspection of data trends within a phase and across phases using criteria described by Kennedy (2005). For example, there had to be a clinically significant increase in correct requesting when intervention was introduced. Second, if relevant, there had to be adequate inter-observer agreement data (i.e., 20% of the sessions and 80% or better agreement). Third, the dependent and independent variables had to be operationally defined. Fourth, the procedures had to be described in sufficient detail to enable replication.

RESULTS

From the 432 studies returned from the search strategies, 421 studies were excluded, leaving 11 studies for summary and analysis. The main reasons for excluding the majority of studies were (a) that the study did not report new data (e.g., review paper), (b) that the study did not include any adult participants, and (c) that it was unclear whether the study included an evaluation of intervention procedures that explicitly aimed to teach the use of a SGD for expressive communication. Table 1 summarizes the participants, target skills, procedures, and main findings for each of the 11 included studies. The final column in Table 1 explains the basis for the study's rating in terms of certainty of evidence.

Participants

Collectively, the 11 studies provided intervention to a total of 15 identified adult participants. Several studies included both adult and adolescent participants (e.g., Wacker, Wiggins, Fowler, & Berg, 1988). Only those participants clearly identified as being of adult age were included in our analysis. One participant in Mechling and Cronin's (2006) study who was aged 17 years 11 months at the beginning of the study was included in the analysis, however, because that person reached 18 years of age during the course of the study.

Settings

Setting descriptions were provided in 9 of the 11 studies (i.e., all except Studies 9 and 11). These studies represented 13 (86%) of the 15 adults. The interventions described in these nine studies were most often undertaken in residential care facilities, classrooms, and vocational settings.

Types of SGDs

Nine different types of SGDs were coded across the 11 included studies. The earliest device described was a microswitch attached to a tape player (i.e., Wacker et al., 1988). Several devices were common to several studies, e.g., WOLF (Adamlab, 1988) and TouchTalker (Prentke Romich Company, nd). The symbols systems installed on the SGDs varied across studies. Examples included the use of Minspeak symbols with TouchTalker devices, Lexigrams, and the English alphabet.

Target Skills

The communication skills targeted for intervention were coded into six pragmatic functions based on the classification system described by Sigafoos et al. (2006): (a) imitative speech, (b) requesting access to preferred stimuli (e.g., food, drinks, toys, or songs), (c) requesting social interaction, (d) naming objects or commenting, (e) receptive language (e.g., respond to requests, answer questions, receptively identify symbols), and (f) respond–recode (e.g., respond to questions/requests and then request information). Another [General] category was used when the communication function was not clearly specified (e.g., use language, enhance nonverbal expression). *Requesting access to preferred stimuli* and the *general* category were most commonly reported communication skills targeted for intervention (3 studies). Two studies targeted *requesting social interaction* and one study targeted *imitative speech, conversation initiations* and *respond-recode*.

Intervention Procedures

Most of the studies (Studies 2, 4, 5, 6, 7, 8, and 10), which collectively involved the majority of participants (n = 11 adults), employed systematic instructional procedures to teach the use of the SGD (Snell & Brown, 2006). The specific instructional tactics typically included some combination

Table 1. Summary of Intervention Studies[1]

Study	Participants	Device	Target Skill	Procedures	Main Findings	Certainty of Evidence
1. Wacker et al. (1988).	Two males and 4 females with profound intellectual disabilities (age range of 13 to 20 years)	Microswitches connected to tape recorders.	Activation of a microswitch to produce tape recorded request to either drink or play.	Phase 1 involved 3 participants. Baseline activities involved the use of a blank tape inserted into player. Participants were asked to "Press this switch" followed by a demonstration of how to press the switch. If participants did not activate the switch, physical prompts were provided. The alternating treatment design involved 4 baseline sessions followed by 8 treatment sessions. During treatment, spontaneous requests for a drink or play were reinforced with provision of a drink or interactive table-top play with the experimenter. Phase 2 involved 6 participants in a simultaneous treatments design. During visits to shopping malls, participants' requests for a specific drink were reinforced by purchasing a drink from a fast food restaurant. Requests for window-shopping were reinforced by the researcher accompanying the participant to view shops.	Phase 1 findings indicated that all participants increased the spontaneity of switch activation. Two participants demonstrated preference for play over a drink. During Phase 2, each participant demonstrated increased requests for either a drink or window shopping. Five of the six participants preferred a drink over window-shopping. Participants requesting a drink also pressed the switch to play "I want a ___ drink" for the cashier at the restaurant. Five of the six participants demonstrated decreases in time taken to order drinks using the microswitches across treatment trials.	Inconclusive. Although comparison of baseline and treatment performance indicated positive treatment effect in Phase 1, no baseline data were provided for Phase 2. Specific ages of each participant were not reported thus making it difficult to determine if individual participants were adults or adolescents.
2. Dattilo & Camarata (1991)	A 36-year-old male (C) with profound intellectual disability and cerebral palsy. A second participant was not considered in this review because his IQ was reported as above average.	Touch Talker with Minspeak software.	Direct selection of Touch Talker symbols to initiate communication by requesting a recreational option (e.g., ball play, music, painting, cards) or snacks.	The baseline phase consisted of training in the operation of the Touch Talker. Five messages were also loaded onto C's device during the first baseline phase. A second baseline phase involved establishment of reliable Touch Talker use (5 times per session). The conversation treatment phase involved the researcher instructing C that he had control of sessions and that his requests would be fulfilled. Prompts included "What do you want?" and "Tell me what you want". Prompts were discontinued after 2 sessions. Participant initiated conversation training continued until C's initiations were 50% for 2 consecutive sessions.	During the first baseline phase, C's mean conversation initiation was 55.4 (SD=15.2) per session. This increased to 110.2 (SD=43.4) during the second baseline phase. C then produced an average of 148.6 (SD=9.3) initiations during conversation initiation training. Probe measures taken at C's residential setting indicated generalization of his increased initiation of conversation.	Inconclusive. The findings provide evidence that the use of an SGD can facilitate increased conversational initiation for an adult with intellectual disability. A multiple baseline design was used with clear definition of the independent and dependent variables. Inter-rater reliability statistics reported a range of 84.5% to 100%, however, authors reported reliability checks made on 12 occasions during the study. It is not clear that 20% of session data were analysed.
3. Adamson, Romski, Deffebach & Sevcik (1992).	Twelve young male adults including two 20 year-olds with severe intellectual disability.	A notebook computer with Voltrax Personal Speech Systems voice synthesizer.	Direct selection of referential and social-regulative lexigrams on the SGD during interaction with communication partners.	A lexigram-embossed computer keyboard with synthesized speech output was introduced to participants. Use of the SGD was encouraged during opportunities for communication. Communication partners were also asked to use the SGD during interaction with participants. A total of 37 observation probes were conducted over 2 years. Conversational transcripts were analysed to determine the device and symbol use for all participants.	The addition of social-regulative lexigrams to the devices did not increase the use of the SGD. The addition of social-regulative lexigrams resulted in greater balance between the use of social-regulative and referential lexigram use.	Inconclusive. A pre-post study design was employed and no individual results were reported. It was therefore impossible to identify the performance of the 2 adults in the group.

Table 1. continued

Study	Participants	Device	Target Skill	Procedures	Main Findings	Certainty of Evidence
4. O'Keefe & Dattilo (1992).	Two females and 1 male, aged from 24-60 years with mild to moderate intellectual disability.	One participant (L) used a Touch Talker with Minspeak software (24 year old female with moderate intelelctual disability). Two participants used communication boards without speech output.	Direct selection of symbols to demonstrate Response-Recode (R-R) linguistic form (i.e., responds to question or request for information (I-O) and then take control of conversation by asking a return question) during interaction with communication partner.	Weekly baseline sessions involved conversation with communication partners around topics such as sports or TV shows. Communication partners provided I-Os or R-Rs (only if participants provided R-R). Weekly training sessions involved communication partners providing explicit instructions (e.g., "After you answer me, I want you to ask me something…" (p. 228).	L did not provide any R-R forms during 6 baseline sessions. During the 10-week intervention, L reached a mean of 9 R-R forms per session. During two post-intervention probes, L produced 15 and 10 R-R forms.	Inconclusive. Although the experimental design and visual inspection of the data are positive indicators for an intervention effect, the findings are considered inconclusive because no reliability data were reported for the baseline or intervention sessions.
5. McGregor et al. (1992).	A 20-year-old male (W) with cerebral palsy and moderate intellectual disability.	Touch Talker with Minspeak software.	Direct selection of Touch Talker symbols (choice of 5) to initiate appropriate task-related communication.	Baseline measurements were taken on W's use of the Touch Talker for communicative purposes. Each instance of communicative use of the Touch Talker was socially reinforced by the teacher. Immediately prior to intervention sessions, W was provided with two "preinstruction" activities. Five buttons with task-specific messages were reviewed with the teacher labeling each message button. W was then asked questions about each button's corresponding message (e.g., "What do you do when you want help?" p. 246). Preinstruction activities were withdrawn once W's independent use of the five message buttons had stablised above 85% for 3 consecutive days. The treatment session involved the teacher creating distance between herself and W to ensure a need for W to use the TouchTalker in order to communicate. Corrective feedback was provided, such as "Use your Touch Talker to tell me what you want" (p.246). Social reinforcement and feedback was provided when W used the Touch Talker to communicate.	Baseline measures revealed low rates of communication initiation using the SGD. Although on 2 of 14 baseline days within a speech clinic room W initiated appropriately on 80% of trials. On the other days his performance was consistently around 0%. W's communication initiation increased to 70% or greater for 2 of the 3 settings (Speech clinic and vocational training room) immediately after introduction of SGD training. W's classroom-based use of the SGD also increased immediately upon introduction of training. However greater variability was observed in this setting. Appropriate communication initiation stablized across all settings after 11 days.	Conclusive. Results from this multiple baseline across settings design study demonstrated a clear intervention effect. Interobserver reliability agreement averaged 98% over 20% of sessions. The study is replicable based in the level of information reported. This study provided conclusive evidence for the use of an SGD with a young adult with mild-to-moderate intellectual disabilities.
6. Soto et al. (1993).	A 22-year-old male with severe/profound intellectual disability and seizure disorder.	WOLF SGD (Adamlab, 1988).	Point to line drawing symbols to request preferred snacks and leisure materials.	During baseline in the leisure activity, S was asked "What do you need/want to draw?" During the snack trials, S was asked "What do you want for a snack?" Correct requests were reinforced by giving him the requested items, but S was not prompted to make a request. Intervention involved an alternating treatments design to compare acquisition of requesting with the picture book versus the electronic device. In addition, a multiple-baseline across settings design was used. During intervention, trials were initiated as in baseline, but S was given praise and the object contingent upon a correct request. In addition, after an incorrect response, the trainer provided verbal feedback ("No, you have to say: I want paper.") and also physically prompted S to point to the correct symbol. After this error correction procedure, S received the requested item. After intervention, a preference assessment was conducted to determine which of the two communication systems would be selected when S was allowed to choose. Maintenance probes were conducted at 1, 2, and 4 week intervals. Generalization probes were also administered in a fast food restaurant.	Correct requests during baseline averaged less than 2%. Rapid acquisition of the requests was obtained with both devices and in both settings within 5 sessions. During the preference assessment, S chose the electronic device 100% of the time. Correct requests decreased somewhat during maintenance. S successfully used the electronic device to order in the restaurant.	Conclusive. The multiple baseline and alternating treatments design provided clear evidence of an intervention effect. Adequate reliability checks were made and achieved a high level of agreement. The study was also described in sufficient detail to enable replication.

Table 1. continued

Study	Participants	Device	Target Skill	Procedures	Main Findings	Certainty of Evidence
7. Spiegel, Benjamin, & Spiegel (1993).	A 19-year-old male (B) with mild to moderate intellectual disability and severe physical impairment.	Touch Talker with Min-speak soft-ware.	Pressing appropriate icon buttons to produce syntactically correct sentences.	Ten grammatically correct sentences with high level of function-ality were selected for training (e.g., "I went to the bank."). Each of the eight training sessions involved two separate phases. The objective of Phase 1 was to teach B to select target sentences on his Touch Talker. The clinician instructed B to "Tell me (target sentence." A model was provided if B provided an incorrect or no response. Phase 2 aimed to teach B to select sentences in response to conversational cues. The clinician introduced topics using modified role play to describe situations in which B could use target sentences. The clinician also used pause and expectant looking to cue B to use target sentences.	Two baseline sessions revealed that B was unable to access the training sentences on his Touch Talker. B's ability to reliably produce syntactically correct sentences increased from 0-10% accuracy during the baseline phase and treatment sessions 1 and 2, to 100% in both Phase 1 and 2. This accuracy was main-tained for two further sessions.	Inconclusive. The results reported indicate an interven-tion effect for B's use of an SGD. These findings however are not conclusive due to the absence of reliability data.
8. Schepis & Reid (1995).	A 23-year-old female (M) with profound intellectual disability and cerebral palsy.	Mega Wolf SGD (Ad-amlab, n.d.).	Pressing appropriate buttons with correspond-ing photograph of desired items.	Baseline observations of M's communication interaction with teacher aides and care facility workers were conducted at 3 time points each day. A 7 p.m. time point was maintained as a control. No SGD was present during baseline observations. Before the SGD was introduced, teacher aides and care staff were provided 15 to 30 min operational training on the Mega Wolf device. Participants were also asked to ensure M had access to her device between 10 a.m. and 4 p.m. No instructions were provided to support communication interaction between staff and M. The SGD was provided to M between 10 a.m. and 4 p.m.	Baseline observations revealed that at Time Point 1 (classroom), communicative interactions were observed between M and communication partners during an average of 21% of observa-tion intervals. At Time Point 2. (residence) interactions averaged 31%. On introduction of the SGD to both settings, interac-tions increased to 63% (class-room) and 86% (residence).	Conclusive. This study pro-vides conclusive evidence that the use of SGD by an adult with profound intellectual disability can increase staff interactions with person with a SGD. An intervention effect was clearly visible and inter-observer reliability figures averaged 88% for interactions and 83% for initiations.
9. Blischak & Lloyd (1996).	A 35-year-old female (K) with physical, visual and intellectual disability.	AllTalk Speech Gener-ating Device (Adap-tive Commu-nication Systems, n.d.)	General functional use of a SGD in a variety of settings and with a variety of communica-tion partners.	Vocabulary was selected for inclusion on four overlays that were fitted to the AllTalk. Each overlay covered one of K's four environments (i.e., care facility, home, community and employment setting) and contained up to 256 selection items. A total of 710 selection items were therefore available on the four overlays. There was considerable repetition of selection items across overlays with 262 vocabulary items present on more than one overlay. K was observed for her spontaneous use of the SGD. The use of the SGD was encouraged as the most functional mode of communication. A variety of intervention approaches were used including modeling, role playing, and line drawing-based scripting. A series of conversation samples were also taken dur-ing the study.	At the conclusion of therapy K was able to self-select overlays and vocabulary. Conversational sampling revealed K used her SGD during an average of 21% of conversations (range = 0% to 80%). Unaided communication occurred during an average of 64% of sampled conversations.	Inconclusive. The evidence provided by this report for SGD use by adults with intel-lectual disability is inconclu-sive. The narrative case study design is pre-experimental and therefore does not provide for certainty of evidence.
10. Mechling & Cronin (2006).	One female with Down syndrome aged 17 years, 11 months at the beginning of study. This participant had moderate intel-lectual impairment Two males with Down syndrome aged 20 and 21 years. One male had severe and the other had moderate intellectual disability.	7-Level Commu-nicator (En-abling Devices, n.d.).	Use of the SGD to place orders at fast food restaurants. Participants were required to point to color photographs on the –Level Communica-tor to request preferred fast food restaurant meal options.	Single subject, multiple-probe design, involving baseline, inter-vention, generalization, and maintenance phases. Participants were exposed to computer-based video instruction (CBVI) sessions to simulate interaction with a cashier at a fast food restaurant. Participants were provided with an SGD to make their requests and respond to questions.	Each participant achieved 100% correct unprompted responses across nine consecu-tive intervention trials before generalization and maintenance probes were administered at fast food restaurants. Participants maintenance of SGD use ranged from 50% to 100% up to 104 days following CBVI	Conclusive. The certainty of evidence provided by this study is conclusive. The multiple baseline design provided clear evidence of an intervention effect. Mean interobserver agreement was 96% across all participants and conditions.

Table 1. continued

Study	Participants	Device	Target Skill	Procedures	Main Findings	Certainty of Evidence
11. Cheslock et al. (2008).	A 30-year-old female (J) with moderate intellectual disability and some intelligible speech.	Dy-navox MT4 (Dy-navox Tech-nologies, n.d.).	The primary focus was on providing instruction to the communication partner with a view to increasing J's use of the SGD.	Two instructional sessions were provided for J's primary com-munication partner, These sessions included: (a) augmented input training; (b) increasing communication opportunities for J; and (c) SGD customization. J's communication partner was asked to maintain a journal to record J's use of the SGD in different envi-ronments and with other communication partners. Pre and post measures of expressive vocabulary and MLU were taken.	There was no increase in expres-sive vocabulary post-SGD. MLU decreased from 1.65 (pre-SGD) to 1.24 (Post-SGD) and then increased to 2.35 (2-years post SGD). Mean lengh of turn in utterances also decreased from pre-SGD level (1.73) to 1-year post-SGD (1.05) then increased to 3.06 2-years post. Overall conversational intel-ligibility rated as 85% pre-SGD then 100% 1 year post-SGD and 94% 2-years post-SGD. Increased responsiveness to questions was also observed (39% pre-SGD to 66% 2-years post SGD).	Inconclusive. The evidence provided by this study is inconclusive. The pre-post/ case study design is pre-experimental and therefore does not provide for certainty of evidence.

[1] Studies are listed in alpha-chronological order by year of publication and then by the first author's surname

of the following operant/behavioral procedures: (a) presenting an opportunity or discriminative stimulus, (b) prompting communicative behavior, and (c) providing reinforcement for appropriate communication.

Study Designs

Study designs were classified as experimental, pre-experimental, or unclear. The experimental designs employed in this set of studies were the multiple-baseline across subjects and settings and the alternating treatments design (Kennedy, 2005). Pre-experimental designs included narrative case study and pre-post designs with no control group.

Follow-Up

Eight studies (Studies 4 to 11) reported on participants' use of the acquired communication skills following intervention. The length of follow-up ranged from 1 week to 2 years. No follow-up information was provided for Studies 1, 2, and 3.

Reliability of Data

Most studies (Studies 1, 2, 3, 5, 6, 8, 10) reported on the reliability of data collection with respect to the dependent variables, such as by collecting inter-observer agreement. Average rates of agreement were reported as high across these studies (greater than 80%).

Outcomes

Outcomes were classified as either showing progress or no progress based on the data presented by the authors. Participant progress in their use of SGDs was demonstrated in each of the 11 studies reported. Although it was impossible to determine if the adults in Wacker et al. (1988) progressed as performance was reported at the group level and the group included adolescent as well as adult participants.

Certainty of Evidence

The certainty of evidence for an intervention effect was rated as conclusive in 4 (36%) of the 11 studies (Studies 5, 6, 8, and 10). For the remaining seven studies, the certainty of evidence for an intervention effect was judged to be inconclusive. These inconclusive ratings stemmed from reliance on pre-experimental designs [Studies 3, 9, and 11] or lack of objective description of methods and failure to present sufficient reliability data [Studies 1, 2, 4, and 7].

DISCUSSION

Our systematic search yielded 11 studies on teaching the use of SGDs to adults with intellectual disabilities. These 11 studies were published between the years 1988 and 2008. Our analysis of these studies suggests that while there is some evidence to support the use of SGD in AAC interventions for adults with intellectual disabilities, the overall evidence base is perhaps best described as promising, but limited. The limitations are evident in terms of the scope and quality of the existing corpus of studies.

In terms of scope, the current database must be considered limited because of the sheer paucity of studies (n = 11) and the relatively small number of adult participants (n = 15). These 15 adults participants were also drawn from fairly narrow age range. Indeed, most of the participants would be described as young adults mainly aged 20-23 years. Only one study (Study 4) included an older adult (60 years of age). Clearly there is a need for research involving larger samples of older adults (i.e., 40+ years of age). This would seem an important gap to fill because AAC intervention for older individuals with intellectual disabilities is likely to be complicated by decreased sensory, memory, and cognitive capabilities associated with aging (Ashman & Suttie, 1996; Balandin & Morgan, 2001).

One might expect the efficacy of AAC interventions involving SGDs to vary depending on the severity and etiology of intellectual disabilities. While plausible, no such interactions were evident from our analysis of these studies with respect to participant progress. This pool of 11 studies included participants with mild to profound intellectual disability and yet progress in the use of SGDs was reported in each of the 11 studies. These positive outcomes suggest that SGDs represent a viable mode of communication for individuals at all levels of intellectual functioning. This conclusion needs to be interpreted with caution, however, given the relatively few participants overall, and the lack of studies specifically designed to compare individuals with differing etiologies and severities of intellectual disabilities. Future research should investigate such issues because it would seem plausible that there might be some important severity/etiology-by-treatment interactions. Recognition of any such interactions would perhaps enable clinicians to decide if, when, and how best to make use of SGDs with adults with varying etiologies and severity of intellectual disability.

In terms of methodological quality, perhaps the most important limitation is that nearly half of the studies appeared to lack a recognized experimental design. This general lack of experimental design, combined with the other methodological limitations that we noted (e.g., lack of procedural detail, limited follow-up, lack of reliability data), meant that the certainty of evidence was inconclusive for seven or 64% of the studies. Thus the reports of positive outcomes in the seven studies that did not include adequate controls must be interpreted with caution.

In terms of the main aim of this paper, the result of this review included a number of sound demonstrations that adults with intellectual disabilities can learn to use SGDs for functional communication. There is thus evidence, albeit limited, to support the use of SGDs in AAC interventions for this population. The evidence further supports an intervention approach that begins by teaching a simple requesting response as recommended by Reichle, York, and Sigafoos (1991). Given that many adults with intellectual disabilities, especially adults with severe to profound intellectual disabilities, are also likely to have additional physical and/or sensory impairments (Sigafoos et al., 2007), it would seem critical to ensure that these skills needed to operate the SGD are within the adult's physical capabilities. For individuals with the extremely limited motor abilities, this will most likely require the clinician to identify some very simple motor act, such as touching a switch. While these recommendations cannot be considered fully empirically validated for this population at the present time, there would seem to be little risk of harm from trying such an approach.

In terms of the second aim of this chapter, which was to identify gaps in the literature, our review has identified several pertinent gaps in terms of the range of procedures evaluated and the range of communication modes and functions targeted for intervention. More specifically, the studies conducted so far have investigated a rather restricted range of procedures and targeted only a few communication modes/functions. Furthermore, none of the studies appeared to have included pre-treatment assessments to inform the intervention. Bridging this latter gap could be critical to developing more effective interventions. A pre-treatment assessment of motor skills may enable clinicians to identify motor acts that the person could use to operate a SGD via assistive technology (Lancioni et al., 2006). While research along these lines might someday yield new and more effective approaches, we conclude that while the use of SGD in AAC interventions for adults with intellectual disabilities is promising, the evidence base supporting this conclusion is limited.

REFERENCES

Abbeduto, L., Evans, J., & Dolan, T. (2001). Theoretical perspectives on language and communication problems in mental retardation and developmental disabilities. *Mental Retardation and Developmental Disabilities Research Reviews*, *7*, 45–55. doi:10.1002/1098-2779(200102)7:1<45::AID-MRDD1007>3.0.CO;2-H

Adamlab. (1988). *WOLF manual*. Wayne, MI.

Adamson, L. B., Romski, M. A., Deffebach, K., & Sevcik, R. A. (1992). Symbol vocabulary and the focus of conversations: Augmenting language development for youth with mental retardation. *Journal of Speech and Hearing Research*, *35*, 1333–1343.

Adaptive Communication Systems (n.d.). *AllTalk*. Clinton, PA: AllTalk.

American Psychiatric Association. (2000). *Diagnostic and statistical manual of mental disorders* (4th ed., Text revision). Washington, DC.

Ashman, A. F., & Suttie, J. (1996). The medical and health status of older people with mental retardation in Australia. *Journal of Applied Gerontology*, *15*, 57–72. doi:10.1177/073346489601500104

Balandin, S., & Morgan, J. (2001). Preparing for the future: Aging and alternative and augmentative communication. *Augmentative and Alternative Communication*, *17*, 99–108.

Bedrosian, J. L. (2003). On the subject of subject selection in AAC: Implications for planning and interpreting efficacy research. In R. W. Schlosser (Ed.), *The efficacy of augmentative and alternative communication: Toward evidence-based practice* (pp. 57-83). Boston: Academic Press.

Beukelman, D. R., & Mirenda, P. (Eds.). (2005). *Augmentative and alternative communication: Supporting children and adults with complex communication needs*. Baltimore: Paul H. Brookes Publishing Co.

Blischak, D. M., & Lloyd, L. L. (1996). Multimodal augmentative and alternative communication: Case study. *Augmentative and Alternative Communication, 12*, 37–46. doi:10.1080/07434619612331277468

Brady, N. C., & Halle, J. W. (2002). Breakdowns and repairs in conversations between beginning AAC users and their partners. In J. Reichle, D. R. Beukelman, & J. C. Light (Eds.), *Exemplary practices for beginning communicators: Implications for AAC* (pp. 323-351). Baltimore: Paul H. Brookes Publishing Co.

Brady, N. C., McLean, J. E., McLean, L. K., & Johnston, S. (1995). Initiation and repair of intentional communicative acts by adults with severe to profound cognitive disabilities. *Journal of Speech and Hearing Research, 38*, 1334–1348.

Carr, A., & O'Reilly, G. (2007). Diagnosis, classification and epidemiology. In A. Carr, G. O'Reilly, P. Noonan Walsh, & J. McEvoy (Eds.), *The handbook of intellectual disability and clinical psychology practice* (pp. 3-49). London: Routledge.

Carter, M., & Iacono, T. (2002). Professional judgments of the intentionality of communicative acts. *Augmentative and Alternative Communication, 18*, 177–191. doi:10.1080/07434610212331281261

Cheslock, M. A., Barton-Hulsey, A., Romski, M. A., & Sevcik, R. A. (2008). Using a speech-generating device to enhance communicative abilities for an adult with moderate intellectual disability. *Intellectual and Developmental Disabilities, 46*, 376–386. doi:10.1352/2008.46:376-386

Dattilo, J., & Camarata, S. (1991). Facilitating conversation through self-initiated augmentative communication treatment. *Journal of Applied Behavior Analysis, 24*, 369–378. doi:10.1901/jaba.1991.24-369

Duker, P. C., van Driel, S., & van de Bracken, J. (2002). Communication profiles of individuals with Down's syndrome, Angelman syndrome, and pervasive developmental disorders. *Journal of Intellectual Disability Research, 46*, 35–40. doi:10.1046/j.1365-2788.2002.00355.x

Dynavox Technologies (n.d.). *Dynavox MT4*. Pittsburgh, PA.

Enabling Devices (n.d.). *7-Level Communicator*. Hastings on Hudson, NY.

Kennedy, C. H. (2005). *Single-case designs for educational research*. Boston: Allyn and Bacon.

Lancioni, G. E., Singh, N. N., O'Reilly, M. F., Sigafoos, J., Oliva, D., & Baccani, S. (2006). Teaching 'Yes' and 'No' responses to children with multiple disabilities through a program including microswitches linked to a vocal output device. *Perceptual and Motor Skills, 102*, 51–61. doi:10.2466/PMS.102.1.51-61

Lloyd, L. L., Fuller, D. R., & Arvidson, H. (1997). *Augmentative and alternative communication: A handbook of principles and practices*. Needham Heights, MA: Allyn & Bacon.

Matson, J. L. (Ed.). (2007). *Handbook of assessment in persons with intellectual disability*. San Diego: Academic Press.

McGregor, G., Young, J., Gerak, J., Thomas, B., & Vogelsberg, R. T. (1992). Increasing functional use of an assistive communication device by a student with severe disabilities. *Augmentative and Alternative Communication, 8*, 243–250. doi:10.1080/07434619212331276233

Mechling, L. C., & Cronin, B. (2006). Computer-based video instruction to teach the use of augmentative and alternative communication devices for ordering at fast-food restaurants. *The Journal of Special Education, 39*, 234–245. doi:10.1177/00224669060390040401

Millar, D. C., Light, J. C., & Schlosser, R. W. (2006). The impact of augmentative and alternative communication intervention on the speech production of individuals with developmental disabilities: A research review. *Journal of Speech, Language, and Hearing Research: JSLHR*, *49*, 248–264.

Mirenda, P., & Brown, K. E. (2009). A picture is worth a thousand words: Using visual supports for augmented input with individuals with autism spectrum disorders. In P. Miranda & T. Iacono (Eds.), *Autism spectrum disorders and AAC* (pp. 303-332). Baltimore: Paul H. Brookes Publishing Co.

Mirenda, P., & Iacono, T. (Eds.) (2009). *Autism spectrum disorders and AAC*. Baltimore: Paul H. Brookes Publishing Co.

O'Keefe, B, M., & Dattilo, J. (1992). Teaching the response-recode form to adults with mental retardation using AAC systems. *Augmentative and Alternative Communication*, *8*, 224–233. do i:10.1080/07434619212331276213

Prentke Romich Company (n.d.). *TouchTalker.* Wooster, OH.

Reichle, J., York, J., & Sigafoos, J. (1991). *Implementing augmentative and alternative communication: Strategies for learners with severe disabilities*. Baltimore: Paul H. Brookes Publishing Co.

Rotholz, D., Berkowitz, S., & Burberry, J. (1989). Functionality of two modes of communication in the community by students with developmental disabilities: A comparison of signing and communication books. *The Journal of the Association for Persons with Severe Handicaps*, *14*, 227–233.

Schepis, M. M., & Reid, D. H. (1995). Effects of a voice output communication aid on interactions between support personnel and an individual with multiple disabilities. *Journal of Applied Behavior Analysis*, *28*, 73–77. doi:10.1901/jaba.1995.28-73

Schepis, M. M., Reid, D. H., & Behrman, M. M. (1996). Acquisition and functional use of voice output communication by persons with profound multiple disabilities. *Behavior Modification*, *20*, 451–468. doi:10.1177/01454455960204005

Schlosser, R. W. (2003). Roles of speech output in augmentative and alternative communication: Narrative review. *Augmentative and Alternative Communication*, *19*, 5–28. doi:10.1080/0743461032000056450

Schlosser, R. W., Belfiore, P. J., Nigam, R., Blischak, D., & Hetzroni, O. (1995). The effects of speech output technology in the learning of graphic symbols. *Journal of Applied Behavior Analysis*, *28*, 537–549. doi:10.1901/jaba.1995.28-537

Schlosser, R. W., & Blischak, D. M. (2001). Is there a role for speech output in interventions for persons with autism? A review. *Focus on Autism and Other Developmental Disabilities*, *16*, 170–178. doi:10.1177/108835760101600305

Schlosser, R. W., Wendt, O., & Sigafoos, J. (2007). Not all systematic reviews are created equal: Considerations for appraisal. *Evidence-based Communication Assessment and Intervention*, *1*, 138–150. doi:10.1080/17489530701560831

Sigafoos, J., Arthur-Kelly, M., & Butterfield, N. (2006). *Enhancing everyday communication for children with disabilities*. Baltimore: Paul H. Brookes Publishing Co.

Sigafoos, J., Didden, R., Schlosser, R. W., Green, V., O'Reilly, M., & Lancioni, G. (2008). A review of intervention studies on teaching AAC to individuals who are deaf and blind. *Journal of Developmental and Physical Disabilities*, *20*, 71–99. doi:10.1007/s10882-007-9081-5

Sigafoos, J., Drasgow, E., Halle, J. W., O'Reilly, M., Seely-York, S., Edrisinha, C., & Andrews, A. (2004). Teaching VOCA use as a communicative repair strategy. *Journal of Autism and Developmental Disorders*, *34*, 411–422. doi:10.1023/B:JADD.0000037417.04356.9c

Sigafoos, J., O'Reilly, M., & Green, V. A. (2007). Communication difficulties and the promotion of communication skills. In A. Carr, G. O'Reilly, P. Noonan Walsh, & J. McEvoy (Eds.), *The handbook of intellectual disability and clinical psychology practice* (pp. 606-642). London: Routledge.

Sigafoos, J., Woodyatt, G., Keen, D., Tait, K., Tucker, M., Roberts-Pennell, D., & Pittendreigh, N. (2000). Identifying potential communicative acts in children with developmental and physical disabilities. *Communication Disorders Quarterly*, *21*, 77–86. doi:10.1177/152574010002100202

Snell, M. E., & Brown, F. (Eds.). (2006). *Instruction of students with severe disabilities* (6th ed.). Upper Saddle River, NJ: Pearson.

Sobsey, D., & Reichle, J. (1989). Components of reinforcement for attention signal switch activation. *Mental Retardation & Learning Disability Bulletin*, *17*, 46–59.

Soto, G., Belfiore, P. J., Schlosser, R. W., & Haynes, C. (1993). Teaching specific requests: A comparative analysis on skill acquisition and preference using two augmentative and alternative communication aids. *Education and Training in Mental Retardation*, *28*, 169–178.

Spiegel, B. B., Benjamin, B. J., & Spiegel, S. A. (1993). One method to increase spontaneous use of an assistive communication device: Case study. *Augmentative and Alternative Communication*, *9*, 111–117. doi:10.1080/07434619312331276491

Wacker, D. P., Wiggins, B., Fowler, M., & Berg, W. K. (1988). Training students with profound or multiple handicaps to make requests via microswitches. *Journal of Applied Behavior Analysis*, *21*, 331–343. doi:10.1901/jaba.1988.21-331

Chapter 11
Synthetic Speech Perception in Individuals with Intellectual and Communicative Disabilities

Rajinder Koul
Texas Tech University, USA

James Dembowski
Texas Tech University, USA

ABSTRACT

The purpose of this chapter is to review research conducted over the past two decades on the perception of synthetic speech by individuals with intellectual, language, and hearing impairments. Many individuals with little or no functional speech as a result of intellectual, language, physical, or multiple disabilities rely on non-speech communication systems to augment or replace natural speech. These systems include Speech Generating Devices (SGDs) that produce synthetic speech upon activation. Based on this review, the two main conclusions are evident. The first is that persons with intellectual and/or language impairment demonstrate greater difficulties in processing synthetic speech than their typical matched peers. The second conclusion is that repeated exposure to synthetic speech allows individuals with intellectual and/or language disabilities to identify synthetic speech with increased accuracy and speed. This finding is of clinical significance as it indicates that individuals who use SGDs become more proficient at understanding synthetic speech over a period of time.

INTRODUCTION

One of the most significant advances in enhancing the communicative abilities of individuals with severe communication impairment has been the development of Speech Generating Devices (SGDs). The use of SGDs for interpersonal communication by individuals with severe communication impairment has increased substantially over the past two decades (Koul, 2003). This increase in the use of SGDs is primarily a result of technological advances in the area of synthetic speech. Most high-end SGDs use text-to-speech synthesis in which graphic symbols, alphabets, words, and digits are entered from an input device, such as touch screen/keyboard/switch/infrared eye tracking technique, and are converted into a speech waveform using a set of mathematical rules. This chapter has three general

DOI: 10.4018/978-1-61520-725-1.ch011

aims. The first aim is to review the literature on the perception of synthetic speech by individuals with language, intellectual, and hearing impairments. The second aim is to use that review to understand the effects of degraded acoustic input on the synthetic speech perception by individuals with developmental communicative and intellectual impairments. The final aim is to present the research on effects of synthetic speech output on acquisition of graphic symbols by individuals with developmental disabilities.

PERCEPTION OF SYNTHETIC SPEECH BY PERSONS WITH INTELLECTUAL DISABILITIES

Data from the United States, Department of Education (2002) indicate that 18.7% of the children ages 6 through 21 who receive services under the Individuals with Disabilities Education Act have a diagnosed speech and/or language impairment and 9.9% have a diagnosed intellectual impairment. Further, about 3.5% and 1.0% of individuals with intellectual impairment fall in the categories of severe and profound impairment respectively (Rosenberg & Abbeduto, 1993). Many individuals with severe-to-profound intellectual disabilities and severe communication impairments are potential candidates for SGDs. Thus, it is critical to investigate the factors that influence synthetic speech perception in individuals with intellectual impairment. Unlike non-electronic communication books and boards, SGDs provide speech output (synthetic or digitized) to the individual user and the communication partner (Church & Glennen, 1992). A retrospective study conducted by Mirenda, Wilk, & Carson, (2000) on the use of assistive technology by individuals with autism and intellectual impairment indicated that 63.6% of the students with severe intellectual impairment used SGDs to augment their communication.

Although substantial research exists on the perception of synthetic speech systems by typical individuals (e.g., Duffy & Pisoni, 1992; Higginbotham & Baird, 1995; Koul & Allen, 1993; Logan, Greene, & Pisoni, 1989; Mirenda & Beukelman, 1987, 1990), limited data are available about the intelligibility and comprehension of synthetic speech by individuals with intellectual disabilities (Koul & Hester, 2006; Koul & Clapsaddle, 2006; Koul & Hanners, 1997; Willis, Koul, & Paschall, 2000). Further, there are differences in aspects of natural language comprehension and information-processing between individuals with intellectual disabilities and mental-age matched typical peers (e.g., Abbeduto, Furman, & Davies, 1989; Abbdeduto & Nuccio, 1991; Berry, 1972; Kail, 1992; Merrill & Jackson, 1992; Rosenberg, 1982; Taylor, Sternberg, & Richards, 1995). Individuals with intellectual disabilities have receptive language delays that exceed their cognitive delays (Abbeduto et al., 1989) and they demonstrate difficulty understanding linguistic information that requires extensive analysis of the acoustic-phonetic aspects of the speaker's words (Abbeduto & Rosenberg, 1992). These differences in language and cognitive domains between typical individuals and individuals with intellectual impairments make it difficult to generalize findings obtained from research in synthetic speech perception with typical individuals to individuals with disabilities. The following sections will focus on perception of synthetic speech by individuals with intellectual disabilities across word, sentence, and discourse tasks.

Single Words

Koul and Hester (2006) examined the perception of synthetic speech by individuals with severe intellectual impairment and severe speech and language impairment using a single-word closed-format task. They reported that individuals with severe intellectual and language impairment (Mean percent correct word identification score =80.95) exhibited significantly greater difficulties than mental age matched typical individuals

(Mean percent correct word identification score =91.19). In contrast, no significant differences were observed between individuals with mild-to-moderate intellectual disabilities and typical individuals on a single word identification task (Koul & Clapsaddle, 2006; Koul & Hanners, 1997). Using an ETI Eloquence synthesizer, Koul & Clapsaddle (2006) reported a mean word identification score of 92% for participants with intellectual disabilities and a mean score of 96% for typical participants. Similar results were obtained by Koul and Hanners (1997). They reported a mean percent single-word accuracy score of 99% and 99% for DECtalk™ male and female voices respectively for typical individuals. Participants with intellectual disabilities in this study obtained a mean percent single-word accuracy score of 98% for each of the DECtalk™ male and female voices.

These results show that perception of single words presented using synthetic speech in a closed-set task by persons with mild-to-moderate intellectual impairment is similar to that of mental-age matched typical peers. However, persons with severe intellectual impairment exhibit greater difficulty in understanding single words presented in synthetic speech in comparison to matched typical individuals.

Sentences

Two studies that have investigated perception of sentences presented in synthetic speech indicate that individuals with mild-to-moderate intellectual disabilities obtain significantly lower accuracy scores than typical individuals on sentence verification and identification tasks (Koul & Hanners, 1997; Koul & Clapsaddle, 2006). Koul and Hanners used a sentence verification task to study perception of synthetic sentences. In this task, participants first had to comprehend a sentence, then make a judgment based on world knowledge as to whether sentence was true (e.g., rain is wet) or false (e.g., bears build houses). Results indicated that sentence verification scores for individuals with intellectual disabilities were significantly lower than those for typical individuals for DECtalk™ male and female voices. Participants with intellectual disabilities obtained mean sentence verification scores of 90% and 85% for DECtalk™ male and female voices respectively. In contrast, typical participants obtained sentence verification scores of 99% and 97% respectively. These results were supported by Koul & Clapsaddle who used a sentence identification task. For this task, the participant heard a series of sentences preceded by a carrier phrase and then pointed to a drawing depicting the sentence. Participants with intellectual disabilities obtained a mean sentence identification score of 80.35 across three trials. Their performance was substantially lower than the performance of typical individuals who obtained a mean score of 89% across three trials. In summary, the current data on perception of three-to-four word sentences presented in synthetic speech indicate that persons with mild-to-moderate intellectual disabilities exhibit greater difficulties in perception of even high-quality synthetic speech (e.g., DECtalk™, ETI Eloquence synthesizer) than matched typical individuals. However, it is important for clinicians and educators to realize that irrespective of the statistically significant differences between persons with intellectual disabilities and typical individuals on sentence perception tasks, the ability of individuals with mild-to-moderate intellectual disabilities to understand 80% to 90% of sentences presented to them in synthetic speech has significant clinical and educational implications. This indicates that people with intellectual impairments who use synthetic speech can understand most, if not all sentences produced by their SGDs.

Discourse

Individuals who use SGDs must correctly identify and derive meaning from all of the words in the sentence or message before the next sentence begins

(Willis, Koul, & Paschall, 2000). Thus, discourse comprehension for a SGD user involves not only deciphering the acoustic and phonetic properties of the speech signal produced by their devices, but also integrating sentences, connecting conversational turns and deriving meaning using linguistic and world knowledge. To facilitate effective interactions between SGD users and their listeners, it is critical that users comprehend the synthetic speech produced by their SGDs for feedback purposes. In the absence of such feedback, SGD users will not be able to sustain conversations as required for effective and efficient communication (Koul, 2003). Although, substantial data exist on the discourse comprehension of synthetic speech by typical individuals (e.g., Higginbotham, Drazek, Kowarsky, & Scally, 1994; Paris, Gilson, Thomas, & Silver, 1995; Ralston, Pisoni, Lively, Greene, & Mullennix, 1991), little research is available on the discourse comprehension of synthetic speech by individuals with intellectual disabilities (Willis, Koul, & Paschall, 2000).

Willis et al. (2000) evaluated the performance of a group of individuals with mild-to-moderate intellectual disabilities on a post-perceptual discourse comprehension task. Three synthetic voices (DECtalk™ Paul, MacinTalk™ Fred, and RealVoice™) were used to present three first grade level passages. The passages were matched for complexity; participants listened to the passages and then responded to multiple choice questions by pointing to pictures on a computer screen. Results revealed superior comprehension scores for DECtalk™ compared to the other two relatively low-quality synthesizers (i.e., RealVoice™ and MacinTalk Fred™). Additionally, authors reported that, like typical individuals persons with intellectual impairment use information from passages together with world knowledge in selecting an answer. Furthermore, the types of errors made in a task involving comprehension of synthetic speech were similar to those involving comprehension of natural speech. These results indicate that strategies used to comprehend conversations or text by individuals with intellectual and communicative disabilities do not differ across natural and synthetic speech.

Practice Effects

A strong body of research indicates that typical listeners become much more adept at correctly recognizing synthetic stimuli as a result of repeated exposure to it (e.g., Greenspan, Nusbaum, & Pisoni, 1988; McNaughton, Fallon, Tod, Weiner, & Neisworth, 1994; Reynolds, Isaacs-Duvall, Sheward, & Rotter, 2000; Rounsefell, Zucker, & Roberts, 1993; Schwab, Nusbaum, & Pisoni, 1985; Venkatagiri, 1994). In contrast, only limited data are available on effects of repeated exposure to synthetic speech in individuals with intellectual and communicative impairments (Koul & Hester, 2006; Koul & Clapsaddle, 2006; Koul & Hanners, 1997, Willis et al., 2000). These data indicate that both individuals with severe intellectual impairment and individuals with mild to moderate intellectual impairment demonstrate significant practice effect as a result of repeated exposure to high quality synthetic speech. Koul and Hester reported that individuals with severe intellectual impairment demonstrated significant reduction in their response latencies for single synthetic words as a result of repeated exposure to synthesized speech produced using DECtalk™ synthesizer. These results are supported by Koul & Clapsaddle who reported that individuals with mild-to-moderate intellectual impairment demonstrate significant improvement in both single word and sentence accuracy scores as a result of repeated listening to synthetic speech produced using ETI Eloquence speech synthesizer. Further, the most interesting finding of the above two reviewed studies with individuals with intellectual impairment was the absence of significant effect for stimulus type (i.e., novel vs. repeated) stimuli. The repeated stimuli were presented across all sessions, whereas a different list of novel stimuli was presented in each listening session. It was anticipated that practice effects for repeated stimuli would be higher than those for novel stimuli because individuals with intellectual impairment may require more redundancy than their typical mental age matched peers to comprehend linguistic stimuli (Haring, McCormick, & Haring, 1994). However, the results of these studies indicate that individuals with intellectual impairment are able to generalize the knowledge of acoustic-phonetic properties of synthetic speech to novel synthetic stimuli. The ability of individuals with intellectual and communicative impairments to generalize to novel synthetic stimuli has significant clinical implications, as SGDs are increasingly being used by these individuals for information transfer and interpersonal communication.

Discussion

Although, only limited data are available on the perception of synthetic speech by individuals with intellectual disabilities, two conclusions are evident. The first is that repeated exposure to synthetic speech allows individuals with intellectual and communicative disabilities to identify synthetic speech with increased speed and accuracy. The second conclusion indicates that as the synthetic speech stimuli or the listening task becomes more complex, the accuracy of responses to such stimuli and/or tasks is reduced and the response latency is increased. The latter conclusion is also true for typical individuals. The difficulty that both typical listeners and listeners with intellectual disabilities experience in processing synthetic speech can be explained through a resource-sharing model of spoken language comprehension (Kintsch & van Dijk, 1978; LaBerge & Samuels, 1974; Moray, 1967). This model proposes that all analyses in the language comprehension system share a limited pool of cognitive resources required for processing information. Thus, according to Koul and Hester (2006) and Duffy and Pisoni (1992), listening to even high-quality synthetic speech may require that a substantial portion of cognitive resources be allocated to deciphering the acoustic-phonetic structure of synthetic speech, leaving fewer resources available for higher level processing such as understanding the word and the semantic content of the message. Persons with intellectual disabilities have reduced cognitive capacity as compared to their typical peers, and their performance seems to rapidly deteriorate as the complexity of the synthetic speech stimuli increases (Haring, McCormick, & Haring, 1994; Hutt & Gibby, 1979; Kail, 1992; Taylor et al., 1995). However, significant practice effects observed in individuals with intellectual disabilities following repeated listening to synthetic speech may be the result of their ability to learn to analyze the acoustic-phonetic structure of synthetic speech in a more efficient manner (Koul & Hester, 2006; Koul & Clapsaddle, 2006). Thus, it can be extrapolated that repeated listening to synthetic speech results in individuals with intellectual disabilities devoting minimal resources to processing the acoustic-phonetic properties of synthetic speech and greater resources to extracting meaning from the synthetic speech signal. The possible shifting of cognitive resources away from processes involved in identifying phonemes, syllables, and words to processes that are involved in extracting semantic content of the message may result in both faster and accurate recognition of synthetic speech stimuli.

PERCEPTION OF SYNTHETIC SPEECH BY INDIVIDUALS WITH HEARING IMPAIRMENT

It is important to investigate perception of synthetic speech in individuals with hearing impairment because many individuals with developmental and acquired disabilities who may benefit from a SGD also demonstrate hearing loss. Twenty percent of individuals with cerebral palsy present with hearing deficits (Robinson, 1973). Hearing loss may also co-occur with neurological disorders, such as

Parkinson's disease, amyotrophic lateral sclerosis (ALS), and aphasia as a consequence of stroke. Further, the communication partners of SGD users may also have hearing impairment. It is estimated that one in three people older than 60 and half of those older than 85 have hearing loss in the United States (National Institute of Deafness and Other Communication Disorders, 2001).

Research addressing perception of synthetic speech in individuals with hearing impairment indicates that hearing loss may not have a detrimental influence on the processing of synthetic speech (Kangas & Allen, 1990; Humes, Nelson, & Pisoni, 1991). Humes et al. (1991) provided evidence that for listeners with hearing impairment, DECtalk™ synthetic speech is as intelligible as natural speech. The authors investigated the performance of three groups of participants: older individuals with hearing impairments; young individuals who listened to natural speech and DECtalk™ speech in the presence of background noise; and young adults who listened to DECtalk ™ speech and natural speech in quiet. Their results indicated that there was no difference in performance on a single word task between elderly hearing-impaired individuals and young adults who listened to DECtalk™ synthetic speech in the presence of background noise (i.e., simulated hearing loss condition).

Kangas and Allen (1990) also reported that in hearing impaired individuals, the ability to recognize single synthetic words was not affected by the degraded acoustic-phonetic properties of the synthesized speech. These authors presented a list of words using DECtalk™ to two groups of older adults: a normal hearing group and a group with acquired sensori-neural hearing loss. Results indicated that intelligibility scores for synthetic speech were significantly lower than those for natural speech across groups. Further, intelligibility scores for individuals with hearing impairment were significantly lower than those for normal hearing listeners across synthetic and natural voices. However, there was no significant interaction between hearing ability and voice type.

DISCUSSION

Current research indicates that hearing impairment affects processing of synthetic and natural speech in an identical manner.

PERCEPTION OF SYNTHETIC SPEECH BY INDIVIDUALS WITH SPECIFIC LANGUAGE IMPAIRMENT

Individuals with specific language impairment (SLI) demonstrate language disorders in the absence of underlying deficits such as intellectual impairment, hearing impairment, motor impairment, emotional disturbance or environmental deprivation (Bishop, 1992). Synthetic speech stimuli have been used to investigate the nature of auditory perceptual deficits in individuals with SLI (Evans, Viele, Kass, & Tang, 2002; Reynolds & Fucci, 1998).Individuals with SLI are not candidates for SGDs and are able to communicate using speech. However, it is critical to understand perception of synthetic speech in people with auditory perceptual deficits because many individuals who either use or are candidates for SGDs may also demonstrate auditory processing disorders.

Previous research suggests that performance of individuals with SLI on tasks that involve processing of synthetic stimuli is significantly lower than matched typical individuals (Evans et al., 2002; Reynolds & Fucci,1998). Reynolds and Fucci observed that response latencies for DECtalk™ synthetic speech were longer than for natural speech for typical children as well as children with SLI. However, there was no significant interaction between group (i.e., typical vs. SLI) and voice (i.e., synthetic speech vs. natural speech). This indicates that synthetic and natural speech may be processed in a similar manner by individuals with SLI. Relatively longer latencies on synthetic speech for both typical children and children with SLI may be due to lack of acoustic phonetic redundancy of synthetic speech. Further, Massey (1988) observed that individuals with language impairment demonstrate greater difficulty understanding synthetic speech than natural speech. However, in contrast to the results obtained by Reynolds and Fucci, no significant differences in accuracy scores between natural and synthetic speech were noted for the typical group. The difference in results between the two above referenced studies may be due to the nature of the experimental task. Reynolds and Fucci used a relatively more sensitive latency task whereas Massey used a less sensitive intelligibility task.

EFFECTS OF SPEECH OUTPUT ON ACQUISITION OF GRAPHIC SYMBOLS

Graphic symbols such as photographs and line drawings have often been used as an alternative form of communication for individuals with little or no functional speech. Further, many SGDs provide in-built software programs that produce synthetic speech upon activation of graphic symbols. Additionally, there are many stand-alone graphic symbol software programs that are compatible with personal computers and allow the user to use those computers as SGDs. One of the variables that has been noted to influence graphic symbol acquisition is iconicity (Brown, 1978). Iconicity can be viewed on a continuum. At one end of the continuum are transparent symbols and at the other end are opaque symbols. Transparent symbols are those that can be easily guessed in the absence of cues such as written words or verbal hints. The opaque symbols are those that bear no relationship to the referents that they represent, and the meaning of opaque symbols cannot be deciphered even when both symbol and referent are presented together. Translucent symbols fall along the middle of the continuum between transparency and opaqueness. The relationship between a translucent symbol and its referent may only be perceived when the symbol and the referent appear together (Bellugi & Klima, 1976; Lloyd & Fuller, 1990). Low translucent symbols like opaque symbols have no to little resemblance to their referents and high translucent symbols like transparent symbols have some resemblance to their referents. A number of studies have been conducted to investigate whether adults with severe to profound intellectual disability learn to associate transparent, translucent, and/or opaque symbols with referents more efficiently with synthetic speech output than without it (Koul & Schlosser, 2004; Romski & Sevcik, 1996; Schlosser, Belfiore, Nigam, Blischak, & Hetzroni, 1995). Schlosser et al. investigated the effects of synthetic speech output on acquisition of opaque symbols in three young adults with severe to profound intellectual disabilities. They observed that the provision of synthetic speech output in association with the selection of a target symbol resulted in a more efficient acquisition of graphic symbols. Also, there were fewer errors in the condition in which synthetic speech output occurred in association with the selection of a graphic symbol in contrast to the condition in which selection of a graphic symbol did not result in the production of a synthesized word representing that symbol.

Koul and Schlosser (2004) examined the effects of synthetic speech output on the learning of symbols high in translucency versus symbols low in translucency. Two adults with little or no functional speech and severe intellectual disabilities served as participants. Both participants learned more low translucent symbols in the synthetic speech output condition. For the non-speech output condition, no consistent across subject differences were obtained. In the speech output condition, the participants' selection of a target symbol resulted in the production of a verbal equivalent of that symbol in synthetic speech. In the non-speech output condition, the synthetic speech output did not accompany selection of a target symbol. The results of this study appear to support the hypothesis that feedback from speech output may facilitate acquisition of low translucent and opaque graphic symbols in adults with severe intellectual and communicative disabilities.

The effects of synthetic speech output on requesting behavior of children with autism was investigated by Schlosser et al., (2007). Participants were trained to request preferred objects using opaque graphic symbols in two conditions. In one condition, the participants heard synthetic speech upon selection of a graphic symbol and in the second condition, the synthetic speech output did not accompany selection of a graphic symbol. The results of this study were mixed. Only two of the five participants requested objects using opaque symbols more effectively with speech output than without it. Two of the remaining three participants did not show any difference in requesting behavior between speech output and non-speech output conditions. One participant did better in the non-speech output condition. The authors indicate that the inconsistency of the results across subjects may have been due to methodological constraints that increased task difficulty beyond a desirable level.

The positive effects of speech output on the acquisition of opaque graphic symbols by individuals with severe intellectual disabilities has also been observed in studies in which synthetic speech output was one of the components of the treatment package (Romski, Sevcik, Robinson, & Bakeman, 1994).

DISCUSSION

In summary, research indicates that synthetic speech output has a positive effect on learning of graphic symbols by individuals with severe speech, language, and intellectual disabilities. Further, synthetic speech output allows the individual with little or no functional speech to compensate for the use of a visually based graphic symbol or orthographic system. The speech output by connecting the visual communication system with an auditory modality facilitates communicative interactions by providing communicative partners, a familiar auditory signal to comprehend the intended message (Romski, Sevcik, Cheslock, & Barton, 2006).

DIRECTIONS FOR FUTURE RESEARCH

Great technological strides have been made in producing text-to-speech systems in the past twenty years. SGDs are being increasingly used to enhance and facilitate the communicative abilities of individuals with a range of developmental and acquired communication disorders. However, there are very little empirical data on the perception of synthetic speech by individuals with little or no functional speech and on the effects of synthetic speech output on the acquisition of symbols and other communicative behaviors such as requesting, choice making, and exchanging information. It is hoped that this chapter will focus the attention of researchers and clinicians on identifying variables that can facilitate clinical and educational applications of synthetic speech.

REFERENCES

Abbeduto, L., Furman, L., & Davies, B. (1989). Relation between the receptive language and mental age of persons with mental retardation. *American Journal of Mental Retardation, 93*, 535–543.

Abbeduto, L., & Nuccio, J. B. (1991). Relation between receptive language and cognitive maturity in persons with intellectual disabilities. *American Journal of Intellectual Disabilities, 96*, 143–149.

Abbeduto, L., & Rosenberg, S. (1992). Linguistic communication in persons with mental retardation. In S. Warren & J. Reichle (Eds.), *Causes and effects in communication and language intervention* (pp. 331-359). Maryland: Paul H. Brookes.

Bellugi, U., & Klima, E. S. (1976). Two faces of sign: Iconic and abstract. *Annals of the New York Academy of Sciences*, *280*, 514–538. doi:10.1111/j.1749-6632.1976.tb25514.x

Berry, B. P. (1972). Comprehension of possessive and present continuous sentences by nonretarded, mildly retarded, and severely retarded children. *American Journal of Mental Deficiency*, *76*, 540–544.

Bishop, D. V. M. (1992). The underlying nature of specific language impairment. *Journal of Child Psychology and Psychiatry, and Allied Disciplines*, *33*, 3–66. doi:10.1111/j.1469-7610.1992.tb00858.x

Brown, R. (1978). Why are signed languages easier to learn than spoken languages? (Part Two). *Bulletin - American Academy of Arts and Sciences. American Academy of Arts and Sciences*, *32*, 25–44. doi:10.2307/3823113

Church, G., & Glennen, S. (1992). *The handbook of assistive technology.* San Diego: Singular Publishing Co.

Duffy, S. A., & Pisoni, D. B. (1992). Comprehension of synthetic speech produced by rule: A review and theoretical interpretation. *Language and Speech*, *35*, 351–389.

Evans, J. L., Viele, K., Kass, R. E., & Tang, F. (2002). Grammatical morphology and perception of synthetic and natural speech in children with specific language impairments. *Journal of Speech, Language, and Hearing Research: JSLHR*, *45*, 494–504. doi:10.1044/1092-4388(2002/039)

Greenspan, S. L., Nusbaum, H. C., & Pisoni, D. B. (1988). Perceptual learning of synthetic speech produced by rule. *Journal of Experimental Psychology. Human Perception and Performance*, *14*, 421–433.

Haring, N. G., McCormick, L., & Haring, T. G. (Eds.). (1994). *Exceptional children and youth* (6th ed.). New York: Merrill.

Higginbotham, D. J., & Baird, E. (1995). Analysis of listeners' summaries of synthesized speech passages. *Augmentative and Alternative Communication*, *11*, 101–112. doi:10.1080/07434619512331277199

Higginbotham, D. J., Drazek, A. L., Kowarsky, K., Scally, C. A., & Segal, E. (1994). Discourse comprehension of synthetic speech delivered at normal and slow presentation rates. *Augmentative and Alternative Communication*, *10*, 191–202. doi:10.1080/07434619412331276900

Humes, L. E., Nelson, K. J., & Pisoni, D. B. (1991). Recognition of synthetic speech by hearing-impaired listeners. *Journal of Speech and Hearing Research*, *34*, 1180–1184.

Hutt, M. L., & Gibby, R. G. (1979). *The mentally retarded child: Development training and education* (4th ed.). Boston: Allyn and Bacon.

Kail, R. (1992). General slowing of information processing by persons with mental retardation. *American Journal of Mental Retardation*, *97*, 333–341.

Kangas, K. A., & Allen, G. D. (1990). Intelligibility of synthetic speech for normal-hearing and hearing-impaired listeners. *The Journal of Speech and Hearing Disorders*, *55*, 751–755.

Kintsch, W., & van Dijk, T. A. (1978). Towards a model for text comprehension and production. *Psychological Review*, *85*, 363–394. doi:10.1037/0033-295X.85.5.363

Koul, R. K. (2003). Synthetic speech perception in individuals with and without disabilities. *Augmentative and Alternative Communication*, *19*, 49–58. doi:10.1080/0743461031000073092

Koul, R. K., & Allen, G. D. (1993). Segmental intelligibility & speech interference thresholds of high-quality synthetic speech in the presence of noise. *Jrnl. of Speech & Hearing Rsrch., 36*, 790–798.

Koul, R. K., & Clapsaddle, K. C. (2006). Effects of repeated listening experiences on the perception of synthetic speech by individuals with mild-to-moderate intellectual disabilities. *Augmentative and Alternative Communication, 22*, 1–11. doi:10.1080/07434610500389116

Koul, R. K., & Hanners, J. (1997). Word identification and sentence verification of two synthetic speech systems by individuals with intellectual disabilities. *Augmentative and Alternative Communication, 13*, 99–107. doi:10.1080/07434619712331277898

Koul, R. K., & Hester, K. (2006). Effects of repeated listening experiences on the recognition of synthetic speech by individuals with severe intellectual disabilities. *Journal of Speech, Language, and Hearing Research: JSLHR, 49*, 1–11.

Koul, R. K., & Schlosser, R. W. (2004). Effects of synthetic speech output in the learning of graphic symbols of varied iconicity. *Disability and Rehabilitation, 26*, 1278–1285. doi:10.1080/09638280412331280299

LaBerge, D., & Samuels, S. L. (1974). Toward a theory of automatic information processing in reading. *Cognitive Psychology, 6*, 293–323. doi:10.1016/0010-0285(74)90015-2

Lloyd, L. L., & Fuller, D. R. (1990). The role of iconicity in augmentative and alternative communication symbol learning. In W. I. Fraser (Ed.), *Key issues in mental retardation research* (pp. 295-306). London: Routledge.

Logan, J. S., Greene, B. G., & Pisoni, D. B. (1989). Segmental intelligibility of synthetic speech produced by rule. *The Journal of the Acoustical Society of America, 86*, 566–581. doi:10.1121/1.398236

Massey, H. J. (1988). Language-impaired children's comprehension of synthesized speech. *Language, Speech, and Hearing Services in Schools, 19*, 401–409.

McNaughton, D., Fallon, D., Tod, J., Weiner, F., & Neisworth, J. (1994). Effects of repeated listening experiences on the intelligibility of synthesized speech. *Augmentative and Alternative Communication, 10*, 161–168. doi:10.1080/07434619412331276870

Merrill, E. C., & Jackson, T. S. (1992). Sentence processing by adolescents with and without intellectual disabilities. *American Journal on Intellectual Disabilities, 97*, 342–350.

Mirenda, P., & Beukelman, D. R. (1987). A comparison of speech synthesis intelligibility with listeners from three age groups. *Augmentative and Alternative Communication, 5*, 84–88.

Mirenda, P., & Beukelman, D. R. (1990). A comparison of intelligibility among natural speech and seven speech synthesizers with listeners from three age groups. *Augmentative and Alternative Communication, 6*, 61–68. doi:10.1080/07434619012331275324

Mirenda, P., Wilk, D., & Carson, P. (2000). A retrospective analysis of technology use patterns of students with autism over a five-year period. *Journal of Special Education Technology, 15*, 5–6.

Moray, N. (1967). Where is capacity limited? A survey and a model. *Acta Psychologica, 27*, 84–92. doi:10.1016/0001-6918(67)90048-0

National Institute of Deafness and Other Communication Disorders. (2001). *About hearing.* Retrieved October 24, 2001 from http://www.nidcd.nih.gov/health

Paris, C. R., Gilson, R. D., Thomas, M. H., & Silver, N. C. (1995). Effect of synthetic voice on intelligibility on speech comprehension. *Human Factors, 37*, 335–340. doi:10.1518/001872095779064609

Ralston, J. V., Pisoni, D. B., Lively, S. E., Greene, B. G., & Mullennix, J. W. (1991). Comprehension of synthetic speech produced by rule: Word monitoring and sentence-by-sentence listening times. *Human Factors*, *33*, 471–491.

Reynolds, M. E., & Fucci, D. (1998). Synthetic speech comprehension: A comparison of children with normal and impaired language skills. *Journal of Speech, Language, and Hearing Research: JSLHR*, *41*, 458–466.

Reynolds, M. E., Isaacs-Duvall, C., Sheward, B., & Rotter, M. (2000). Examination of the effects of listening practice on synthesized speech comprehension. *Augmentative and Alternative Communication*, *16*, 250–259. doi:10.1080/07434610012331279104

Robinson, R. O. (1973). The frequency of other handicaps in children with cerebral palsy. *Developmental Medicine and Child Neurology*, *15*, 305–312.

Romski, M. A., & Sevcik, R. A. (1996). *Breaking the speech barrier: Language development through augmented means.* Baltimore: Brookes.

Romski, M. A., Sevcik, R. A., Cheslock, M., & Barton, A. (2006). The System for Augmenting Language: AAC and emerging language intervention. In R. J. McCauley & M. Fey (Eds.), *Treatment of language disorders in children* (pp. 123-147). Baltimore: Paul H. Brookes Publishing Co.

Romski, M. A., Sevcik, R. A., Robinson, B., & Bakeman, R. (1994). Adult-directed communications of youth with intellectual disabilities using the system for augmenting language. *Journal of Speech and Hearing Research*, *37*, 617–628.

Rosenberg, S. (1982). The language of the mentally retarded: Development, processes, and intervention. In S. Rosenberg (Ed.), *Handbook of applied psycholinguistics: Major thrusts of research and theory* (pp.329-392). Hillsdale, NJ: Erlbaum.

Rosenberg, S., & Abbeduto, L. (1993). *Language & commun. in mental retardation: Development, processes, and intervention.* Hillsdale, NJ: Erlbaum.

Rounsefell, S., Zucker, S. H., & Roberts, T. G. (1993). Effects of listener training on intelligibility of augmentative and alternative speech in the secondary classroom. *Education and Training in Mental Retardation*, *12*, 296–308.

Schlosser, R. W., Belfiore, P. J., Nigam, R., Blischak, D., & Hetzroni, O. (1995). The effects of speech output technology in the learning of graphic symbols. *Journal of Applied Behavior Analysis*, *28*, 537–549. doi:10.1901/jaba.1995.28-537

Schlosser, R. W., Sigafoos, J., Luiselli, J. K., Angermeier, K., Harasymowyz, U., Schooley, K., & Belfiore, P. J. (2007). Effects of synthetic speech output on requesting and natural speech production in children with autism: A preliminary study. *Research in Autism Spectrum Disorders*, *1*, 139–163. doi:10.1016/j.rasd.2006.10.001

Schwab, E. C., Nusbaum, H. C., & Pisoni, D. B. (1985). Some effects of training on the perception of synthetic speech. *Human Factors*, *27*, 395–408.

Taylor, R. L., Sternberg, L., & Richards, S. B. (1995). *Exceptional children: Integrating research and teaching* (2nd ed.). San Diego: Singular.

U. S. Department of Education. (2002). *Implementation of the Individuals with Disabilities Education Act: Twenty-first annual report to congress*. Washington, DC: Author.

Venkatagiri, H. S. (1994). Effects of sentence length and exposure on the intelligibility of synthesized speech. *Augmentative and Alternative Communication*, *10*, 96–104. doi:10.1080/07434619412331276800

Willis, L., Koul, R., & Paschall, D. (2000). Discourse comprehension of synthetic speech by individuals with mental retardation. *Education and Training in Mental Retardation and Developmental Disabilities*, *35*, 106–114.

Chapter 12
The Use of Synthetic Speech in Language Learning Tools:
Review and a Case Study

Oscar Saz
University of Zaragoza, Spain

Eduardo Lleida
University of Zaragoza, Spain

Victoria Rodríguez
Vienna International School, Austria

W.-Ricardo Rodríguez
University of Zaragoza, Spain

Carlos Vaquero
University of Zaragoza, Spain

ABSTRACT

This chapter aims to bring up a discussion on the use of Computer Synthesized Speech (CSS) in the development of Computer-Aided Speech and Language Therapy (CASLT) tools for the improvement of the communication skills in handicapped individuals. CSS is strongly required in these tools for two reasons: Providing alternative communication to users with different impairments and reinforcing the correct pronunciation of words and sentences. Different possibilities have arisen for this goal, including pre-recorded audio, embedded Text-to-Speech (TTS) devices or talking faces. These possibilities are reviewed and the implications of their use with handicapped individuals are commented, showing the experience of the authors in the development of tools for Spanish speech therapy. Finally, a preliminary study in the use of computer-based tools for the teaching of Spanish to young children showed how the synthetic speech feature in the language learning tool was sufficient to maintain the possibilities of the tool as a valuable language teaching element in the absence of other visual elements.

DOI: 10.4018/978-1-61520-725-1.ch012

INTRODUCTION

Different development, sensorial or physical impairments like Down's syndrome, hearing loss or cerebral palsy, among others, are also associated to mid-severe speech disorders like dysarthria or dysglossia. These disorders are characterized by affections on the central nervous system that prevent from a correct control of the articulation organs (dysarthria) or by morphological affections on those organs like left clip and palate (dysglossia). Other disorders at the speech and language level arise from functional or hearing disabilities that produce a delay in the normal process of language acquisition in the student. In other cases, traumatic situations like surgery can make the patient lose the phonation and articulation abilities and force for a language re-training.

The main effect of these disorders is the degradation of the acoustic and lexical properties of the patient's speech compared to the normal healthy speech, creating a wide barrier to the communication of these individuals with the surrounding environment. These speakers produce a speech whose intelligibility is much lower than that of unimpaired speakers, in some severe cases of dysarthria leading to a totally unintelligible speech; or, in other cases, they change or delete phonemes in words during their speech production, leading to semantic and syntactic misunderstandings and inaccuracies.

Speech therapy allows, in many occasions, the reduction of the pernicious effects of these disorders and provides these patients with a more effective communication, favoring the social inclusion of these individuals. Unfortunately, it is usually the case that there are not sufficient resources to provide this therapy in the way in which speech therapists would like to. Speech therapy activities are usually very time-demanding for the therapists as they have been traditionally based in the direct interaction between patient and educator, limiting the possibilities of carrying out an extensive program with several patients in the same time period or for the patients to continue and extend the therapy at their homes.

The interest in fulfilling these necessities has produced, in the latest years, a great deal of research in speech technologies for the development of computer-based tools that can provide an effective support for the semi-automation of speech therapy oriented to the speech handicapped community. These Computer-Aided Speech and Language Therapy (CASLT) tools are part of the whole effort put in the development of Computer-Aided Language Learning (CALL) tools, where CASLT tools are included as well as tools oriented to other target users, like Second Language (L2) learning tools for non-native foreign students.

The bigger effort about these tools has been focused in studying and understanding how novel acoustic analysis techniques, Automatic Speech Recognition (ASR) systems and pronunciation evaluation algorithms could provide a correct and accurate feedback to the users for the improvement of their oral proficiency. The increase in the capabilities of these tools has been significant during this time, and now most of these tools can detect with high accuracy pronunciation mistakes of the speaker, difficulties in reading, distortion in the speech and problems in the acquisition of the native or a foreign language.

However, there is little information on the use of Computer Synthesized Speech (CSS) in these tools, as most of the authors take for granted that any kind of CSS can be the optimal solution for the presentation of the audio prompt to the user. While most of the CALL tools take advantage of the possibilities of computerized speech to present the activities or to provide feedback to the user, it is not well known how the presence of this oral reinforcement affects the performance of the students to improve their communication or how students perceive this oral output, especially in the cases of severely handicapped individuals, whose perception of CSS can be extremely different compared to the unimpaired users.

This chapter, hence, aims to bring up a comprehensive view of the use of CSS in CASLT tools. A literature review will be carried out with that aim to understand how different approaches are taken to deal with the different needs of each case. The effort for the development of these tools for the Spanish language in "Comunica" will be presented, focusing on the use of CSS, and the conditions that shaped this use of computerized speech in the present versions of the tools. Finally, a small case study with one of these CALL tools will be reviewed, focusing in the interaction between the target students and the CSS output and how it affected their capability to improve their pronunciation skills with the help of the tool.

BACKGROUND

As stated in the introduction, recent years have seen how speech researchers have put their eyes into translating the knowledge in several speech facets to the development of CALL tools. Authors like (Cucchiarini et al., 2008) have shown that this has to be a major goal for the governments and industry nowadays as more and more people are on the verge of exclusion due to the lack of language abilities, either due to their speech impairments or because of their lack of knowledge of the new language in the case of the migrant population.

CALL tools can be divided in several groups attending to their target population or the facet of language that they aim to train: Those tools oriented to the training of patients with language difficulties, acquisition delays or speech impairments in their own language are gathered in CASLT tools; while tools specifically designed for the acquisition of a second by a foreign speaker belong to the group of L2 learning tools. According to which feature of language the tools are prepared to train, Computer Assisted Pronunciation Training (CAPT) tools focus only on improving the phonological and phonetic abilities of the target user (whether a native or a non-native speaker); while, on the other hand, reading tutors aim for upper linguistic levels like grammar, semantics and syntax, as well as reading proficiency. The objective of this Section is, hence, to provide an overview of the different tools existing, providing remarkable examples of all of them, before analyzing the relevance of CSS in them.

A major boost in the European countries for the development of CASLT tools for the language impaired community occurred within the 5th Framework Program of the European Union (1998-2002), which contained a thematic program under the subject of "Quality of life and management of living resources". Several projects appeared under this program or in related programs like the Orto-Logo-Paedia project (Öster et al., 2002); the ISAEUS consortium (García-Gómez et al., 1999), SPECO (Vicsi et al., 1999) or the ISLE project (Atwell et al., 2003).

Orto-Logo-Paedia (Öster et al., 2002, Hatzis et al., 2003), and its predecessor Optical-Logo-Therapy (Hatzis et al., 1997; Hatzis, 1999) aimed for the training of different phonetic features by the use of phonetic maps. These phonetic maps presented the phonetic space divided in the different phonemes according to several properties like voiceness, roundness, fricativeness, etc...; when the user was asked to utter a certain phoneme, the application displayed in the map where the user's utterance was located according to this features and, hence, showed how far or close the user had been from the canonic pronunciation of the phoneme.

SPECO (Vicsi et al., 1999) and ISAEUS (García-Gómez et al., 1999) were oriented in a similar way to the training of designated phonemes like vowels or fricatives. Their novel interest was their ability to produce the tools in several language of the European Union like Spanish, German and French in ISAEUS or Hungarian, Slovenian, Swedish and English in SPECO. These tools, and other studies like (Öster, 1996) were mainly aimed to the hearing impaired community; as hearing difficulties are a main origin in many speech disorders, as the hearing feedback is of main relevance in the process of speech acquisition.

The possibilities of CASLT tools since them have been translated to many other cases like the patients of full larynx removal in (Kornilov, 2004) or young adults with language difficulties (Granström, 2005), as well as users with pronunciation difficulties (Witt & Young, 1997) or severely handicapped people (Cole et al., 2007). Further tools oriented to other special groups of students like preliterate children have been also developed within the Tball project (Black et al., 2008), or to patients with stuttering problems (Umanski et al., 2008). However, the number of existing tools and research groups working in speech assessment and speech rehabilitation is great and their areas of interest are wide.

The efforts for the development of L2 tools have been many in the recent years as these tools are arising recently as a key interest for researchers in CALL tools. Although they are not oriented for the handicapped community, their study is of major interest as many of the results in pronunciation training can be directly translated between the two groups of users. Tools for the learning of English pronunciation are being developed targeted to European countries like Italy and Germany in the ISLE project (Atwell et al., 2003) or to Asian speakers like the Ya-Ya language box (Chou, 2005) or Chelsea (Harrison et al., 2008), oriented to the Chinese community, among others. Asiatic countries are being nowadays a great consumer of L2 tools for English with a big number of products appearing for this purpose.

While traditionally, most of the research has been conducted for the training of English as a second language, new languages are getting introduced to these tools like Dutch in the "New neighbors" framework (Neri et al., 2006) or Japanese (Tsurutami et al., 2006; Wang & Kawahara, 2008) and many others. This latest system (Wang & Kawahara, 2008) is an example of novel approaches not only acting as CAPT but also aimed to train grammar and syntax in the foreign student who is in the process of learning the new language.

Finally, reading tutors are appearing nowadays as a result of the increased capabilities of Natural Language Processing (NLP) to understand and decode natural and conversational human speech. These tools are oriented to the training of the upper linguistic features. Their aim is to work in children and young adults with language difficulties (reading problems or language disorders like Specific Language Impairment (SLI)) for the rehabilitation of these disorders that can suppose a major communication barrier too although the subject's speech is correct from the phonetic point of view.

Several works like the SPACE project (Cleuren et al., 2006; Duchateau et al., 2007), Tball (Tepperman et al., 2006, Gerosa & Narayanan, 2008) or others (Strik et al., 2008) have been oriented to this area. As a small summary, these applications, and those similar, work presenting a text to the student to be read aloud while the application detects the reading proficiency of the speaker, measuring the number of pronunciation mistakes, the rate of pauses or the velocity of reading to evaluate the overall abilities of the student. Afterwards, some of these tools present some questions to the student about the text. With the answers to these questions, either by speech or text, the application can measure the ability of the student to understand long texts or the semantic and syntactic level of the student.

Computer Synthesized Speech in Call Tools

Oral output is a very common feature in all CALL tools for presenting the tool's activities, as well as for providing the results and the final feedback. There are three main reasons for the use of synthetic speech in them: First, to make the interface more attractive for potential users, who can be in many cases children or handicapped individuals; second, to provide audio as an Augmentative and

Alternative Communication (AAC) system for users with sensorial or development disabilities; and finally, and not the less important, because audio reinforcement is of capital relevance in the process of speech and language acquisition. Infants start uttering the first sounds by repetition of their environment, and the process of phonological acquisition is mostly based on repetition too.

A major development issue in CALL tools is whether the application is intended for hearing impaired individuals or not. Hearing impairments are a major source of speech difficulties, as most of the language acquisition is done by listening to the surrounding environment. In these cases, the use of CSS can be of little or no use, and the tools have to focus on substituting this audio feedback by and enhanced visual feedback. This is the case of many tools reviewed in the literature like SPECO (Vicsi et al., 1999; García-Gómez et al., 1999; Öster, 1996) that are oriented either completely or in part to the hearing impaired community.

The way in which CALL tools provide this CSS output can be found in the literature as very varied and depending strongly on the objectives of each tool. Three main lines will be reviewed in this Section as a summary of all possibilities: Pre-recorded audio, Text-to-Speech (TTS) devices and talking heads. As it is well known that handicapped individuals are extremely sensitive to the quality of the synthesized speech (Koul, 2003), especially in children (Massey, 1998), the design of the oral output is of extreme relevance in the tools which are oriented to the handicapped.

Recorded Audio

The use of pre-recorded audio is the simplest way of including CSS in a CALL tool. This audio can be sound and music, correct speech from the speech therapists or a third person or the oral emissions from the own student. The implications of the use of any of these three modalities are widely different.

The simple use of sounds or music can be used to provide feedback to the patient on the resolution on the speech therapy activity. This is especially recommended for basic tools that train the basic articulatory skills of the patient in preliterate children. In this stage, previous to speech, no speech reinforcement is needed, but this audio feedback can provide a motivational and useful environment. One of the first and most successful commercial systems, IBM's Speech Viewer (Adams et al., 1989), made use of this feature. Moreover, most tools oriented to children include this in addition to other techniques to attract the young students.

Speech recorded from the speech therapist, or a third person, allows for the reinforcement of healthy correct speech to the patient. This option is the closest one to the traditional interaction between patient and therapist, where the therapist can perform the reinforcement in the desired way, deciding where to focus the learning of the student. However, this technique becomes unacceptable when the number of audio signals to record (words, sentences or different activities) increases, because it demands plenty of time and effort from the therapist.

Finally, recording the patient's own speech to play it back after the activity is another possibility with a great deal of interest in CAPT tools. When patients of speech therapy can hear their own speech and compare to the speech from the therapist like in (Ringeval et al., 2008; Hatzis, 1999; Vicsi et al., 1999), it is useful for them to learn from those differences and improve their proficiency.

Text-to-Speech Devices

TTS synthesizers are, nowadays, a state-of-the-art technology for the introduction of an oral output interface in any system. Their main capability is to produce a waveform of speech uttering the text introduced by the user. TTS systems are used nowadays in many dialogue systems which are part of everyday's life like call centers or hands-free devices.

Their main use in CALL tools is to provide a speech signal for all possible activities or words to be trained by the speech therapy patient. TTS is fully versatile compared to recording manually all these possible words and provides a reasonable quality output speech, depending on the selected TTS system. However, the main drawback when using TTS devices is their possible lack of naturalness and how this might affect users with special development capabilities, whose perception of synthetic speech can be much different from that of unimpaired users (Koul, 2003).

TTS devices are embedded in tools like the AzAR system by (Jokisch & Hoffmann, 2008) or in most of previously mentioned systems that create dynamically words, sentences or activities for language training like in (Chou, 2005; Wang & Kawahara, 2008; Tepperman et al., 2006, Gerosa & Narayanan, 2008; Strik et al., 2008) and many others.

Talking Heads

Talking heads (or talking faces) are becoming the new paradigm in multimodal user interaction, as part of avatars in computer interfaces. The basis of the talking head is the integration of a TTS system into a moving 2D or 3D image representing the face or head of the avatar. This face has to produce gestures and control the movement of the different elements of the face (lips, teeth or jaw) accordingly to the varying acoustic and articulatory characteristics of the synthesized speech signal. Synchronization is, hence, the main issue in the development of talking heads, as well as the correct modeling of the speech production model and the vocal tract shapes.

The interest in talking heads appears as it is well known that a big deal of information in the human communication is in paralinguistic features like lip movement or gestures. They also provide an enhanced interface for individuals with hearing difficulties, who complete with lip reading the information that they are missing due to their impairments. Anyways, there is a big deal of research in understanding how this knowledge of lip and tongue movement can really be helpful in speech perception like it was shown on (Engwall & Wik, 2009).

With all of this, many recent CALL tools are embedding talking heads as one of their main interaction elements. "Box of Tricks", final result of the SPECO project (Vicsi et al., 1999) used a talking head to show patients how to position the vocal tract for the generation of different sounds. ARTUR, in (Granström, 2005), VILLE in (Wik et al., 200), and other works like (Massaro, 2008) showed that talking heads could have a useful role for this task.

AN EXPERIENCE OF CSS IN THE DEVELOPMENT OF CASLT TOOLS

The development of CASLT tools for the handicapped community has been a major line of research for the authors of this Chapter during the latest years. These tools have been gathered under the framework of "Comunica" (Saz et al., 2009a; Rodríguez, W.-R. et al., 2008a) and comprehend three tools for the training of three different linguistic levels: "PreLingua" (Rodríguez, W.-R. et al., 2008b) for the training of phonatory skills in small children; "Vocaliza" (Vaquero et al., 2008) for the pronunciation training of disordered speech users; and "Cuéntame" for the language therapy at the semantic and pragmatic levels.

"Comunica" is a major effort for providing resources to speech therapists in Spain and Latin America. It was born in collaboration with educational institutions like the Public School for Special Education (CPEE) "Alborada", and it counted with the work and review from their speech therapists and educators for the designing of the tools and activities. The spirit of "Comunica" is based in the development of these tools, completely free-licensed, as they want to be the answer to the needs of an important group of handicapped individuals who are suffering a serious social gap due to their speech and language disorders.

These tools make an extensive use of AAC systems to allow full accessibility of patients with very different development and sensorial capabilities. The presentation and prompting of the different activities in "Vocaliza" and "Cuéntame" is always based on the use of the following elements:

- Text, which allows users with reading capabilities to directly read aloud the word, sentence or scene to be performed in the activity.
- Images, which allow users with reading difficulties due to development disorders or mid visual impairments to access the content of the activity. Images are a primary element in AAC devices like communication boards, and for that reason are included in the tools.
- Audio/speech, which allows users with visual impairments to access the different activities. It also reinforces the correct pronunciation of the prompted word or sentence. Audio, in the form of attractive sounds, is also used in "PreLingua" to motivate the activities with young children.

The main research effort for study in "Comunica" have been the possibilities of ASR for handicapped individuals, and how it relates to their speech proficiency (Vaquero et al., 2008) and the development of pronunciation verification algorithms for individuals with speech disorders to be used within the tools (Saz et al., 2009a, Saz et al., 2009b, Yin et al., 2009); all this research conducted over a novel speech corpus of speech from impaired children (Saz et al., 2008). However, all the tools in "Comunica" count with specific interfaces for their target users, created in collaboration with the people from the CPEE "Alborada". And, as it is the objective of this Section, the inclusion of an appropriate oral output interface also provided a very interesting discussion between speech researchers and speech therapists about the needs and requirements of these special users.

"Vocaliza" was the first tool developed in "Comunica". TTS synthesis was initially chosen as the only speech output for the prompting of the different activities (words, riddles and sentences). The first TTS device embedded in the application was based on diphone concatenation, this is, units that model the boundary between two consecutive phonemes; this is, the final part of the first phoneme with the initial part of the next phoneme. The first approach to this system by speech therapists and users was, anyways, rather negative. All their opinions pointed out this TTS voice as excessively "robotic", with very low naturalness and sometimes unintelligible, which made it unable for its use within "Vocaliza".

It was seen then, that a more natural TTS system was requested; otherwise the application would risk to be totally rejected by the potential users. A review on novel TTS systems shown that those based on the concatenation of large units are providing nowadays the best voices for speech synthesis; however, the best state-of-the-art systems like LoquendoTTS (Baggia et al., 2006) require a license that has to be purchased from the developer for the use in one exclusive computer. "Comunica" aims to provide free licensed tools for speech therapists, and the inclusion of an expensive license for the TTS systems would have broken this rule. Finally, a license-free system was included on "Vocaliza", the Spanish voices of the Lernout & Hauspie TTS3000 system.

The system provided an enhanced TTS voice, with more configuration features than the previous voice. Figure 1 shows the TTS adjustments window in "Vocaliza" where different elements can be modified like:

Figure 1. Control of TTS features in "Vocaliza"

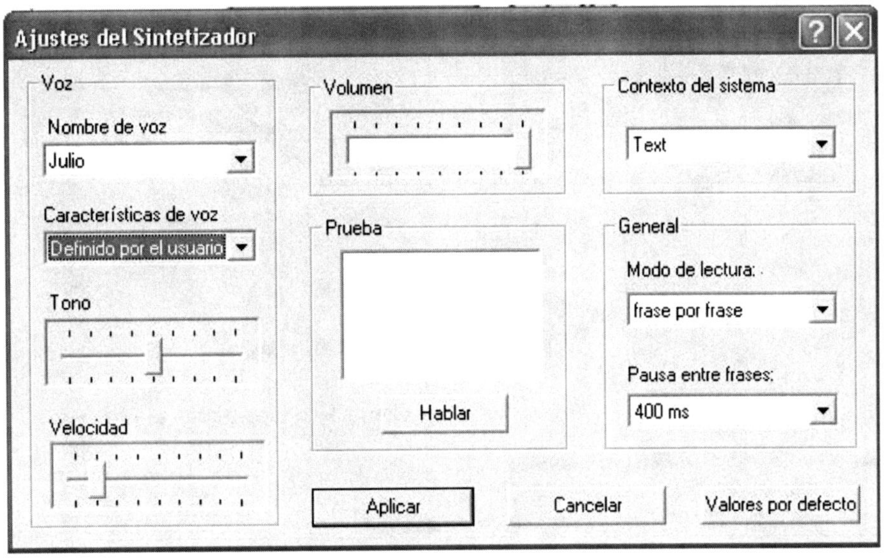

- **Gender:** A male (Julio) or a female (Carmen) voice can be selected.
- **Pitch:** The fundamental frequency of the voice can be modified from the original standard pitch value.
- **Speaking rate:** The speaking rate can be modified to make the voice speak faster or slower.
- **Volume:** The volume of the output voice can be decided.

After the initial trials, this new voice was preferred by the speech therapists and students, although it was considered that the voice had a high speaking rate, and was sometimes hard to follow by the speakers with more difficulties. To avoid this, the default value of the speaking rate that the application use was lowered until it was finally accepted by all users.

However, speech therapists felt that still this could not fulfill their needs. Children with severe development disorders still had difficulties to understand the synthetic speech and, furthermore, speech therapists did not find the synthetic speech as versatile as their own speech for one reason: Usually, when speech therapist and patient work together the therapist emphasizes that part of the utterance in which the patient has to put more effort (this can be done by raising volume or pitch or pronouncing slower the desired segment). The TTS voice embedded in "Vocaliza" allows for the modification of these properties of speech, but only at the utterance level, and not in different parts of the utterance; so, this feature of interaction in speech therapy was not possible with the TTS voice.

After evaluating all possibilities, it was decided that the TTS voice could be substituted by pre-recorded audio when the speech therapist decided so. For this reason, when a new activity is introduced in "Vocaliza" (word, riddle or sentence), the window shown in Figure 2 allows to choose between TTS synthesis (option "Sintentizar Voz" in the window) or recording the therapist's own speech to reproduce that recording each time the activity is presented (option "Reproducir grabación" in the window).

The own application allows for the self-recording of the therapist, who can verify the quality of the recorded speech to accept or discard the recording. When finally the therapist accepts a recording, it gets stored in the application for its posterior use in the activities.

Figure 2. Introducing new words in "Vocaliza": Selection of TTS or recorded audio

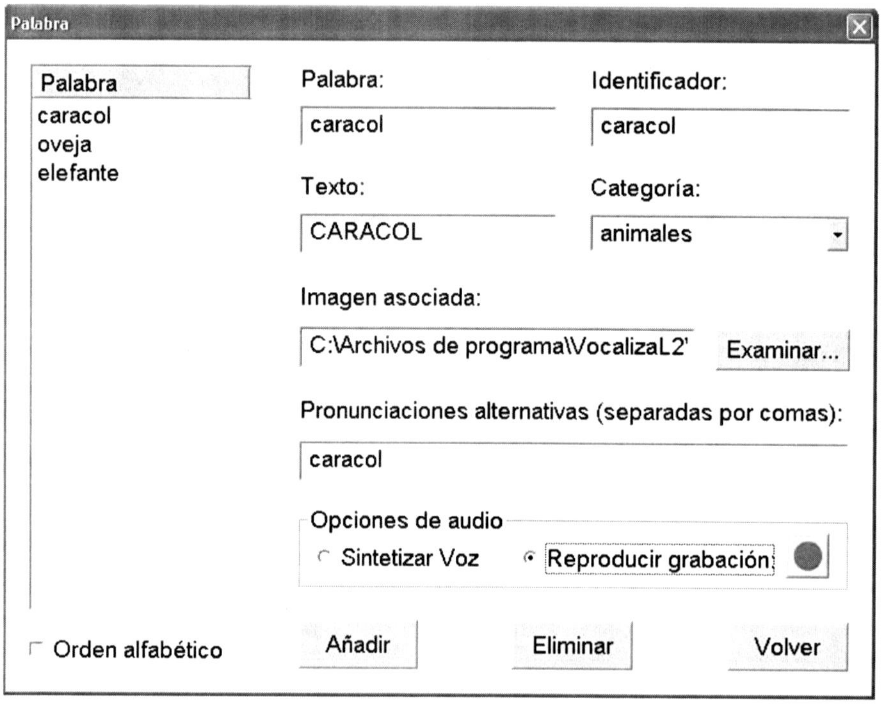

With all these functionalities, the application achieved the desired versatility in terms of the speech output. For requirements of users with special needs, speech therapists can record their own speech at their wish; or, on the contrary, rely on TTS to provide all the CSS in the application.

A CASE STUDY ON THE USE OF CSS IN CALL TOOLS

A real-environment study was carried out for the evaluation of the CAPT tools developed in "Comunica". This study intended to evaluate the ability of the tools to accurately provide feedback to a group of students on their oral proficiency and to know how these students interacted with the application interface.

The experimental case was set up at the Vienna International School (VIS). This institution aims to provide a multicultural education to their students, with language teaching as one of the pillars. English and German are the official languages at VIS, and students also study their mother tongue and another language (French or Spanish) of their choice when they reach the 6th grade.

This experimental study, part of the extensive work in (Rodríguez, V., 2008), aimed to provide the results of the work with "Vocaliza" during a set of sessions with 12 students of this institution. Five sessions of 45 minutes length each one were programmed, where each student had 10 minutes to work with the application in 10 predefined words, with 2 different trials per word. The 12 students were 6th graders of 11 years old with 8 boys and 4 girls in the group. They all were in their first year of Spanish classes and their mother tongues were as different as English, German, French, Swedish, Dutch, Icelandic, Tamil and Urdu, with English as the language in which classes were taught.

The application used for the study was a novel version of "Vocaliza", which provided a phonetic-level feedback on the quality of the student's speech. The application also provided a word-level evaluation based on the averaged values of all the phonemes in the word. The phonetic evaluation was based on a confidence scoring system and a novel score normalization system similar to the one used in (Saz et al., 2009c). This system showed a reliable ability for phoneme pronunciation verification in the disordered speech task.

The evaluation of the tool was made in two different ways: On one hand, opinions from the students were collected after each session to know how they had felt during the work with the application and their likes and dislikes about it. On the other hand, the scores given by the tool for all the phonemes and words of each student were stored for a posterior analysis in terms of the speaker proficiency of the students, and how it varied depending on the different words and sessions.

Full evaluation results of the experience can be found in (Rodríguez, V., 2008) and (Saz et al., 2009b), but what is of relevance for this Chapter are the results concerning the use of CSS for the prompting of the words to be pronounced by the students. The most interesting feature of the evaluation regarding CSS is that in the fourth session, text prompting was eliminated and the students had to work on the application relying only on the audio prompt (with the only help of the pictogram), after being using the audio-visual prompting during the first 3 sessions. The differences between presenting only the audio prompting or not could be, hence, studied.

Results of the Experimental Study

Concerning the opinions of the students about the oral prompt, most of them (8 out of the 12 students) remarked the lack of naturalness of the embedded TTS voice, Lernout & Hauspie TTS3000 as mentioned before. These young students showed off their great sensitivity to the quality of the synthetic speech used by the application, this situation being aggravated by the fact that they were not accustomed to hear the Spanish language. Even if it is not the same case, certain similarities could be expected between the way in which non-native speakers perceive a TTS voice in a new language (Axmear et al., 2005) and heavily impaired individuals do, as both groups present characteristics that make them unable to understand the new voice consistently.

Furthermore, when it came to the fourth session, they mostly indicated that it had been harder than the three previous sessions, despite they were more used to the application, due to the lack of the text presenting the word and having to rely only on synthetic speech. However, even when the synthetic voice was considered unnatural for many of the students, they could go along with it and kept working relying only in the oral prompt.

However, this major difficulty shown by the students in the fourth session had to be confirmed by an objective measure. Regarding this objective performance of the students with the tool, all the scores achieved at the word level by the students were averaged to obtain a final score per session (this score could indicate the proficiency of the students in Spanish during the session). The four values for the four sessions can be seen in Figure 3. Although the lack of more data and the impossibility to count with labeled data, make the study less significant than it could be, some discussion can be made from these results.

Scores achieved by the students increased from session 1 to session 2 and from session 2 to session 3, indicating that students were getting more and more used to the application and more comfortable with it. However a dropout in the scores was seen at session 4, the session where the text prompting had been eliminated. This dropout is consequent with the opinions from the students, where they had indicated that the session had been more difficult for them than the previous ones. But, in no case, this decrease could be considered significant, as the average score achieved by the students was similar to the score of the second session where text and audio prompt were available.

Figure 3. Average word evaluation by sessions

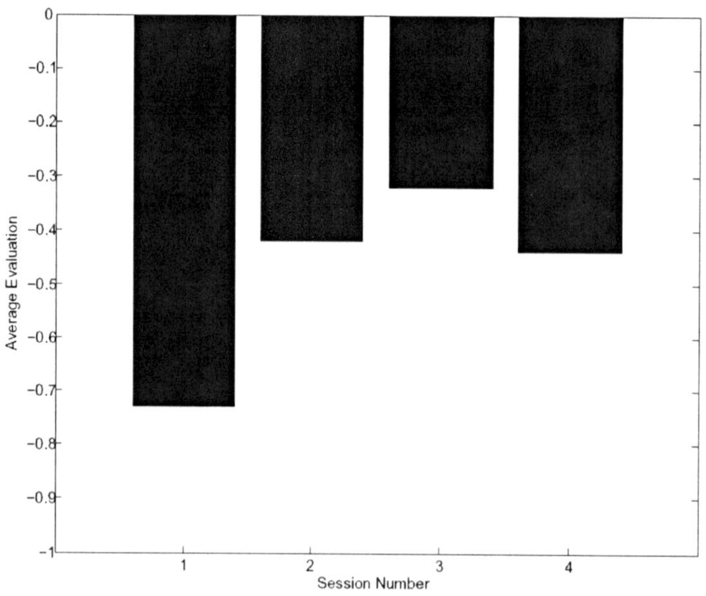

From the results of this experience, it was seen how oral prompt is actually helpful in a CALL tool, even when students might find it "poor" or "unnatural" in a subjective opinion, although if the TTS voice cannot provide sufficient quality, it is necessary to work with other AAC elements to provide full functionality.

FUTURE RESEARCH DIRECTIONS

The results of the experimental study and the experience gained in the development of CASLT tools have pointed up the necessity of enhancing the study of the use of CSS in the new applications that will be developed by the researchers in the following years. Once that it has been seen how CALL tools can really help and provide an effective feedback to the users, it is time to take all these tools to the real world in an extensive way. For this, all the interface elements have to be especially prepared and taken care of to make these tools attractive, interesting and useful for the potential users.

The requirements of patients and therapists have been already set and are well known (Eriksson et al., 2005), but it has been still not possible to provide a full adaptation to them. The lack of naturalness of synthetic speech still limits all the possibilities that these technologies can provide for novel tools. This area of research involves all specialists in the development of TTS devices, who have to work to increase the intelligibility and naturalness of their voices

From all the reviewed techniques, talking heads are the most novel and offer a wide range of possibilities to developers, as they can fulfill all the needs in CASLT tools: First, giving an entertaining and attractive interface; second, prompting activities and words with an audio reinforcement; and, finally, showing the positioning of all the elements in the vocal tract for further therapy elements. Development of talking heads is already the state-of-the-art for many CALL tools, where the articulatory abilities of the patient need to be trained. However, they still require research to provide more naturalness in the TTS voice embedded in the talking head and in the 3D avatars design.

From the technical point of view, talking heads can be enhanced by novel vocal tract normalization techniques that allow detecting the positioning of the vocal tract elements in the end user/student to show them in the talking head and compare them to the correct positioning as made by the therapist. This vocal tract normalization like in (Rodríguez & Lleida, 2009) is strongly required when dealing with children' speech, because their vocal tract shapes are smaller than those of adults and vary according to the height or age of the child. Without this normalization, it is usually the case that formant detection algorithm, for instance, obtain mistaken results.

CONCLUSION

As a conclusion to this Chapter, it was seen how CSS is an extremely important design issue in the development of CASLT tools for the handicapped. Although speech researchers in the field of speech-based aids for the handicapped are working to enhance this audio interface with state-of-the-art techniques like TTS devices or talking heads, more studies have to be conducted to understand which CSS possibility is more appropriate for the different target users of the different CASLT tools developed or to be developed in the future.

The maximum configurability in this subject has to be provided, because the many different and special characteristics of the handicapped community do not allow for knowing in advance which option will be better for any users. While some users might easily accept the technologically novel forms of CSS like TTS synthesis or talking faces, some others will find them unacceptable and the possibility of providing digitally recorded audio has to be given to them. This effect was shown during the development of CASLT tools in Spanish under the "Comunica" framework, where in the end, two different CSS possibilities, recorded audio from the therapist and a TTS voice, were embedded in "Vocaliza" for the posterior selection by the therapist according to the special needs of each patient.

In all ways, this Chapter wants to encourage a further study in the effect of oral prompting in CALL tools, the preliminary research here has shown how this feature can boost the student's ability in pronunciation, but it is necessary to avoid that users might have and a priori bad experience with the computer synthesized voice. This happened in the experience shown in this Chapter with a Spanish tool for L2 learning, where students pointed out some negative remarks about the synthetic voice embedded in the application, but they showed up to perform accurately during the activities when the audio prompt was the only feedback and the textual prompting was removed.

ACKNOWLEDGMENT

This work was supported by the national project TIN2008-06856-C05-04 from MEC of the Spanish government.

The authors want to thank Pedro Peguero, José Manuel Marcos and César Canalís from the CPEE "Alborada" for their fruitful discussion in this work, and Antonio Escartín for his work.

REFERENCES

Adams, F.-R., Crepy, H., Jameson, D., & Thatcher, J. (1989). *IBM products for persons with disabilities.* Paper presented at the Global Telecommunications Conference (GLOBECOM'89), Dallas, TX, USA.

Atwell, E., Howarth, P., & Souter, C. (2003). The ISLE Corpus: Italian and German Spoken Learners' English. *ICAME JOURNAL - Computers in English Linguistics, 27*, 5-18.

Axmear, E., Reichle, J., Alamsaputra, M., Kohnert, K., Drager, K., & Sellnow, K. (2005). Synthesized speech intelligibility in sentences: a comparison of monolingual English-speaking and bilingual children. *Language, Speech, and Hearing Services in Schools, 36*, 244–250. doi:10.1044/0161-1461(2005/024)

Baggia, P., Badino, L., Bonardo, D., & Massimino, P. (2006). *Achieving Perfect TTS Intelligibility.* Paper presented at the AVIOS Technology Symposium, SpeechTEK West 2006, San Francisco, CA, USA.

Black, M., Tepperman, J., Kazemzadeh, A., Lee, S., & Narayanan, S. (2008). *Pronunciation Verification of English Letter-Sounds in Preliterate Children.* Paper presented at the 10th International Conference on Spoken Language Processing (ICSLP - Interspeech), Brisbane, Australia.

Chou, F.-C. (2005). *Ya-Ya Language Box - A Portable Device for English Pronunciation Training with Speech Recognition Technologies.* Paper presented at the 9th European Conference on Speech Communication and Technology (Eurospeech-Interspeech), Lisbon, Portugal.

Cleuren, L., Duchateau, J., Sips, A., Ghesquiere, P., & Van Hamme, H. (2006). *Developing an Automatic Assessment Tool for Children's Oral Reading.* Paper presented at the 9th International Conference on Spoken Language Processing (ICSLP - Interspeech), Pittsburgh, PA, USA.

Cole, R., Halpern, A., Ramig, L., van Vuuren, S., Ngampatipatpong, N., & Yan, J. (2007). A Virtual Speech Therapist for Individuals with Parkinson Disease. *Journal of Education Technology, 47*(1), 51–55.

Cucchiarini, C., Lembrechts, D., & Strik, H. (2008). *HLT and communicative disabilities: The need for co-operation between government, industry and academia.* Paper presented at the LangTech2008, Rome, Italy.

Duchateau, J., Cleuren, L., Van Hamme, H., & Ghesquiere, P. (2007). *Automatic Assessment of Children's Reading Level.* Paper presented at the 10th European Conference on Speech Communication and Technology (Eurospeech-Interspeech), Antwerp, Belgium.

Engwall, O., & Wik, P. (2009). *Are real tongue movements easier to speech read than synthesized?* Paper presented at the 11th European Conference on Speech Communication and Technology (Eurospeech-Interspeech), Brighton, UK.

Eriksson, E., Bälter, O., Engwall, O., & Öster, A.-M. (2005). *Design Recommendations for a Computer-Based Speech Training System Based on End-User Interviews.* Paper presented at the 10th International Conference Speech and Computer (SPECOM), Patras, Greece.

García-Gómez, R., López-Barquilla, R., Puertas-Tera, J.-I., Parera-Bermúdez, J., Haton, M.-C., Haton, J.-P., et al. (1999). *Speech Training for Deaf and Hearing Impaired People: ISAEUS Consortium.* Paper presented at the 6th European Conference on Speech Communication and Technology (Eurospeech-Interspeech), Budapest, Hungary.

Gerosa, M., & Narayanan, S. (2008). *Investigating Assessment of Reading Comprehension in Young Children.* Paper presented at the International Conference on Acoustics, Speech and Signal Processing (ICASSP), Las Vegas, NV, USA.

Granström, B. (2005). *Speech Technology for Language Training and e-Inclusion.* Paper presented at the 9th European Conference on Speech Communication and Technology (Eurospeech-Interspeech), Lisbon, Portugal.

Harrison, A.-M., Lau, W.-Y., Meng, H., & Wang, L. (2008). *Improving mispronunciation detection and diagnosis of learners' speech with context-sensitive phonological rules based on language transfer.* Paper presented at the 10th International Conference on Spoken Language Processing (ICSLP - Interspeech), Brisbane, Australia.

Hatzis, A. (1999). *Optical Logo-Therapy: Computer-Based Audio-Visual Feedback Using Interactive Visual Displays for Speech Training.* Unpublished doctoral dissertation, University of Sheffield, United Kingdom.

Hatzis, A., Green, P., Carmichael, J., Cunningham, S., Palmer, R., Parker, M., & O'Neill, P. (2003). *An Integrated Toolkit Deploying Speech Technology for Computer Based Speech Training with Application to Dysarthric Speakers*. Paper presented at the 8th European Conference on Speech Communication and Technology (Eurospeech-Interspeech), Geneva, Switzerland.

Hatzis, A., Green, P.-D., & Howard, S.-J. (1997). *Optical Logo-Therapy (OLT): A Computer-Based Real Time Visual Feedback Application for Speech Training*. Paper presented at the 5th European Conference on Speech Communication and Technology (Eurospeech-Interspeech), Rhodes, Greece.

Jokisch, O., & Hoffmann, R. (2008). *Towards an Embedded Language Tutoring System for Children*. Paper presented at the Workshop on Child, Computer and Interaction, Chania, Greece.

Kornilov, A.-U. (2004). *The Biofeedback Program for Speech Rehabilitation Of Oncological Patients After Full Larynx Removal Surgical Treatment*. Paper presented at the 9th International Conference Speech and Computer (SPECOM), Saint Petersburg, Russia.

Koul, R.-K. (2003). Synthetic Speech Perception in Individuals with and without Disabilities. *Augmentative and Alternative Communication, 19*, 49–58. doi:10.1080/0743461031000073092

Massaro, D.-W. (2008). *Just in Time Learning: Implementing Principles of Multimodal Processing and Learning for Education of Children with Special Needs*. Paper presented at the Workshop on Child, Computer and Interaction, Chania, Greece.

Massey, J.-H. (1988). Language-Impaired Children's Comprehension of Synthesized Speech. *Language, Speech, and Hearing Services in Schools, 19*, 401–409.

Neri, A., Cucchiarini, C., & Strik, H. (2006). *Improving Segmental Quality in L2 Dutch by Means of Computer Assisted Pronunciation Training With Automatic Speech Recognition*. Paper presented at the CALL 2006, Antwerp, Belgium.

Öster, A.-M. (1996). *Clinical Applications of Computer-Based Speech Training for Children with Hearing Impairment*. Paper presented at the 4th International Conf. on Spoken Language Processing (ICSLP-Interspeech), Philadelphia, PA, USA.

Öster, A.-M., House, D., Protopapas, A., & Hatzis, A. (2002). *Presentation of a new EU project for speech therapy: OLP (Ortho-Logo-Paedia)*. Paper presented at the XV Swedish Phonetics Conference (Fonetik 2002), Stockholm, Sweden.

Ringeval, F., Chetouani, M., Sztahó, D., & Vicsi, K. (2008). *Automatic Prosodic Disorders Analysis for Impaired Communication Children*. Paper presented at the Workshop on Child, Computer and Interaction, Chania, Greece.

Rodríguez. V. (2008). *El uso de herramientas multimedia para la práctica de la pronunciación en clases de ELE con adolescentes*. Unpublished master dissertation, Antonio de Nebrija University, Spain.

Rodríguez, W.-R., & Lleida, E. (2009). *Formant Estimation in Children's Speech and its Application for a Spanish Speech Therapy Tool*. Paper presented at the Workshop on Speech and Language Technologies in Education (SLaTE), Abbey Wroxall State, UK.

Rodríguez, W.-R., Saz, O., Lleida, E., Vaquero, C., & Escartín, A. (2008a). *COMUNICA - Tools for Speech and Language Therapy*. Paper presented at the Workshop on Child, Computer and Interaction, Chania, Greece.

Rodríguez, W.-R., Vaquero, C., Saz, O., & Lleida, E. (2008b). *Speech Technology Applied to Children with Speech Disorders*. Paper presented at the 4th Kuala Lumpur International Conference on Biomedical Engineering, Kuala Lumpur, Malaysia.

Saz, O., Lleida, E., & Rodríguez, W.-R. (2009c). *Avoiding Speaker Variability in Pronunciation Verification of Children' Disordered Speech.* Paper presented at the Workshop on Child, Computer and Interaction, Cambridge, MA.

Saz, O., Rodriguez, V., Lleida, E., Rodríguez, W.-R., & Vaquero, C. (2009b). *An Experience with a Spanish Second Language Learning Tool in a Multilingual Environment.* Paper presented at the Workshop on Speech and Language Technologies in Education (SLaTE), Abbey Wroxall State, UK.

Saz, O., Rodríguez, W.-R., Lleida, E., & Vaquero, C. (2008). *A Novel Corpus of Children's Impaired Speech.* Paper presented at the Workshop on Child, Computer and Interaction, Chania, Greece.

Saz, O., Yin, S.-C., Lleida, E., Rose, R., Rodríguez, W.-R., & Vaquero, C. (2009a). Tools and Technologies for Computer-Aided Speech and Language Therapy. *Speech Communication, 51*(10), 948–967. doi:10.1016/j.specom.2009.04.006

Strik, H., Neri, A., & Cucchiarini, C. (2008). *Speech Technology for Language Tutoring.* Paper presented at the LangTech 2008, Rome, Italy.

Tepperman, J., Silva, J., Kazemzadeh, A., You, H., Lee, S., Alwan, A., & Narayanan, S. (2006). *Pronunciation Verification of Children's Speech for Automatic Literacy Assessment.* Paper presented at the 9th International Conf. on Spoken Language Processing (ICSLP - Interspeech), Pittsburgh, PA.

Tsurutami, C., Yamauchi, Y., Minematsu, N., Luo, D., Maruyama, K., & Hirose, K. (2006). *Development of a Program for Self Assessment of Japanese Pronunciation by English Learners.* Paper presented at the 9th International Conference on Spoken Language Processing (ICSLP - Interspeech), Pittsburgh, PA.

Umanski, D., Kosters, W., Verbeek, F., & Schiller, N. (2008). *Integrating Computer Games in Speech Therapy for Children who Stutter.* Paper presented at the Workshop on Child, Computer and Interaction, Chania, Greece.

Vaquero, C., Saz, O., Lleida, E., & Rodríguez, W.-R. (2008). *E-Inclusion Technologies for the Speech Handicapped.* Paper presented at the International Conference on Acoustics, Speech and Signal Processing (ICASSP), Las Vegas, NV.

Vicsi, K., Roach, P., Öster, A., Kacic, P., Barczikay, P., & Sinka, I. (1999). *SPECO: A Multimedia Multilingual Teaching and Training System for Speech Handicapped Children.* Paper presented at the 6th European Conference on Speech Communication and Technology (Eurospeech-Interspeech), Budapest, Hungary.

Wang, H., & Kawahara, T. (2008). *A Japanese CALL system based on Dynamic Question Generation and Error Prediction for ASR.* Paper presented at the 10th International Conference on Spoken Language Processing (ICSLP - Interspeech), Brisbane, Australia.

Wik, P., Hincks, R., & Hirschberg, J. (2009). *Responses to Ville: A virtual language teacher for Swedish.* Paper presented at Speech and Language Technology for Education Workshop, Wroxall Abbey Estate, UK.

Witt, S., & Young, S.-J. (1997). *Computer-Assisted Pronunciation Teaching based on Automatic Speech Recognition.* Paper presented at the International Conference on Language Teaching, Language Technology, Groningen, The Netherlands.

Yin, S.-C., Rose, R., Saz, O., & Lleida, E. (2009). *A Study of Pronunciation Verification in a Speech Therapy Application.* Paper presented at the International Conference on Acoustics, Speech and Signal Processing (ICASSP), Taipei, Taiwan.

ADDITIONAL READING

Ball, M.-J. (1993). *Phonetics for Speech Pathology.* London, UK: Whurr Publishers.

Bax, S. (2003). CALL: Past, Present and Future. *System, 31*(1), 13–28. doi:10.1016/S0346-251X(02)00071-4

Enderby, P.-M. (1983). *Frenchay Dysarthria Assessment.* London, UK: College Hill Press.

Enderby, P.-M., & Emerson, J. (1995). *Does Speech and Language Therapy Work?* London, UK: Whurr Publishers.

Eskenazi, M. (2009). An overview of spoken language technology for education. *Speech Communication, 51*(10), 832–844. doi:10.1016/j.specom.2009.04.005

Ferguson, C.-A., Menn, L., & Stoel-Gammon, C. (Eds.). (1992). *Handbook of Child Language Acquisition.* Lutherville Timonium (MD), USA: York Press.

Huang, X., Acero, A., & Hon, H.-W. (1993). *Spoken Language Processing.* Upper Saddle River (NJ), USA: Prentice Hall.

Hubbard, P. (Ed.). (2008). *Computer Assisted Language Learning: Critical Concepts in Linguistics, Volumes I-IV.* London, UK: Routledge.

Jakobson, R. (1968). *Child Language, Aphasia and Phonological Universals.* Den Haag, The Netherlands: Mouton.

Kirk, U. (Ed.). (1983). *Neuropsychology of Language, Reading, and Spelling.* New York (NY), USA: Academic Press.

Morley, J. (1994). *Pronunciation Pedagogy and Theory: New View, New Directions.* Alexandria (VA), USA: TESOL Publications.

Oller, D.-K., & Eilers, R.-E. (1988). The Role of Audition in Infant Babbling. *Child Development, 59*, 441–449. doi:10.2307/1130323

Shriberg, L.-D., & Kwiatkowski, J. (1994). Developmental Phonological Disorders I: A Clinical Profile. *Journal of Speech and Hearing Research, 37*, 1100–1126.

Strik, H., Truong, K., de Wet, F., & Cucchiarini, C. (2009). Comparing different approaches for automatic pronunciation error detection. *Speech Communication, 51*(10), 832–844. doi:10.1016/j.specom.2009.05.007

Winitz, H. (1969). *Articulatory Acquisition and Behavior.* New York (NY), USA: Appleton Century Crofts.

KEY TERMS AND DEFINITIONS

Augmentative and Alternative Communication: Techniques for providing enhanced communication to individuals with sensorial and development disabilities.

Computer Aided Language Learning: The process of acquiring a first or second language with the help of a computer application.

Language Acquisition: The natural process in which a student learns all the processes of language, starting in babbling as an infant and finishing in the functional language as a child.

Speech and Language Therapy: The corrective treatment, carried by a specialist in speech pathology, for the improvement in oral communication of patients with different language disorders.

Speech Assessment: The process of determining, in an objective or subjective way, the quality of a subject's speech.

Speech Disorder: Any functional or morphological alteration in the speech processes that leads to a difficulty or inability in speech.

Speech Technologies: Engineering techniques for the simulation of different parts of the oral communication like speech recognition or speech synthesis.

Talking Head: An avatar whose lips, tongue and jaws movement are synchronized to the articulatory properties of the output speech.

Text-to-Speech Devices: Systems that create an audio waveform that automatically translates a given text to an oral utterance.

Section 4
Social Factors

Chapter 13
Attitudes toward Computer Synthesized Speech

John W. Mullennix
University of Pittsburgh at Johnstown, USA

Steven E. Stern
University of Pittsburgh at Johnstown, USA

ABSTRACT

This chapter reviews an emerging area of research that focuses on the attitudes and social perceptions that people have toward users of computer synthesized speech (CSS). General attitudes toward people with speech impairments and AAC users are briefly discussed. Recent research on people's attitudes toward speaking computers is reviewed, with the emphasis on the similarity in the way that people treat computers and humans. The research on attitudes toward CSS and whether persuasive appeals conveyed through CSS indicates that, in general, people view CSS less favorably than natural human speech. However, this tendency is reversed when people know that the user is speech impaired. It also appears that people's attitudes are modified by the situation which CSS is used for. Overall, the findings present an intriguing perspective on attitudes toward people with speech impairments who use CSS and will serve to stimulate further research in this area.

INTRODUCTION

Over the years, attitudes in society regarding individuals possessing severe communication impairments have shifted from financially reimbursing people for loss of function to attempts to re-establish normal speech to attempts at using communication alternatives (Beukelman, 1991). In recent years, communication alternatives have benefited greatly from technological advancements in the area of alternative and augmentative communication (AAC). These advancements have provided encouraging news for those suffering from hearing loss, stuttering, speech impairments, language disorders and autistic spectrum disorders. A variety of different techniques have been developed to assist adults and children, with unaided communication techniques (consisting of manual signs and gestures) and aided communication techniques (consisting of external devices) both proving useful (Mirenda, 2003). The

DOI: 10.4018/978-1-61520-725-1.ch013

goal of using AAC techniques is to develop and enhance communicative competence (Beukelman, 1991; Light, 1996). As Light (1996) puts it, "Communication is the essence of human life" (p. 61). We communicate to express needs and wants, to establish and maintain our social relationships with friends and family, to share information with each other and to fulfill the normative conventions of social interaction (Light, 1996). The inability to communicate can be potentially devastating to an individual. In terms of AAC being able to assist individuals with communication disorders, as Beukelman (1991) puts it, "For someone who is unable to speak to "talk' and someone who is unable to write to place words on paper or computer screen… it is magical" (p. 2).

In the present chapter, our focus is on speech impaired individuals and the use of AAC devices designed to provide them with spoken voice output. In the research literature, these devices are called voice output communication aids (VOCAs) or speech generating devices (SGDs). VOCAs are portable electronic devices that produce synthetic or digitized speech output (Mirenda, 2003, p. 210). In the research reviewed below, we focus specifically on VOCAs that produce computer synthesized speech (CSS). CSS is often bundled together in text-to-speech systems, which are systems that take typed text and convert it into synthesized speech output. The famed astrophysicist Stephen Hawking, who suffers from amyotrophic lateral sclerosis (ALS), has been using a text-to-speech system for years to communicate with others and deliver his lectures. In fact, at one point Dr. Hawking became so attached to his American accented synthetic voice that he refused to switch to a newer system with a British accent.

Our concern is with how other people view a speech impaired individual who is using CSS as a speaking aid. Much of the cognitive psychological research on CSS has focused on intelligibility of CSS compared to natural speech (e.g., Fucci, Reynolds, Bettagere, & Gonzales, 1995; Koul & Allen, 1993; Logan, Greene, & Pisoni, 1989; Mirenda & Beukelman, 1987, 1990), the attentional requirements of processing CSS (Luce, Feustel, & Pisoni, 1983), and the degree to which comprehension of CSS is affected by its impoverished quality (Duffy & Pisoni, 1992; Ralston, Pisoni & Mullennix, 1995). In general, the increased cognitive processing demands of perceiving and comprehending CSS, in comparison to natural human speech, are well documented. However, one area of research on the use of CSS that has been neglected is how social psychological factors affect people's reactions to speech coming from a CSS user. When considering the effect that a speaker has on a listener, we know that there is a close relationship between language, perceptions held about the speaker and social influence (Stern, 2008). Research on a speaker's influence on the listener has typically focused on issues of credibility, trustworthiness and attractiveness, as well as issues related to the content of the message (Stern, 2008). There are a whole host of issues related to how the listener views a speech impaired CSS user that may be just as important as determining the intelligibility and comprehensibility of CSS. Does the listener believe that the CSS user is competent and trustworthy? Does the listener believe that the message from the CSS user is accurate? Does the listener have any negative attitudes toward the CSS user? If the CSS user is attempting to persuade or influence the listener, are they effective or ineffective? These issues are very important in terms of practical applications for a speech impaired user of CSS. In this chapter, we attempt to review some research that addresses some of these issues.

ATTITUDES TOWARD SPEECH DISABILITY

As with physical disabilities, there is evidence that people with speech disabilities are stigmatized (Weitzel, 2000). Interestingly, there is evidence that people with speech disabilities are less accepted and less liked in comparison to people with physical disabilities (Anderson & Antonak, 1992). People with communication disabilities find themselves excluded from participating in activities that involve communicating and experience a highly debilitating loss of power and leverage in the speaking world (Simmons-Mackie & Damico, 2007). They also have fewer social contacts than able-bodied people (Cruice, Worrall, & Hickson, 2006; Hilari & Northcott, 2006).

However, somewhat counter intuitively, there is also empirical support for a positive prejudice toward people with disability (Carver, Glass, & Katz, 1978; Elliot & Frank, 1990; Makas, 1988) or a reverse discrimination effect (Harber, 1998). In some research studies, people with a disability are often rated more favorably than people without a disability. These positive evaluations may be attributed to social desirability concerns, including political correctness (Wolsko, Park, Judd & Wittenbrink, 2000) or an over-correction bias that can occur when we are trying to account for information that may or may not be consistent with existing stereotypes (Wegener & Petty, 1997). Furthermore, some authors suggest that positive prejudice may be attributed to earnest beliefs that people with disabilities have to overcome great obstacles to achieve their successes (Carver et al., 1978).

There is the potential, as documented by Heinemann (1990), for a simple inconsistency in how people believe they should act toward people with physical disabilities and how they automatically react, or implicitly feel. In his research, participants evaluated confederates with physical disabilities more positively than people without disabilities in an adjective checklist task, yet expressed more behaviors reflecting non-verbal uneasiness and chose greater interpersonal distance when making personal contact. Furthermore, listening to a confederate with a disability elicited greater electrodermal activity (measured by skin resistance; a physiological measure of arousal) than listening to a confederate without a disability.

Attitudes of children toward disability (Harper, 1999; Sigelman, Adams, Meeks, & Purcell, 1986) also help us to better understand the ambiguity of reactions toward disability finding regarding children's reactions to physical disability. Young children show more interest than aversion toward adults with disabilities, while avoiding children with disabilities for more functional purposes as not being able to play with them. Older children show more aversion, yet are more positive verbally, indicating an understanding of the social desirability of behaving appropriately toward people with disability.

ATTITUDES TOWARD AAC USERS

Attitudes of people towards users of augmentative and alternative communication (AAC) aids are an important factor in judging the effectiveness of AAC for facilitating communication. Negative attitudes about AAC users can have significant impact on their social interactions, education and employment success. McCarthy and Light (2005) found that, in general, females have more positive attitudes towards AAC users than males. They also found that individuals who had prior experience with disabled people reported more positive attitudes toward AAC users. As well, the perceived similarity of an individual to an AAC user may affect attitudes, with ratings of high similarity resulting in more positive attitudes (Gorenflo & Gorenflo, 1997).

The research on attitudes toward AAC users is of particular interest when examining children's attitudes toward speech impaired children who use AAC. Children with communication disabilities tend to interact less with peers, be less liked and experience general social difficulty (Fujiki, Brinton, Isaacson, & Summers, 2001; Gertner, Rice, & Hadley, 1994). Their teachers may possess negative attitudes toward the children, believing that their academic ability and social skills are lower and resulting in less interaction with the student

(Bennet & Runyah, 1982; Popich & Alant, 1997; Rice, Hadley, & Alexander, 1993; Ruscello, Stutler, & Toth, 1983). However, negative attitudes toward the children using AAC can be attenuated through various intervention techniques such as information about disabilities and role-playing (Beck & Fritz-Verticchio, 2003). It is interesting that the predisposition for females to possess more favorable attitudes toward children using AAC than males is present at a very early age (Beck & Dennis, 1996; Blockberger, Armstrong, O'Connor, & Freeman, 1993; Lilienfeld & Alant, 2002).

ATTITUDES TOWARD SPEAKING COMPUTERS

Nass and colleagues have proposed a framework called the Social Responses to Communication Technologies (SRCT) paradigm that suggests in many circumstances social reactions to computers are similar to social reactions to people (see Nass & Moon, 2000; Reeves & Nass, 1996; Sundar & Nass, 2000). For example, people appear to gender stereotype male and female voices coming from a computer (Nass, Moon & Green, 1997), they exhibit similar psychological responses to "computer personalities" as they would human personalities (Moon & Nass, 1996; Nass & Lee, 2001), they view computers as acceptable teammates (Nass, Fogg, & Moon, 1996), and they are positively affected by the caring orientation of a computer-mediated agent (Lee et al., 2007). In this research, the similarity of social responses that people exhibit to both computers and humans suggests that human-computer interaction is guided by many of the same social communicative principles and guidelines that human-human interaction is guided by (Reeves & Nass, 1996).

The issue of whether social responses to computers are similar to humans is of particular interest when considering the use of computer technologies in AAC, especially when dealing with synthetic speech generated on a computerized AAC device. The question is that of how a listener reacts to speech coming from the device. Do they attribute the same qualities to a CSS speaker as they do a human speaker? Is the content of the message processed in the same way?

One avenue of research pursued by Nass and colleagues focuses on reactions to CSS when it is mixed with human speech or presented with human faces (Gong & Lai, 2003; Gong & Nass, 2007; Nass & Brave, 2005). Gong and Lai (2003) conducted a study where they examined participants' task performance interacting with a telephone-based virtual assistant system. They compared a situation where only CSS messages were heard over the phone to a situation where both CSS and a pre-recorded natural human voice were mixed together in messages heard over the phone. They found that task performance was better in the CSS only condition. Gong and Lai (2003) suggested that the consistency of processing the same type of speech output was more conducive to the cognitive processing of the speech information, even though the CSS output sounded less natural than pre-recorded human speech. In other words, CSS is treated in the same way as human speech but only if CSS is the only type of speech that you hear in a situation.

Another study indicating the importance of consistency in a human-computer interface using CSS was conducted by Gong and Nass (2007). In their study, they examined computer-generated anthropomorphic faces and speech. Participants were shown videos of "talking heads" in various combinations of real or computer-generated human faces and recorded human speech or CSS. Participants were told they were testing a prototype interviewing system and they were asked to type in answers in response to self-disclosure questions asked by the animated talking computer agent. Trust in the computer agent was assessed by a self-disclosure index and a trust scale. Their results showed that when the face and voice matched (e.g., if a computer-generated face was paired with CSS, or a human face was paired with human speech), participants formed judgments more quickly, they disclosed more personal information about themselves and they reported greater trust in the agent.

The research of Gong and Lai (2003) and Gong and Nass (2007) shows that the manner in which CSS is used and presented to listeners (in terms of consistency) is important in terms of ease of cognitive processing and social factors such as trust. Their work suggests that CSS and human speech may be treated in a similar fashion, but only if the listener is exposed to CSS in a situation where CSS is not mixed with human voice or human faces. In order to probe further the issue of consistency and social perceptions of CSS, a study was conducted in our laboratory (Stern, Mullennix, & Yaroslavsky, 2006). We decided to examine social perceptions of CSS as measured by attitudes toward the message and speaker as well as a measure of how persuasive the message was. In this study, a long passage was used that consisted of a persuasive message about comprehensive college exams (Petty & Cacioppo, 1986). Consistency was examined by manipulating the type of speech (human or CSS) and the source (human or computer), with consistent conditions (human voice spoken by a person and CSS spoken by a computer) compared to inconsistent conditions (human voice spoken by a computer and CSS spoken by a human). The experimental conditions were arranged by manipulating instruction sets. When the source was human, participants were told that a student was delivering a speech and they listened to either human speech or CSS through a tape recorder. When the source was a computer, participants were told that the speech was being delivered by a computer and they listened to human speech or CSS while watching a computer monitor display the sound waveform.

The results of Stern et al. (2006) indicated that the consistency of source (human or computer) and type of speech (human or CSS) interacted. When the human source was paired with CSS, listeners viewed the speaker more negatively. They rated the speaker as less credible, less competent and less stimulating compared to a human speaking naturally. When the computer was paired with CSS, the attitudes toward the computer speaking with CSS were about the same as attitudes toward the computer speaking with a human voice. This latter result was contrary to what we might expect from the findings of Gong and Lai (2003), in that a computer speaking with (consistent) CSS was not viewed more favorably than a computer speaking with a (inconsistent) human voice.

The results of Stern et al. (2006) also provide some insight into whether reactions to a speaking computer are driven by social group processes. Tajfel (1978) discusses how people naturally fall into different social categories and how some people are viewed as "in-group" members of a socially defined group and how some are viewed as "out-group" members. There is evidence indicating that in-group members are evaluated and viewed differently than out-group members, which can lead to a phenomenon called the Black Sheep Effect (Marques, Yzerbyt, & Leyens, 1988). The Black Sheep Effect refers to a situation where members of the ingroup judge a fellow member more harshly than a person who is a member of the outgroup when exhibiting a negative (non-normative) behavior. The reason that the Black Sheep Effect exists is to preserve the overall integrity of the group. When someone in the ingroup behaves in a way that is out of line with the normal behavior of the group, then they are "punished" by other members of the group in terms of distancing the offender from the rest. This creates pressure to conform to ingroup norms. Conversely, when a member of the ingroup behaves in a way that is consistent with ingroup norms, they are evaluated more favorably than someone who exhibits the same behavior from the outgroup. This also preserves group integrity.

In terms of Stern et al.'s (2006) findings, the situation could be viewed through the lens of ingroup/outgroup belongingness and the Black

Sheep Effect. The analogy works in the following manner: In the person as source condition, the person is viewed as a member of the ingroup. In the computer as source condition, the computer is viewed as a member of the outgroup. When the person is using their human voice, this is a normative situation in the ingroup and the person is judged favorably. However, when the person uses CSS, this is an atypical behavior that goes against the ingroup norm. Thus, the person using CSS is judged harshly. This is the pattern of results that we found, with the person in the person as source condition rated much more negatively when using CSS compared to when the person was using (normative) human speech. In the computer as source condition, i.e. the outgroup, the computer speaker was judged about the same when using either CSS or human speech. Thus, in the computer outgroup, the pattern of reward and punishment in terms of the voice fitting normative behavior does not occur, which is to be expected in terms of outgroup processes (Marques et al., 1988).

The classification of the source of speech into ingroups and outgroups obviously has ramifications for how the speech from impaired users of CSS is viewed. One factor in determining how likely these social group processes play a role is the experience that the normal speaking person has with computers and with CSS systems. If a person has little experience with either, perhaps they would be more likely to treat a computer source as a member of an outgroup. However, if a person has extensive computer and/or CSS experience, perhaps to them treating a computer like a person is normal and it would not be unusual to hear speech from a computerized device. In this latter case, perhaps they would treat the computer source as an ingroup member.

People's tendency to classify others into ingroups and outgroups may also affect how they view speech impaired persons. When a normal speaking person encounters a speech impaired CSS user, do they assign them status as an ingroup member to which they both belong to, or does the person assign them status as an outgroup member because of their disability? If they are considered to be a member of the ingroup, then normal hearing people may judge the CSS user more harshly because they are exhibiting behavior (using a computer to speak) which is not normative for the group. This would suggest that people's reactions to CSS will be negative and may impact the value of what the CSS user is attempting to communicate. On the other hand, if a normal speaking person assigned the speech impaired person to the outgroup, perhaps they be more forgiving of the use of CSS.

ATTITUDES TOWARD CSS USERS

The work of Stern et al. (2006) suggests that attitudes toward a CSS user are more negative than attitudes toward a normal speaker. To some degree, perhaps negative attitudes arise because there is an increased need for the listener to pay more attention to the somewhat unnatural and acoustically impoverished CSS, compared to natural speech, which could result in a certain degree of frustration. In a test of the relationship of ease of processing and attitudes toward CSS, Gorenflo, Gorenflo and Santer (1994) assessed attitudes toward four different CSS systems that varied in "ease of listening." They prepared a series of videotapes that depicted an augmented communicator interacting with a non-disabled person. The script consisted of a social dialog between the two people, with the two acting as acquaintances meeting after a period of time who discussed topics such as the weather, jobs and families. Four different CSS systems were used for the augmented communicator's speech across conditions. These systems varied in their quality and intelligibility. To assess attitudes toward the CSS user, participants were given the Attitudes Towards Nonspeaking Persons Scale (ATNP, from Gorenflo & Gorenflo, 1991). Overall, they found that attitudes toward the CSS user were more favorable when the quality of the speech from the CSS system was higher. Thus, they demonstrated that there was a significant relationship between difficulty of cognitive processing of CSS and favorability ratings and attitudes toward the CSS user.

Over the last few years, we have conducted a series of studies in our laboratory designed to examine attitudes toward the CSS user in more detail than in previous research (Mullennix, Stern, Wilson, & Dyson, 2003; Stern, 2008; Stern, Dumont, Mullennix, & Winters, 2007; Stern & Mullennix, 2004; Stern, Mullennix, Dyson, & Wilson, 1999; Stern, Mullennix & Wilson, 2002; Stern et al., 2006). In this research, we have focused on the social perceptions that listeners have about a speaker and the degree to which the listener is convinced by a persuasive message uttered by the speaker. The key comparison is to assess social perceptions and persuasiveness for passages spoken by a person using their natural voice and for passages spoken by a CSS system. In our line of research, the basic paradigm consists of listeners receiving a persuasive appeal on the topic of comprehensive exams in college (Petty & Cacioppo, 1986). After the passage is heard, listeners rate a number of items on a semantic differential scale designed to assess the listener's perception of the speaker, the message, the effectiveness of the message and various attributes of the speaker's voice (items such as competent-incompetent, qualified-unqualified, monotone-lively, effective-ineffective, etc.). The persuasiveness of the message is assessed by a pre-test/post-test measure attitudinal measure (Rosselli, Skelly, & Mackie, 1995) that measures attitude change for the comprehensive exam issue discussed in the persuasive appeal as well as three control topics measuring attitudes on animal rights, environmentalism and college tuition raises.

In all these studies, attitudes and persuasion are assessed for recorded natural human speech and CSS. The CSS system we used was DECtalk, a fairly high-quality, high-intelligibility system which at the time was the standard system used in most VOCA devices. In all studies, listeners received either a natural speech passage or a CSS passage.

First, we will summarize our findings on social perceptions and attitudes that listeners exhibit toward the persuasive message. In general, people rate natural human speech more favorably than CSS. Generally speaking, listeners find the natural human speaker to be more knowledgeable, more truthful, and more involved than the CSS speaker. They also find the message from the human speaker to be more convincing, more stimulating and more accurate than the message from the CSS speaker (Mullennix et al., 2003; Stern et al., 1999; Stern et al., 2002). There are also differences in listeners' ratings of speech qualities, with listeners finding CSS more "accented," more nasal, and less lively than human speech. The differences in speech qualities were not unexpected, due to more impoverished nature and less natural sound of CSS produced by rule in the DECtalk system. Thus, these results indicate that negative attitudes toward the CSS user are held by nondisabled listeners, suggesting that the content being conveyed by the CSS user is viewed in a less positive light.

Most of these studies were conducted with a male CSS speaker. In light of this, Mullennix et al. (2003) decided to test both a male CSS voice and a female CSS voice, since some speech impaired users of CSS will choose female voice for their mode of voice output. Comparing male and female voices also allowed us to examine whether gender stereotyping of voice occurred for CSS, a phenomenon observed by Nass et al. (1997) for computers. Overall, as in our previous studies, the ratings of attitudes toward natural speech were higher than CSS. In terms of the attitudes of male and female listeners toward male and female voices, the pattern of ratings was similar for natural voices and CSS voices. In other words, the gender of the synthetic speaker did not result in different attitudes toward the speech and supported the idea that CSS voices were gender stereotyped in a manner similar to human voices. However, there was a slight tendency for female listeners to rate male voices more favorably than male listeners. There was also a slight tendency to rate male CSS more favorably than female CSS on effectiveness of the message. Overall, these results are similar to what was observed by Gorenflo et al. (1994), who found little evidence that gender of listener interacted with gender of CSS voice to affect attitudes towards an augmented communicator using CSS.

In the studies described so far, listeners simply listened to the natural speech and CSS passages and they were not provided with any information related to using CSS as an aid for speech impairment. Stern et al. (2002) decided to examine the effects of perceived disability on attitudes toward CSS in an experimental paradigm incorporating disability status of the speaker as an explicit variable. To accomplish this, a trained male actor was videotaped. In one scenario, the actor read the persuasive appeal. In another scenario, the actor pretended to type on a keyboard as if he was using a text-to-speech system, with the CSS passage was dubbed over the video. Instruction set was also manipulated. In the nondisabled condition, disability was not mentioned to listeners. In the disabled condition, if the actor was using CSS, participants were told that the actor had a speech impairment. If the actor was reading the passage, then participants were told that he had a speech impairment and he was in the process of losing his ability to speak. The results for the nondisabled condition were similar to what we found previously, in that rated attitudes toward natural speech were more favorable than attitudes toward CSS. However, in the disabled condition this difference diminished, with CSS speech rated about the same as natural speech. This finding suggested that the knowledge that a person is speech impaired and is using CSS as a speaking aid predisposes people to view the speaker, the message, and the effectiveness of the message in a more positive light compared to a situation where no information about the reason for CSS being used was provided.

The results of Stern et al. (2002) are very important. They indicate that the negative attitudes people may hold against unnatural sounding CSS are attenuated when they feel that the person using CSS needs it in order to communicate. This finding is consistent with other work regarding positive reactions to users of CSS who have a disability (Gorenflo & Gorenflo, 1997; Lasker & Beukelman, 1999; Romski & Sevcik, 2000). This has important ramifications for the use of CSS as a speaking aid, a point that will be returned to later.

Further examination of these reactions to CSS in persuasive appeals (Stern, Dumont, Mullennix, & Winters, 2007) has illuminated the relationship between perceptions of disability and the use of CSS. In Stern et al. (2007) study, some participants were told that the CSS user was engaged in the socially undesirable task of conducting a telephone campaign. When this variable was taken into consideration, the positive reaction toward the user with a disability (observed by Stern et al. 2002) reversed and the person without a disability who used CSS was rated more favorably than the user with the disability. These findings suggest that CSS is a salient disability cue. In Western society, where prejudice toward people with disabilities is socially unacceptable, the CSS cue provokes a positive reaction that can be considered as a positive prejudice. On the other hand, when a situational factor is present that permits some ambiguity such as the use of the technology for an unpleasant motive (e.g., telephone campaign; see also earlier research on stigma and disability, Snyder, Kleck, Strenta, & Mentzer, 1979), prejudice and discrimination toward people with disabilities can be unwittingly yet openly expressed. Crandall and Eshleman (2003) conceptualize this in terms of a Justification Suppression Model. This model suggests that prejudices may exist at a deep emotional level and that the emotional expression of a prejudice may be suppressed for reasons such as empathy toward a target of prejudice, social desirability and enhancing one's self-image. However, people may seek out "justifications" to express the underlying prejudice. If they can find a suitable justification, such as the person is behaving badly, then the prejudice then may be released and expressed. Thus, in the situation concerning an aversive telephone campaign solicitation, the campaigner is engaged in an activity the listener views as negative and thus the underlying prejudice against the person with a disability comes out. Given these situations, it is entirely possible that situational variables modify the effect of knowledge of disability by the listener.

So far, we have focused on attitudes expressed toward CSS. However, the other variable studied in our research program was the degree of persuasion induced by the persuasive appeal communicated by the CSS user. The primary issue is whether CSS is as persuasive as normal speech when attempting to communicate a persuasive appeal on a topic. Overall, the results on persuasion are mixed. Mullennix et al. (2003) and Stern et al. (1999) found no difference in persuasion between natural speech and CSS, while Stern et al. (2002) found that natural speech was more persuasive than CSS. Thus, at best, natural speech is only weakly more persuasive than CSS, meaning that a speech impaired CSS user should be as persuasive as a non impaired speaker using natural speech.

CONCLUSION

In this chapter, we reviewed an area of research relevant to the general issue of how people react to CSS. The reactions we focused on are social psychological in nature, including people's attitudes toward the CSS speaker, their attitudes toward the spoken message being conveyed, whether they believed the message was effective and whether they were persuaded by the message. When people are not informed about the disability status of the CSS speaker, then they rate natural speech more favorably than CSS. They trust the natural speaker more, they believe the natural speaker is more knowledgeable, they believe that the natural message is more convincing, etc., etc. They don't like CSS very much and they express negative attitudes toward CSS.

However, when the disability status of the CSS speaker is made overt, then attitudes on the part of listeners change (Stern et al., 2002). As mentioned above, a positive prejudice or a reverse discrimination effect may account for the reversal of attitudes toward CSS. In contrast to everyday situations where CSS in used in such applications as telephone interfaces, talking terminals, warning systems, voice mail, library retrieval, weather forecasts, etc. (Syrdal, 1995), when a listener is aware that a person is using a CSS system to speak because they have a disability, their reactions to CSS change dramatically. This is very important as a practical matter for individuals using VOCAs as AAC aids. Assuming that the attitude shifts observed in the laboratory extend to real-life situations, then the news for speech impaired users of CSS is good, in that listeners have a positive attitude towards them and the content of their utterances.

But it also appears that this "forgiveness" of CSS as used by a person with a disability can disappear under certain conditions. Stern et al. (2007) demonstrated that when a listener hears CSS from a person they know is disabled, negative attitudes toward CSS reappear if the CSS speaker is engaged in an activity people don't like (i.e., a telephone campaign). Most people do not like being solicited for money and bothered on the phone. As Stern et al. (2007) speculated, the prejudice and stereotyping of people with a disability that may exist in a person is allowed to re-emerge when there is a reason not to like the CSS user. Thus, situational variables may eliminate the positive prejudice effect Stern et al. (2002) observed. In future research, a variety of situational variables should be examined in order to form a more complete picture of the situations where speech from a CSS user with a disability is viewed negatively. This would be valuable information for users of CSS to possess.

In terms of the potential persuasiveness of CSS utterances, our research indicates that there is a tendency for CSS to be somewhat less persuasive than natural speech when measuring degree of persuasion as induced by a persuasive appeal. However, the difference is small and for all practical purposes not significant. This is an important finding because it suggests that a CSS user can be just as persuasive as a natural voice speaker when using CSS in such situations as business, industry and government, where one's job may include giving presentations that are designed to influence or convince people of an argument or issue. However, persuasion needs to be studied in situations that are more ecologically valid than hearing standard persuasive appeals in the laboratory. If similar results are found, then again this is positive news for disabled CSS users.

In this chapter, we also drew upon research examining people's general reactions to computers in order to place the issue of reactions to CSS and AAC into a larger context. Most VOCAs are bundled up in a computerized device of some sort. The work of Nass and his colleagues indicates that in many circumstances people view computers as similar to people in various ways, to the point of attributing human-like qualities to them (Lee et al., 2007; Moon & Nass, 1996; Nass & Lee, 2001). In terms of attitudes toward the CSS user, the question is whether people view CSS as emanating from the computer (the VOCA device) or whether they view CSS as emanating from the disabled person. In other words, to what degree is the impoverished quality and unnaturalness of CSS attributed to the user and not the device, or vice-versa? This is an issue that needs to be delineated. And in terms of social group processes, it is also possible that ingroup/outgroup processes are at work in terms of processing the social situation where a disabled CSS user interacts with a normal speaker (Stern et al., 2006). Further research on group processes and how they affect attitudes toward CSS would be fruitful to pursue.

In summary, to return to Light's (1996) assertion about communication being the essence of human life, there is no question that communication is a central part of our human existence. Communicative competence is critical to human development, interaction and the ability to enjoy life to its fullest. It is clear that there are also social psychological factors that affect how people on the receiving end of AAC speech output treat the speech from the user. Ultimately, these factors may prove just as important as the ability of the speech output from a VOCA to be highly intelligible and natural sounding, in terms of the usability issues for a person with a speech impairment who uses speech disabled user of CSS.

AUTHOR NOTE

Parts of the research discussed here were funded by grants to the author from the University of Pittsburgh Central Research and Development Fund and from the University of Pittsburgh at Johnstown Faculty Scholarship Grant Program.

REFERENCES

Anderson, R. J., & Antonak, R. F. (1992). The influence of attitudes and contact on reactions to persons with physical and speech disabilities. *Rehabilitation Counseling Bulletin*, *35*, 240–247.

Beck, A., & Dennis, M. (1996). Attitudes of children toward a similar-aged child who uses augmentative communication. *Augmentative and Alternative Communication*, *12*, 78–87. doi:10.1080/07434619612331277528

Beck, A. R., & Fritz-Verticchio, H. (2003). The influence of information and role-playing experiences on children's attitudes toward peers who use AAC. *American Journal of Speech-Language Pathology, 12*, 51–60. doi:10.1044/1058-0360(2003/052)

Bennett, W., & Runyah, C. (1982). Educator's perceptions of the effects of communication disorders upon educational performance. *Language, Speech, and Hearing Services in Schools, 13*, 260–263.

Beukelman, D. R. (1991). Magic and cost of communicative competence. *Augmentative and Alternative Communication, 7*, 2–10. doi:10.1080/07434619112331275633

Blockberger, S., Armstrong, R., O'Connor, A., & Freeman, R. (1993). Children's attitudes toward a nonspeaking child using various augmentative and alternative communication techniques. *Augmentative and Alternative Communication, 9*, 243–250. doi:10.1080/07434619312331276661

Carver, C. S., Glass, D. C., & Katz, I. (1978). Favorable evaluations of blacks and the handicapped: Positive prejudice, unconscious denial, or social desirability. *Journal of Applied Social Psychology, 8*, 97–106. doi:10.1111/j.1559-1816.1978.tb00768.x

Crandall, C. S., & Eshleman, A. (2003). A justification-expression model of the expression and experience of prejudice. *Psychological Bulletin, 119*, 414–446. doi:10.1037/0033-2909.129.3.414

Cruice, M., Worrall, L., & Hickson, L. (2006). Quantifying aphasic people's social lives in the context of non-aphasic peers. *Aphasiology, 20*, 1210–1225. doi:10.1080/02687030600790136

Duffy, S. A., & Pisoni, D. B. (1992). Comprehension of synthetic speech produced by rule: A review and theoretical interpretation. *Language and Speech, 35*, 351–389.

Elliot, T., & Frank, R. (1990). Social and interpersonal reactions to depression and disability. *Rehabilitation Psychology, 35*, 135–147.

Fucci, D., Reynolds, M. E., Bettagere, R., & Gonzales, M. D. (1995). Synthetic speech intelligibility under several experimental conditions. *Augmentative and Alternative Communication, 11*, 113–117. doi:10.1080/07434619512331277209

Fujiki, M., Brinton, B., Isaacson, T., & Summers, C. (2001). Social behaviors of children with language impairments on the playground: A pilot study. *Language, Speech, and Hearing Services in Schools, 32*, 101–113. doi:10.1044/0161-1461(2001/008)

Gertner, B., Rice, M., & Hadley, P. (1994). Influence of communicative competence on peer preferences in a preschool classroom. *Journal of Speech and Hearing Research, 37*, 913–923.

Gong, L., & Lai, J. (2003). To mix or not to mix synthetic speech and human speech? Contrasting impact on judge-rated task performance versus self-rated performance and attitudinal responses. *International Journal of Speech Technology, 6*, 123–131. doi:10.1023/A:1022382413579

Gong, L., & Nass, C. (2007). When a talking-face computer agent is half-human and half-humanoid: Human identity and consistency preference. *Human Communication Research, 33*, 163–193.

Gorenflo, C. W., & Gorenflo, D. W. (1991). The effects of information and augmentative communication technique on attitudes toward nonspeaking individuals. *Journal of Speech and Hearing Research, 34*, 19–26.

Gorenflo, C. W., Gorenflo, D. W., & Santer, S. A. (1994). Effects of synthetic voice output on attitudes toward the augmented communicator. *Journal of Speech and Hearing Research, 37*, 64–68.

Gorenflo, D. W., & Gorenflo, C. W. (1997). Effects of synthetic speech, gender, and perceived similarity on attitudes toward the augmented communicator. *Augmentative and Alternative Communication, 13*, 87–91. doi:10.1080/07434619712331277878

Harber, K. (1998). Feedback to minorities: Evidence of a positive bias. *Journal of Personality and Social Psychology, 74*, 622–628. doi:10.1037/0022-3514.74.3.622

Harper, D. C. (1999). Social psychology of difference: Stigma, spread, and stereotypes in childhood. *Rehabilitation Psychology, 44*, 131–144. doi:10.1037/0090-5550.44.2.131

Heinemann, W. (1990). Meeting the handicapped: A case of affective-cognitive inconsistency. In W. Stroebe & M. Hewstone (Eds.) *European review of social psychology,* (Vol.1, pp. 323-335). London: John Wiley.

Hilari, K., & Northcott, S. (2006). Social support in people with chronic aphasia. *Aphasiology, 20*, 17–36. doi:10.1080/02687030500279982

Koul, R. K., & Allen, G. D. (1993). Segmental intelligibility & speech interference thresholds of high-quality synthetic speech in the presence of noise. *Jrnl. of Speech & Hearing Rsrch., 36*, 790–798.

Lasker, J., & Beukelman, D. R. (1999). Peers' perceptions of storytelling by an adult with aphasia. *Aphasiology, 12*, 857–869.

Lee, J. R., Nass, C., Brave, S. B., Morishima, Y., Nakajima, H., & Yamada, R. (2007). The case for caring colearners: The effects of a computer-mediated colearner agent on trust and learning. *The Journal of Communication, 57*, 183–204. doi:10.1111/j.1460-2466.2007.00339.x

Light, J. (1996). "Communication is the essence of human life": Reflections on communicative competence. *Augmentative and Alternative Communication, 13*, 61–70. doi:10.1080/07434619712331277848

Lilienfeld, M., & Alant, E. (2002). Attitudes of children toward an unfamiliar peer using an AAC device with and without voice output. *Augmentative and Alternative Communication, 18*, 91–101. doi:10.1080/07434610212331281191

Logan, J. S., Greene, B. G., & Pisoni, D. B. (1989). Segmental intelligibility of synthetic speech produced by rule. *The Journal of the Acoustical Society of America, 86*, 566–581. doi:10.1121/1.398236

Luce, P. A., Feustel, T. C., & Pisoni, D. B. (1983). Capacity demands in short-term memory for natural and synthetic speech. *Human Factors, 25*, 17–32.

Makas, E. (1988). Positive attitudes toward disabled people: Disabled and nondisabled persons' perspectives. *The Journal of Social Issues, 44*, 49–62.

Marques, J. M., Yzerbyt, V. Y., & Leyens, J. P. (1988). The "black sheep effect": Extremity of judgments towards ingroup members as a function of group identification. *European Journal of Social Psychology, 18*, 1–16. doi:10.1002/ejsp.2420180102

McCarthy, J., & Light, J. (2005). Attitudes toward individuals who use augmentative and alternative communication: Research review. *Augmentative and Alternative Communication, 21*, 41–55. doi:10.1080/07434610410001699753

Mirenda, P. (2003). Toward functional augmentative and alternative communication for students with autism: Manual signs, graphic symbols, and voice output communication aids. *Language, Speech, and Hearing Services in Schools, 34*, 203–216. doi:10.1044/0161-1461(2003/017)

Mirenda, P., & Beukelman, D. R. (1987). A comparison of speech synthesis intelligibility with listeners from three age groups. *Augmentative and Alternative Communication, 5*, 84–88.

Mirenda, P., & Beukelman, D. R. (1990). A comparison of intelligibility among natural speech and seven speech synthesizers with listeners from three age groups. *Augmentative and Alternative Communication*, *6*, 61–68. doi:10.1080/07434619012331275324

Moon, Y., & Nass, C. (1996). How "real" are computer personalities? Psychological responses to personality types in human-computer interaction. *Communication Research*, *23*, 651–674. doi:10.1177/009365096023006002

Mullennix, J. W., Stern, S. E., Wilson, S. J., & Dyson, C. (2003). Social perception of male and female computer synthesized speech. *Computers in Human Behavior*, *19*, 407–424. doi:10.1016/S0747-5632(02)00081-X

Nass, C., & Brave, S. (2005). *Wired for speech: How voice activates and advances the human-computer relationship*. Cambridge, MA: MIT Press.

Nass, C., Fogg, B. J., & Moon, Y. (1996). Can computers be teammates? *International Journal of Human-Computer Studies*, *45*, 669–678. doi:10.1006/ijhc.1996.0073

Nass, C., & Lee, K. M. (2001). Does computer-synthesized speech manifest personality? Experimental tests of recognition, similarity-attraction, and consistency-attraction. *Journal of Experimental Psychology. Applied*, *7*, 171–181. doi:10.1037/1076-898X.7.3.171

Nass, C., & Moon, Y. (2000). Machines and mindlessness: Social responses to computers. *The Journal of Social Issues*, *56*, 81–103. doi:10.1111/0022-4537.00153

Petty, R. E., & Cacioppo, J. T. (1986). *Communication and persuasion*. New York: Springer.

Popich, E., & Alant, E. (1997). Interaction between a teacher and the non-speaking as well as speaking children in the classroom. *The South African Journal of Communication Disorders*, *44*, 31–40.

Ralston, J. V., Pisoni, D. B., & Mullennix, J. W. (1995). Perception and comprehension of speech. In A. Syrdal, R. Bennet, & S. Greenspan (Eds.), *Applied speech technology* (pp. 233-288). Boca Raton, FL: CRC Press.

Reeves, B., & Nass, C. (1996). *The media equation: How people treat computers, television, and new media like real people and places*. New York: Cambridge University Press/CSLI.

Rice, M., Hadley, P., & Alexander, A. (1993). Social bases towards children with speech and language impairments: A correlative causal model of language limitations. *Applied Psycholinguistics*, *14*, 445–471. doi:10.1017/S0142716400010699

Romski, M. A., & Sevcik, R. A. (2000). Children and adults who experience difficulty with speech. In D. Braithwaite & T. Thompson (Eds.), *Handbook of communication and people with disabilities: Research and application* (pp. 439-449). Hillsdale, NJ: Erlbaum.

Rosselli, F., Skelly, J. J., & Mackie, D. M. (1995). Processing rational and emotional messages: The cognitive and affective mediation of persuasion. *Journal of Experimental Social Psychology*, *31*, 163–190. doi:10.1006/jesp.1995.1008

Ruscello, D., Stutler, S., & Toth, D. (1983). Classroom teachers' attitudes towards children with articulatory disorders. *Perceptual and Motor Skills*, *57*, 527–530.

Sigelman, C. K., Adams, R. M., Meeks, S. R., & Purcell, M. A. (1986). Children's nonverbal responses to a physically disabled person. *Journal of Nonverbal Behavior*, *10*, 173–186. doi:10.1007/BF00987614

Simmons-Mackie, N. N., & Damico, J. S. (2007). Access and social inclusion in aphasia: Interactional principles and applications. *Aphasiology*, *21*, 81–97. doi:10.1080/02687030600798311

Snyder, M. L., Kleck, R. E., Strenta, A., & Mentzer, S. J. (1979). Avoidance of the handicapped: An attributional ambiguity analysis. *Journal of Personality and Social Psychology*, *37*, 2297–2306. doi:10.1037/0022-3514.37.12.2297

Stern, S. E. (2008). Computer-synthesized speech and the perceptions of the social influence of disabled users. *Journal of Language and Social Psychology*, *27*, 254–265. doi:10.1177/0261927X08318035

Stern, S. E., Dumont, M., Mullennix, J. W., & Winters, M. L. (2007). Positive prejudice towards disabled persons using synthesized speech: Does the effect persist across contexts? *Journal of Language and Social Psychology*, *26*, 363–380. doi:10.1177/0261927X07307008

Stern, S. E., & Mullennix, J. W. (2004). Sex differences in persuadability of human and computer-synthesized speech: Meta-analysis of seven studies. *Psychological Reports*, *94*, 1283–1292. doi:10.2466/PR0.94.3.1283-1292

Stern, S. E., Mullennix, J. W., Dyson, C., & Wilson, S. J. (1999). The persuasiveness of synthetic speech versus human speech. *Human Factors*, *41*, 588–595. doi:10.1518/001872099779656680

Stern, S. E., Mullennix, J. W., & Wilson, S. J. (2002). Effects of perceived disability on persuasiveness of computer synthesized speech. *The Journal of Applied Psychology*, *87*, 411–417. doi:10.1037/0021-9010.87.2.411

Stern, S. E., Mullennix, J. W., & Yaroslavsky, I. (2006). Persuasion and social perception of human vs. synthetic voice across person as source and computer as source conditions. *International Journal of Human-Computer Studies*, *64*, 43–52. doi:10.1016/j.ijhcs.2005.07.002

Sundar, S. S., & Nass, C. (2000). Source orientation in human-computer interaction: Programmer, networker, or independent social actor? *Communication Research*, *27*, 683–703. doi:10.1177/009365000027006001

Syrdal, A. K. (1995). Text-to-speech systems. In A.K. Syrdal, R. Bennet, & S. Greenspan (Eds.), *Applied speech technology* (pp. 99-126). Boca Raton, FL: CRC Press.

Tajfel, H. (1978). *Differentiation between groups: Studies in the social psychology of intergroup relations*. London: Academic Press.

Wegener, D. T., & Petty, R. E. (1997). The flexible correction model: The role of naive theories of bias in bias correction. In M. P. Zanna (Ed.) *Advances in experimental social psychology* (Vol 29, pp. 141-208). New York: Academic Press.

Weitzel, A. (2000). Overcoming loss of voice. In D. O. Braithwaite & T. L. Thompson, (Eds.), *Handbook of communication and people with disabilities: Research and application,* (pp. 451-466). Mahwah, NJ: Erlbaum.

Wolsko, C., Park, B., Judd, C. M., & Wittenbrink, B. (2000). Framing interethnic ideology: Effects of multicultural and colorblind perspectives of judgments of groups and individuals. *Journal of Personality and Social Psychology*, *78*, 635–654. doi:10.1037/0022-3514.78.4.635

Chapter 14
Stereotypes of People with Physical Disabilities and Speech Impairments as Detected by Partially Structured Attitude Measures

Steven E. Stern
University of Pittsburgh at Johnstown, USA

John W. Mullennix
University of Pittsburgh at Johnstown, USA

Ashley Davis Fortier
University of Pittsburgh at Johnstown, USA

Elizabeth Steinhauser
Florida Institute of Technology, USA

ABSTRACT

Partially Structured Attitude Measures (PSAMs) are non-reaction-time based measures of implicit attitudes. Participants' attitudes are measured by the degree to which they react toward ambiguous stimuli. The authors developed a series of PSAMs to examine six stereotypes of people with disabilities: asexual, unappealing, isolated, dependent, entitled, and unemployable. In two studies, they found that PSAMs detected implicit endorsements of stereotypes toward people with a physical disability, speech impairment, or combination of the two. Compared to people without disabilities, stereotypes were endorsed for people with disabilities, with unappealing, dependent and unemployable being more prominent for physically disabled targets and dependent, entitled and isolated being more prominent for speech disabled targets. Implications for understanding the stereotyping of people with physical and speech disabilities are discussed.

DOI: 10.4018/978-1-61520-725-1.ch014

INTRODUCTION

Disability has been long recognized as a stigmatized condition in our society (Goffman, 1963; Green, Davis, Karshmer, Marsh, & Straight, 2005). There is anecdotal as well as experimental evidence that people are prone to avoid, physically distance themselves from, speak down to, and experience psychological discomfort when interacting with people with physical disabilities (Comer & Piliavin, 1972; Crawford & Ostrove, 2003; Hart & Williams, 1995; Hebl & Kleck, 2000; Hebl, Tickle, & Heatherton, 2000; Olkin & Howson, 1994; Snyder, Kleck, Strenta, & Mentzer, 1979). The psychological discomfort can manifest itself in motoric inhibition (Comer & Piliavin, 1972; Kleck, Ono, & Hastorf, 1966), verbal inhibition (Kleck, Ono, & Hastorf, 1966), and arousal as detected by Galvanic Skin Response (Kleck, Ono, & Hastorf, 1966). Able bodied and people with disabilities report that interactions between the two are often awkward and unbalanced (Hebl, Tickle, & Heatherton, 2000; Makas, 1988) and people with disabilities report that they are frequently treated as if they were invisible (Crawford & Ostrove, 2003). Some people with disabilities report able bodied people respond to them with oversolicitiousness (Hart & Williams, 1995), which is tantamount to being treated as a permanent child (Phillips, 1985).

Speech impairment is also stigmatized (Weitzel, 2000). Interestingly, there is evidence that people with speech impairments are less accepted and less liked in comparison to the people with physical disabilities (Anderson & Antonak, 1992). People with communication disabilities find themselves excluded from participating in activities that involve communicating and experience a highly debilitating loss of power and leverage in the speaking world (Simmons-Mackie & Damico, 2007). They also have fewer social contacts than able-bodied people (Cruice, Worrall, & Hickson, 2006; Hilari & Northcott, 2006).

Stigmatized groups that are relegated to outgroup status are frequently subjected to stereotyping. The influential social and personality psychologist, Gordon Allport (1958) among others stressed that people tend to categorize themselves and others like themselves into ingroups and people unlike themselves into outgroups. In turn, members of an outgroup tend to be seen as sharing similar psychological and physical attributes with each other. This process of automatic categorization and subsequent generalizations can be seen as a heuristic or mental shortcut that makes it possible to make quicker decisions regarding people based upon their group membership (Fiske, 2005).

As with many heuristics, stereotyping becomes more likely when a person is cognitively busy (Gilbert & Hixon, 1991). Of particular importance when considering the experience of computer synthesized speech (CSS) users, there is evidence that listening to CSS involves using more cognitive resources on the part of the listener (Luce, Feustel, & Pisoni, 1983; Ralston, Pisoni, & Mullennix, 1995). Taken together, these findings suggest that while CSS is designed to aid people with speech impairments to communicate more effectively, it might simultaneously and unintentionally promote stereotyping by the listener.

The present study is focused on the specific stereotypes that able bodied persons hold toward people with disabilities. While much research on attitudes toward the disabled has focused on the measurement of global attitudes toward disability (e.g., Yuker & Block, 1986) or the distinction between affective, cognitive, and behavioral components of attitudes toward the disabled (Findler, Vilchinsky, & Werner, 2007), there has been less of a concerted effort to examine the specific stereotypes that are frequently applied toward people with disabilities, particularly people with physical disabilities. In the present research, we identified specific stereotypes in the disability literature, selected six that were particularly prominent, and used both measures of explicit and measures of implicit attitudes to detect these stereotypes.

STEREOTYPES OF DISABLED PERSONS

Although few studies have catalogued specific stereotypes of people with disabilities, a review of the literature reveals numerous stereotypes that are commonly held about people with physical disabilities. We have grouped those that we believe to be synonymous. We focused on six stereotypes that were prominent in the literature.

- Socially isolated or lonely (Fichten & Amsel, 1986; Fichten, Robillard, Judd, & Amsel, 1989; Schwartz, 1999)
- Asexual (Crawford & Ostrove, 2003 Fichten, Robillard, & Judd, 1989; Fine & Asch, 1988; Howland & Rintala, 2001; Schwartz, 1999)
- Unemployable or likely to pose difficulties in the workplace (Colella & Varma, 1999; Gouvier, Sytsma-Jordan, & Mayville, 2003; Louvet, 2007; Schwartz, 1999; Stone & Colella, 1996)
- Dependent or helpless (Abrams, Jackson & St. Claire, 1990; Fichten & Amsel, 1986; Fine & Asch, 1988; Phillips, 1985)
- Self pitying or having a sense of entitlement (Fichten & Bourdon, 1986; Fine & Asch, 1988; Furnham & Thompson, 1994; Phillips, 1985)
- Unappealing (Fichten & Amsel, 1986; Fine & Asch, 1988; Schwartz, 1999)

There were other stereotypes that were identified that we did not examine, but are worth noting.

- Weak (Phillips, 1985)
- Passive (Phillips, 1985)
- Incompetent (Crawford & Ostrove, 2003; Fiske, Cuddy, Glick, & Xu, 2002)
- Mentally challenged (Crawford & Ostrove, 2003)
- Depressed (Elliott, et al., 1990; Fichten & Amsel, 1986)
- Silent (Fichten & Amsel, 1986)

It should also be noted that although we are focusing on negative stereotypes, some researchers have identified positive stereotypes that people have toward those with disabilities. Fichten and Amsel (1986) identified six positive stereotypes: quiet, honest, gentle hearted, softhearted, non-egotistical and undemanding. These stereotypes are consistent with the Stereotype Content Model (Fiske et al, 2002) which suggests that people with disabilities are viewed as incompetent yet warm. In contrast, Gregory (1998) reported that people with disabilities are sometimes stereotyped as super capable owing to their assumed capacity to overcome adversity.

PARTIALLY STRUCTURED ATTITUDE MEASURES AS MEASURES OF IMPLICIT ATTITUDES

During the last several years, researchers have made numerous advancements in the measurement of implicit attitudes, particularly attitudes such as prejudice and stereotyping, which are not considered socially acceptable (Crandall & Eshleman, 2003), and in turn, are highly inhibited (Maas, Castelli, & Arcuri, 2000) because they are inconsistent with other values (e.g., egalitarianism) that people hold important (Rudman, 2004). While many measures of implicit attitudes, such as the Implicit Attitude Test citation (IAT; Greenwald, McGhee, & Schwartz, 1998) are dependent upon sensitive measurements such as reaction time, it is possible to measure underlying attitudes without complex technological apparatus. Vargas, von Hippel and Petty (2004) reintroduced Cook and Selltiz's (1964) Partially Structured Attitude Measure (PSAMs). According to the logic of the PSAM, participants are presented with ambiguous

Figure 1. Illustration of expected responses for implicit PSAM responses versus explicit measure responses.

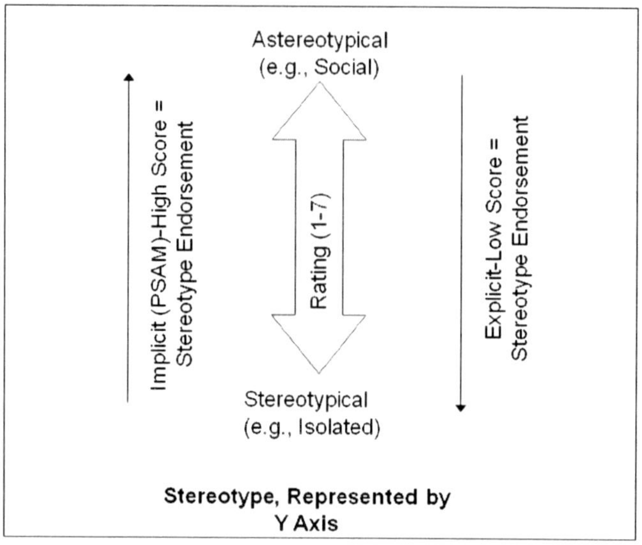

stimuli and the dependent measure becomes the degree to which they react against it.

For example, in the work described here, participants were presented with a photograph of a person with a physical disability while a recorded audio statement was played. The audio statements were ambiguous in terms of stereotype-relevant information, containing both stereotype consistent information (suggesting "isolated") and stereotype inconsistent information (suggesting "social"). Then participants were asked to rate the person with a disability on a semantic differential scale anchored at "social" and "isolated." It was expected that if the person holds the stereotype that people with disabilities are more isolated than people without disabilities, they will react to the stereotype inconsistent information (social) and rate the person with a disability as more social than they would rate a person without a disability. It is as if they are rating him to be social *for* a person with a disability. Figure 1 is an illustration of what is expected from PSAM responses versus explicit responses.

As an implicit measure, PSAMs are different from many other implicit measures in that they are not dependent upon reaction time. There are a number of qualities that a test could have that would lead one to consider it to be implicit instead of explicit. De Houwer and Moors (2007) have suggested that a measure is implicit if it examines a construct "by virtue of processes that are uncontrolled, unintentional, goal-independent, purely stimulus-driven, autonomous, efficient, or fast" (p. 14). Consistent with this definition, PSAMs measure processes that are goal-independent and unintentional. In other words, when attitudes are examined using PSAMs, participants are not fully aware of the motivation behind their response. In their examination of PSAMs, Vargas et al. (2004) found that they were useful in the prediction of behavior when social desirability was an issue, and only moderately correlated to explicit measures, as we would expect with most implicit measures of attitudes.

THE PRESENT STUDIES

We conducted two experiments in which PSAMs were employed to examine six stereotypes of people with disabilities: being asexual, unappealing, dependent, isolated, unemployable, and having a sense of entitlement. We examined whether they would be endorsed implicitly with ratings in the opposite direction of the stereotype. We also examined how they applied to physical disability as well as speech disability.

More specifically, we examined closely the content of stereotypes held for people with disabilities and how different types of disability are viewed. By including an assessment of six different stereotypes in one study, we present a comprehensive approach to the issue. This is in contrast to more exploratory studies examining a more diverse selection of impressions people have toward those with disabilities. Furthermore, our design allows us to examine two types of disability separately and in combination. Stereotypes of people with disabilities may vary with the perceived level of disability or may vary substantially based on attributions people make when seeing a person in a wheelchair versus using an assistive aid to speak. It is important to determine the nature of any differences that exist in attitudes expressed toward different disabilities.

Figure 2. Sample photographs of target in disabled and non-disabled conditions used in both studies.

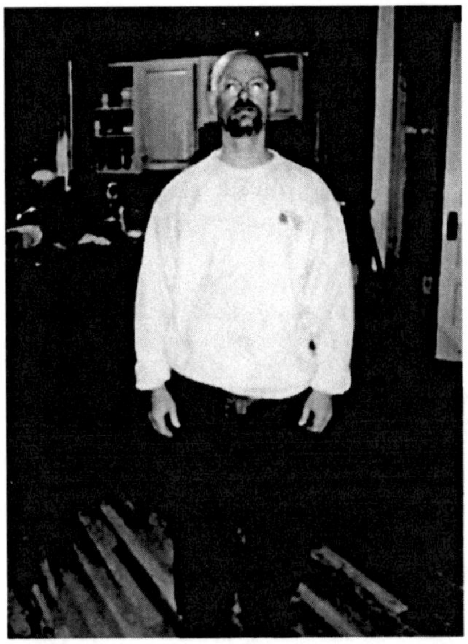

(a)

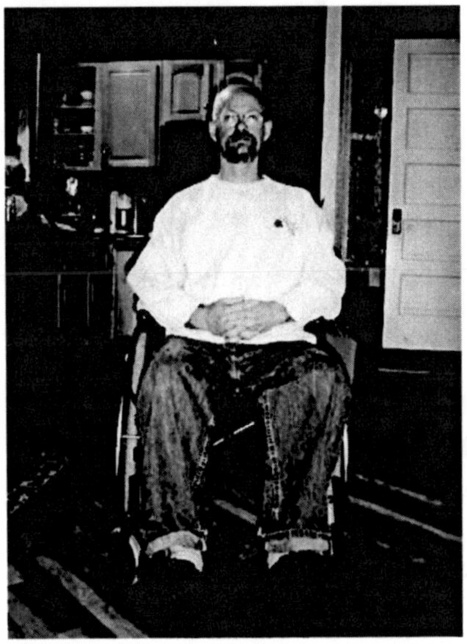

(b)

Study 1

In Study 1 we examined the utility of PSAMs to assess stereotypes toward people with disabilities. The design allowed us to examine how participants react to disabled targets compared to non-disabled targets. We also compared an explicit measure of stereotyping with the implicit PSAM data. It was hypothesized that, for each of the disability-related stereotypes, there would be an interaction whereby (a) in the explicit condition, targets' disability status (i.e., disabled or non-disabled) would make little difference in the ratings while (b) in the implicit (PSAM) conditions disabled targets would be rated with stronger endorsements of stereotypes than non-disabled targets.

A total of 102 undergraduates (70 males; 32 females; mean age = 18.51) undergraduates participated in the first study. The stimuli included audio stimuli and photographs. All human voice samples were recorded using SoundForge, a high-end sound recording and editing program. Four photographs of two male targets, each posing as both able-bodied and disabled, were taken with commercially available digital cameras (see Figure 2 for sample photographs of one of the targets

Table 1. Stereotype ambiguous and stereotype irrelevant statements used in all three studies (Stereotype ambiguous statements are italicized)

ASEXUAL/DOES NOT HAVE SEX
My mother makes the best chicken and broccoli casserole, and her carrot cake is delicious.
I spend time mostly with relatives and friends. Sheryl has become my closest friend for the last two months. I'm thinking of asking her out, although I've never had a long-term girlfriend.
Christmas is my favorite holiday. My neighborhood looks very beautiful when it's all lit up.
UNAPPEALING
I enjoy listening to music. I like almost every type of music.
I often question my attractiveness. I feel as though I'm not handsome, but women have told me they find me cute.
I have one sister and one brother. I'm the middle child.
DEPENDENT
I enjoy reading. My favorite author is Stephen King.
My parents often given me money and cook my meals, although I really can take care of myself and always make sure to pay them back.
I enjoy playing trivia games and playing cards.
ENTITLED
I like to watch football on Sundays.
I can complete most takes without any assistance but when someone needs helps, I think other people should help them out.
My favorite movie is War of the Worlds. The special effects are really awesome.
ISOLATED
I enjoy looking up at the starts on a clear night. I always thought it would be neat to learn astronomy.
I often go out to dinner with family and go to the mall with friends, but it seems like I spend most of my time alone.
I am not a big fan of fast-food. I prefer home cooked meals.
UNEMPLOYABLE
I enjoy watching snow fall. It fascinates me how every snowflake is different.
I have recently gotten a job, but I've been unemployed for most of my life. Finding a job was a difficult task and I really hope I can keep it.
I can complete most tasks without any assistance but when someone needs help, I think other people should help them out.

in the disabled and non-disabled conditions). All audio and visual materials were presented to participants on IBM-PC compatible computers. E-Prime software was used to present experimental materials to the participants as well as to collect responses and demographic data.

For this research we created six statements, each pertaining directly to one of the six stereotypes. These statements were designed specifically to be ambiguous, in terms of stereotype-relevant information. Twelve neutral statements were created as well. For each stereotype, the ambiguous stereotype-relevant statement was sandwiched in between two neutral statements. All statements were recorded by a male speaker. Table 1 displays all of the statements used in the study.

First, the slide show introduced the target of evaluation. After participants were introduced to the target, in order to better activate stereotypes of people with physical disabilities, participants were requested to spend one minute imagining a day in the life of the target (see Gilbert & Hixon, 1991). During this one minute interval, the keyboard was not functional. Participants in the disabled condition were also told that the target had suffered from a stroke. This change was intended to strengthen the disability status manipulation.

Next, for each of the six stereotypes, the slideshow presented audio clips of statements while showing a still image of the target, followed by a semantic differential scale pertaining directly to the stereotype related to the recorded statement. The six scales were as follows: does not have sex-has sex, unappealing-appealing, dependent-independent, entitled-satisfied, isolated-social, unemployable-employable.

The first study was a 2 (status of target: non-disabled vs. disabled) X 2 (ambiguous statement: absent vs. present) design with six separate dependent variables. The purpose of the ambiguous statement variable was to ascertain that the reverse pattern of stereotyping expected from the partially structured stimuli (PSAM's) was different than how participants responded normally to the target.

For each participant, the target as well as the target's disability status was held constant. In the first slide of the slideshow, the participant viewed a picture of the target who is introduced as Jamie Ryan, a 35 year old male. Depending upon the condition, he is either portrayed as a person with a physical disability (appearing in a wheelchair) or able bodied, with no other information given.

For each of the six stereotypes, participants were presented with a photograph of the target and depending upon condition heard either all three statements pertaining to the stereotype (stereotype ambiguous statement sandwiched in between two neutral statements) or just the two neutral statements. All participants were debriefed as to the nature of the study after they completed the tasks.

As shown by comparing Figure 3a (implicit endorsements) to Figure 3b (explicit endorsements), the study provided substantial support that the presence of the ambiguous statement led participants to react against the stereotype inconsistent information. In focused contrasts (*t*s) comparing the pattern of means between participants in the explicit conditions (that did not have the ambiguous statements) and the participants in the implicit conditions (who did have the ambiguous statements), there was a significant effect in the predicted direction for four of the six dependent variables (see Table 2). Specifically, participants who had read the PSAM statements implicitly endorsed the stereotypes while participants who did not have the ambiguous PSAM statements explicitly endorsed the stereotypes or simply rated the disabled targets the same as the non-disabled targets.

Table 2. Focused comparisons (ts) testing hypothesized difference between explicit and implicit conditions in Study 1.

	$t_{contrast}$	*p(one-tailed)**	*r*
Does Not Have Sex	5.89	<.001	.51
Unappealing	1.19	>.05,n.s.	.12
Dependent	7.15	<.001	.59
Entitled	5.01	<.001	.45
Isolated	.08	>.05,n.s.	.01
Unemployable	2.02	.02	.20

*Degrees of freedom and mean square error term are taken from entire ANOVA design

Study 2

Having established the expected pattern of implicit responding to PSAMs in the detection of stereotypes of physically disabled targets, we designed Study 2 to expand the scope of disability.

Figure 3. (a) Implicit PSAM ratings of stereotype endorsement for disabled and non-disabled targets (Study 1); (b) Explicit ratings of stereotype endorsement for disabled and non-disabled targets (Study 1).

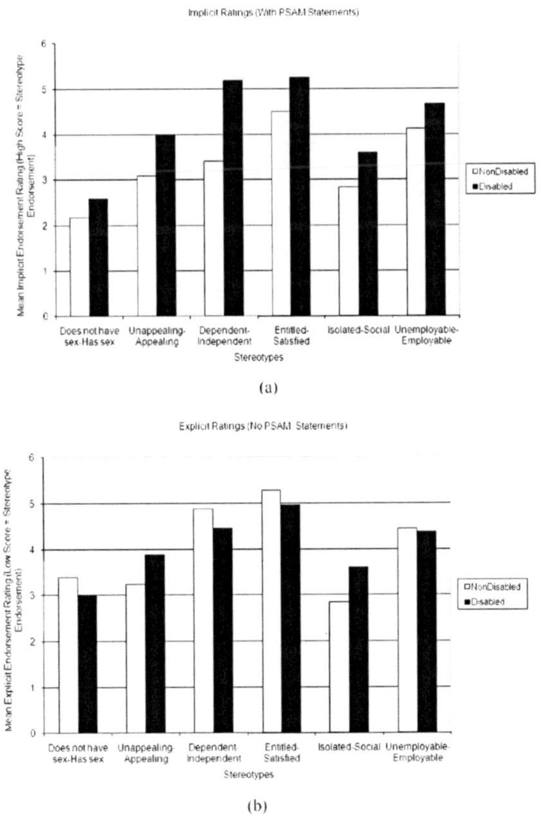

We examined whether the stereotypes endorsed for a physically disabled target in a wheelchair found in Study 1 would also apply to a speech impaired target and a target with both speech and physical disabilities. Unlike Study 1, we did not examine explicit endorsement of the stereotypes. We hypothesized that implicit endorsements of the stereotypes would be stronger for each of the three types of disabled targets (speech disabled, physically disabled, both speech and physically disabled) compared to the non-disabled targets. For the sake of simplicity, at this point we are using the terms speech impairment and speech disability interchangeably.

A total of 178 undergraduates (69 males; 109 females; mean age = 19.66) participated in this study. To create realistic speech disability and full disability (speech and physical disability combined) conditions, we added stimuli produced with DecTalk, a professional level computerized speech synthesizer typically used by people with speech disabilities. In the photographs used in the speech disability conditions (see Figure 4), the target is wearing a LightWRITER device on a strap around his neck. LightWRITER is a frequently used keyboard like interface designed for disabled users of synthetic speech. In the full disabled condition, the target is sitting in a wheelchair as well as wearing a LightWRITER.

Study 2 was an extension Study 1, inasmuch as in Study 1 only physical disablement (as illustrated by a person sitting in a wheelchair) was examined. In Study 2, a speech disabled condition was added, where the target was wearing a synthetic speech interface and the statements were presented using synthetic speech. And a "fully disabled" condition was added, where the target was sitting in a wheelchair and using synthetic speech. Because Study 1 had demonstrated that stereotypes of the disabled could be detected with PSAMs, all of the conditions contained the ambiguous statements.

Study 2 was a 2 (physical disability: disabled vs. non-disabled) X 2 (speech disability: disabled vs. non-disabled) design. This resulted in four conditions: a non-disabled condition, a physically disabled only condition, a speech disabled only condition, and a condition where the target had both types of disabilities.

Figure 4. Sample photographs of target in speech disabled and fully (physically and speech disabled) conditions used in Study 2.

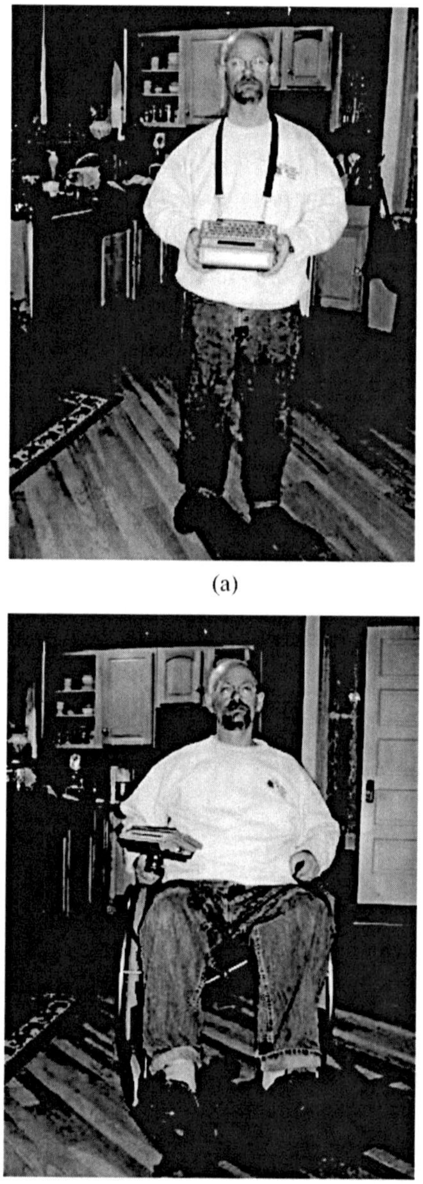

(a)

(b)

Study 2 extended Study 1 by comparing reactions to the non-disabled target to three disabled targets representing physical disability, speech disability, or the combination of the two. A series of 2 (physical disability: disabled vs. non-disabled) X 2 (speech disability: disabled vs. non-disabled) ANOVAs revealed that participants endorsed the stereotypes more for the disabled targets than the non-disabled targets. Table 3 details the outcomes of the significance tests.

An examination of the main effects for physical disability showed that at or near statistically significant levels, stereotypes were implicitly endorsed more for the physically disabled targets than non-physically disabled targets for three of six dependent variables: unappealing (F (1, 174) = 4.00, p = .05, *eta* = .15), dependent (F (1, 174) = 3.42, p = .07, *eta* = .14), and unemployable (F (1, 174) = 6.37, p = .01, *eta* = .19).

The main effects for speech disability showed that three of the six stereotypes were implicitly endorsed more for the speech disabled targets than the non-speech disabled targets: dependent (F (1, 174) = 10.73, p = .001, *eta* = .24), entitled (F (1, 174) = 6.82, p = .01, *eta* = .19), and isolated (F (1, 174) = 4.58, p = .03, *eta* = .16).

There were significant interactions between the two variables for three of the six dependent measures: entitled, isolated, and unemployable. For all three of these variables, as shown in Figure 5, stereotypes were more strongly endorsed for speech disabled targets than for fully (with both disabilities) disabled targets. For one stereotype, unemployable, stereotypes were endorsed for both the physically and speech disabled targets than for the fully disabled targets.

To specifically test the hypothesis that each of the three types of disabled targets (physically

Table 3. Significance tests for main effects and interactions for Study 2.

	Main Effect for Physical Disability			Main Effect for Speech Disability			Interaction		
	F	p	r	F	p(one-tailed)	r	F	p(one-tailed)	r
Does Note Have Sex	.04	>.05,n.s.	.02	.21	>.05,n.s.	**.03**	1.37	>.05,n.s.	.09
Unappealing	4.00	.05	.15	2.17	>.05,n.s.	**.11**	1.80	>.05,n.s.	.10
Dependent	3.42	.07	.14	10.73	.001	**.24**	2.01	>.05,n.s.	.10
Entitled	.68	>.05,n.s.	.06	6.82	.01	**.19**	9.23	.003	.22
Isolated	.54	>.05,n.s.	.06	4.58	.03	**.16**	6.75	.01	.19
Unemployable	6.37	.01	.19	.06	>.05,n.s.	**.02**	17.17	<.001	.30

Table 4. Simple effects tests (contrast ts) examining difference between non-disabled and diabled targets.

	NonDisabled vs. Physically Disabled			NonDisabled vs. Speech Disabled			NonDisabled vs. Both Disabilities		
	t	p	r	t	p	r	t	p	r
Does Not have Sex	1.05	>.05,n.s	.08	1.29*	.10	**.10**	.48	>.05,n.s.	.04
Unappealing	2.63	.005	.20	2.20	.01	**.16**	2.70	.004	.20
Dependent	2.56	.006	.19	3.69	<.001	**.27**	4.05	<.001	.29
Entitled	3.09	.001	.23	4.48	<.001	**.32**	2.73	.003	.20
Isolated	2.68	.004	.20	3.76	<.001	**.27**	2.28	.01	.17
Unemployable	5.30	<.001	.37	3.48	<.001	**.26**	2.20	.01	.16

*Marginally Significant in opposite of predicted directions

Figure 5. Implicit PSAM ratings of stereotype endorsement for non-disabled, physically disabled, speech disabled, and full-disabled (Study 2).

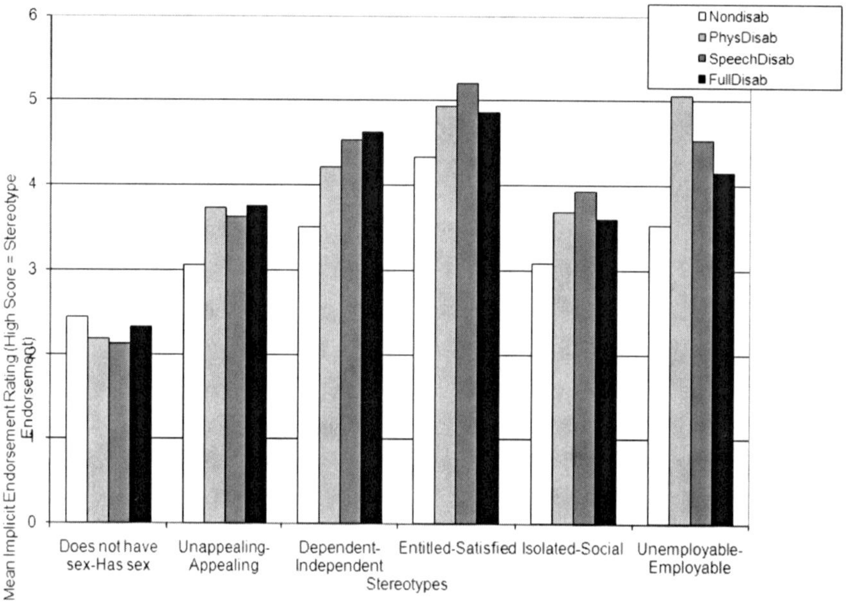

disabled, speech disabled, and both physically and speech disabled) would garner stronger endorsements of the stereotypes, for each stereotype we conducted simple effects tests comparing the non-disabled group to each of the three other groups. As shown in Table 4, except for asexual, stereotypes were endorsed significantly higher for each of the three disabled targets in comparison to the non disabled targets.

CONCLUSION

In this series of studies, we detected evidence for six specific implicit stereotypes of disability that had been documented in the previous literature. More specifically, we demonstrated that our participants expected a disabled target to be more asexual, isolated, dependent, unappealing, entitled, and unemployable than a non-disabled target. We further demonstrated that these stereotypes held for both speech and physical disability.

While not hypothesized, it is interesting to note that different patterns of stereotyping emerged for people with physical and speech disabilities. This raises interesting questions that merit further attention. Our data suggests, for instance, that people with speech disabilities may be stereotyped as more isolated than people with physical disabilities while the reverse pattern may hold true for stereotyping of unemployability. These are issues that beget further examination for a more complete understanding of stereotypes of disabled persons.

The PSAMs we developed detected the presence of a stereotype in our population. We cannot, however, assert that the PSAMs, predict explicit attitudes or behavior of participants. This is a criticism that has been held for numerous implicit measures.

How people perceive and potentially stereotype people with disabilities can have wide ranging implications. Although there is increasing societal and legal concern with the fair treatment of people with disabilities (e.g., the Americans with Disabilities Act in the U.S.), perceptions of how people with specific types of disability may fit into specific occupations still affect how employees are hired and evaluated at their jobs (Colella & Varma, 1999; Gouvier, Sytsma-Jordan,& Mayville, 2003; Louvet, 2007). Hence a more informed understanding of stereotypes of specific disabilities may help to better understand and ameliorate these issues in occupational and other settings.

This research has focused mainly on the content of stereotypes of people with disabilities. We have not examined issues regarding the processes by which they are stereotyped, and to recognized that these processes have an effect on the content of stereotypes. The content of stereotypes is subject to change over the course of time (Fiske et al., 2002). Stereotypes based upon race (e.g., African American) or religion (e.g., Jewish) have changed immensely during the last century. These are encouraging issues to consider, inasmuch as we can see that these types of potentially harmful attitudes are neither immutable nor inevitable.

It is important to consider that our understanding of stereotyping of people with disabilities is limited in comparison with how well we understand stereotyping of people based upon other characteristics such as race, gender, and nationality. This is partially because less attention has been paid to stereotypes of people with disabilities. There are, however, some factors that make it difficult to infer that the same processes involved in racial stereotyping are involved in stereotyping of people with disabilities. Unlike race, for instance, level of disability can change during our lives, disability can be temporary or long lasting, disability can be more easily masked in some cases. It is also possible that for many people with disabilities, their disabled status may not engender a group identity.

In the research discussed here, we have focused mainly on negative stereotypes. Whether stereotypes are negative (e.g., unemployable) or positive (e.g., gentlehearted) they can be problematic for the target of these attitudes. Inasmuch as stereotypes are frequently blanket generalizations, they are prone to inaccuracy when applied to individual. Furthermore, stereotypes can run the risk of being both descriptive, describing how people are viewed, and prescriptive, describing how people are expected to behave. When people with disabilities are not only seen in terms of limitations, but are expected to remain limited, the potential repercussions are particularly negative.

Combined with the results from our research on attitudes toward CSS users (see Chapter 13, this volume), the work presented here can help us understand, if not predict and work to change peoples' reactions to people with disabilities. In both bodies of research we have found evidence that people can hold negative attitudes toward people with disabilities that they are not necessarily aware of. This finding is clearly corroborated by the abundant reports from people with disabilities that they are treated differently than people without disabilities, and are frequently avoided.

And with respect to specific issues concerning CSS users with speech impairments, the present findings suggest that people with speech impairments are subject to stereotyping, with stereotypes related to dependency, entitlement and isolation perhaps even stronger than what one would see with a person with a non-speech related physical disability. In terms of people's attitudes toward CSS users, this stereotyping is an important factor that should be understood by CSS users, their family, their caretakers and the professionals who work with them. People need to understand the social dynamics at work that may influence a person's interactions with a CSS user who is using CSS as an AAC speaking aid. And people need to realize that a person interacting with an AAC user may not be consciously aware of stereotypes they may unwittingly apply toward the CSS user. The more we understand about the social factors that affect these interactions, the better we can help the CSS user be effective at communicating.

ACKNOWLEDGMENT

We would like to express our gratitude to the Pennsylvania Assistive Technology Lending Library at Temple University for loaning us an augmentative communications system, and the courteous and helpful staff at the Hiram G. Andrews Center in Johnstown, PA for their consistent support of our efforts. Numerous undergraduate students, including Ben Grounds, Donald Horvath, Robert Kalas, Eric May, and Brian Tessmer provided invaluable assistance to us. We are also grateful to the people who posed for the target photographs. This research was funded by grants from both the University of Pittsburgh and the University of Pittsburgh at Johnstown.

REFERENCES

Abrams, D., Jackson, D., & St. Claire, L. (1990). Social identity and the handicapping functions of stereotypes: Children's understanding of mental and physical handicap. *Human Relations*, *43*, 1085–1098. doi:10.1177/001872679004301103

Allport, G. W. (1958). *The nature of prejudice*. Garden City, NY: Doubleday.

Anderson, R. J., & Antonak, R. F. (1992). The influence of attitudes and contact on reactions to persons with physical and speech disabilities. *Rehabilitation Counseling Bulletin*, *35*, 240–247.

Colella, A., & Varma, A. (1999). Disability-job fit stereotypes and the evaluation of persons with disabilities at work. *Journal of Occupational Rehabilitation*, *9*, 79–95. doi:10.1023/A:1021362019948

Comer, R. J., & Piliavin, J. A. (1972). The Effects of Physical Deviance upon Face-to Face Interaction: The Other Side. *Journal of Personality and Social Psychology*, *23*, 33–39. doi:10.1037/h0032922

Cook, S. W., & Selltiz, C. (1964). A multiple-indicator approach to attitude measurement. *Psychological Bulletin*, *62*, 36–55. doi:10.1037/h0040289

Crandall, C. S., & Eshleman, A. (2003). A justification-suppression model of the expression and experience of prejudice. *Psychological Bulletin*, *129*, 414–446. doi:10.1037/0033-2909.129.3.414

Crawford, D., & Ostrove, J. M. (2003). Representations of Disability and the Interpersonal Relationships of Women with Disabilities. *Women & Therapy*, *26*, 179–194. doi:10.1300/J015v26n03_01

Cruice, M., Worrall, L., & Hickson, L. (2006). Quantifying aphasic people's social lives in the context of non-aphasic peers. *Aphasiology*, *20*, 1210–1225. doi:10.1080/02687030600790136

DeHouwer, J., & Moors, A. (2007). How to define and examine the implicitness of implicit measures. In B. Wittenbrink & N. Schwarz (eds.) *Implicit measures of attitudes: Procedures and controversies*. New York: Guilford Press (pp. 179-194).

Elliot, T., & Frank, R. (1990). Social and interpersonal reactions to depression and disability. *Rehabilitation Psychology*, *35*, 135–147.

Fichten, C. S., & Amsel, R. (1986). Trait Attributions about College Students with a Physical Disability: Circumplex Analyses and Methodological Issues. *Journal of Applied Social Psychology*, *16*, 410–427. doi:10.1111/j.1559-1816.1986.tb01149.x

Fichten, C. S., & Bourdon, C. V. (1986). Social Skill Deficit or Response Inhibition: Interaction between Disabled and Nondisabled College Students. *Journal of College Student Personnel*, *27*, 326–333.

Fichten, C. S., Robillard, K., Judd, D., & Amsel, R. (1989). College students with physical disabilities: Myths and realities. *Rehabilitation Psychology*, *34*, 243–257.

Findler, L., Vilchinsky, N., & Werner, S. (2007). The multidimensional attitudes scale toward persons with disabilities (MAS): Construction and validation. *Rehabilitation Counseling Bulletin, 50*, 166–176. doi:10.1177/00343552070500030401

Fine, M., & Asch, A. (1988). *Women with disabilities: Essays in psychology, culture, and politics*. Temple University Press: Philadelphia.

Fiske, S. T. (2005). Social cognition and the normality of prejudgment. In J. F. Dovidio, P. Glick, & L. A. Rudman (Eds.), *Reflecting on "The Nature of Prejudice,"* (pp. 36-53). Malden, MA: Blackwell.

Fiske, S. T., Cuddy, A. J. C., Glick, P., & Xu, J. (2002). A model of (often mixed) stereotype content: Competence and warmth respectively follow from status and competition. *Journal of Personality and Social Psychology, 82*, 878–902. doi:10.1037/0022-3514.82.6.878

Furnham, A., & Thompson, R. (1994). Actual and perceived attitudes of wheelchair users. *Counselling Psychology Quarterly, 7*, 35. doi:10.1080/09515079408254133

Gilbert, D. T., & Hixon, J. G. (1991). The trouble of thinking: Activation of stereotypic beliefs. *Journal of Personality and Social Psychology, 60*, 509–517. doi:10.1037/0022-3514.60.4.509

Goffman, E. (1963). *Stigma: Notes on the management of spoiled identity*. Englewood Cliffs, NJ: Prentice Hall.

Gouvier, W. D., Sytsma-Jordan, S., & Mayville, S. (2003). Patterns of discrimination in hiring job applicants with disabilities: The role of disability type, job complexity, and public contact. *Rehabilitation Psychology, 48*, 175–181. doi:10.1037/0090-5550.48.3.175

Green, S., Davis, C., Karshmer, E., Marsh, P., & Straight, B. (2005). Living stigma: The impact of labeling, stereotyping, separation, status loss, and discrimination in the lives of individuals with disabilities and their families. *Sociological Inquiry, 75*, 197–215. doi:10.1111/j.1475-682X.2005.00119.x

Greenwald, A. G., McGhee, D. E., & Schwartz, J. L. K. (1998). Measuring individual differences in implicit cognition: The Implicit Association Test. *Journal of Personality and Social Psychology, 74*, 1464–1480. doi:10.1037/0022-3514.74.6.1464

Gregory, D. (1998). Reactions to Ballet with Wheelchairs: Reflections of Attitudes toward People with Disabilities. *Journal of Music Therapy, 35*(4), 274–283.

Hart, R. D., & Williams, D. E. (1995). Able-Bodied Instructors and Students with Physical Disabilities: A Relationship Handicapped by Communication. *Communication Education, 44*, 140–154. doi:10.1080/03634529509379005

Hebl, M., & Kleck, R. E. (2000). The social consequences of physical disability. In T. F. Heatherton, R. E. Kleck, J. Hull, & M. R. Hebl, J. G. Hull (Eds.), *The social psychology of stigma* (pp. 88-125). New York: Guilford Press.

Hebl, M., Tickle, J., & Heatherton, T. (2000). Awkward moments in interactions between nonstigmatized and stigmatized individuals. In T. F. Heatherton, R. E. Kleck, J. Hull, & M. R. Hebl, J. G. Hull (Eds.), *The social psychology of stigma* (pp. 88-125). New York: Guilford Press.

Hilari, K., & Northcott, S. (2006). Social support in people with chronic aphasia. *Aphasiology, 20*, 17–36. doi:10.1080/02687030500279982

Howland, C. A., & Rintala, D. H. (2001). Dating behaviors of disabled women. *Sexuality and Disability, 19*, 41–70. doi:10.1023/A:1010768804747

Kleck, R., Ono, H., & Hastorf, A. H. (1966). The Effects of Physical Deviance upon Face-to-Face Interaction. *Human Relations*, *19*, 425–436. doi:10.1177/001872676601900406

Louvet, E. (2007). Social judgment toward job applicants with disabilities: Perceptions of personal qualities and competencies. *Rehabilitation Psychology*, *52*, 297–303. doi:10.1037/0090-5550.52.3.297

Luce, P. A., Feustel, T. C., & Pisoni, D. B. (1983). Capacity demands in short-term memory for synthetic and natural speech. *Human Factors*, *25*, 17–32.

Maas, A., Castelli, L., & Arcuri, L. (2000). Measuring prejudice: Implicit versus explicit techniques. In D. Capozza & R. Brown (Eds.) *Social identity processes: Trends in theory and research*. London: Sage (pp. 96-116).

Makas, E. (1988). Positive attitudes toward disabled people: Disabled and nondisabled persons' perspectives. *The Journal of Social Issues*, *44*, 49–62.

Olkin, R., & Howson, L. (1994). Attitudes Toward and Images of Physical Disability. *Journal of Social Behavior and Personality*, *9*(5), 81–96.

Phillips, M. J. (1985). "Try Harder": The Experience of Disability and the Dilemma of Normalization. *The Social Science Journal*, *22*, 45–57.

Ralston, J. V., Pisoni, D. B., & Mullennix, J. W. (1995). Perception and comprehension of speech. In A. Syrdal, R. Bennett, & S. Greenspan (Eds.), *Applied speech technology* (pp. 233-287). Boca Raton, FL: CRC Press.

Rudman, L. A. (2004). Sources of implicit attitudes. *Current Directions in Psychological Science*, *13*, 79–82. doi:10.1111/j.0963-7214.2004.00279.x

Schwartz, L. L. (1999). *Psychology and the media: A second look*. Washington, DC: American Psychological Society.

Simmons-Mackie, N. N., & Damico, J. S. (2007). Access and social inclusion in aphasia: Interactional principles and applications. *Aphasiology*, *21*, 81–97. doi:10.1080/02687030600798311

Snyder, M. L., Kleck, R. E., Strenta, A., & Mentzer, S. J. (1979). Avoidance of the handicapped: An attributional ambiguity analysis. *Journal of Personality and Social Psychology*, *37*, 2297–2306. doi:10.1037/0022-3514.37.12.2297

Stone, D. L., & Colella, A. (1996). A framework for studying the effects of disability on work experiences. *Academy of Management Review*, *21*, 352–401. doi:10.2307/258666

Vargas, P., von Hippel, W., & Petty, R. E. (2004). Using "partially structured" attitude measures to enhance the attitude-behavior relationship. *Personality and Social Psychology Bulletin*, *30*, 197–211. doi:10.1177/0146167203259931

Weitzel, A. (2000). Overcoming loss of voice. In D. O. Braithwaite & T. L. Thompson, (Eds.), *Handbook of communication and people with disabilities: Research and application* (pp. 451-466). Mahwah, NJ: Erlbaum.

Yuker, H. E., & Block, J. R. (1986). *Research with the Attitude Toward Disabled Persons Scales (ATDP): 1960-1985*. Hempstead, NY: Center for the Study of Attitudes Toward Persons with Disabilities, Hofstra University.

Section 5
Case Studies

Chapter 15
A Tale of Transitions:
The Challenges of Integrating Speech Synthesis in Aided Communication

Martine Smith
Trinity College Dublin, Ireland

Janice Murray
Manchester Metropolitan University, England

Stephen von Tetzchner
University of Oslo, Norway

Pearl Langan
Trinity College Dublin, Ireland

ABSTRACT

Many aided communicators have used low-tech communication boards for extended periods of time when they receive a voice output device. Integrating sophisticated technology into conversational interactions draws on a range of skills for both the aided communicator and their speaking partners. A range of individual and environmental factors influences the transition from low-tech to hi-tech communication aids. This chapter considers the impact of these factors on intervention and the developmental course of two individuals, Niall and Cara. The potential benefits of synthetic speech are clearly illustrated in the stories of Niall and Cara and by the literature. However, the scaffolding needed to support effective use of voice output must be carefully constructed, if these benefits are to be realized in ways that lead to genuine social inclusion and to meaningful, positive changes in the communication experiences of aided communicators.

INTRODUCTION

The course of language development in people who lack the ability to speak and therefore have to express themselves with alternative means of communication, differs in significant ways from ordinary speech development (von Tetzchner & Grove, 2003), even in those who have good comprehension of spoken language (for a description of different groups of users, see von Tetzchner and Martinsen, (2000). Somewhat uniquely, these individuals may

DOI: 10.4018/978-1-61520-725-1.ch015

hear one form of language as input (speech), but produce a very different form of language for expressive output. The production process itself may be far less automatic, and require different and potentially greater cognitive resources than speech articulation. One important characteristic of *aided language development* (i.e., the development of expressive language with manual and electronic communication aids) is a discontinuity in production and form. Individuals who develop aided language typically change graphic systems, vocabulary organization structures and expressive communication modes, often several times across the lifespan (Williams, Krezman, & McNaughton, 2008) due to changes in intervention practice as well changes and innovations in technology (Arvidson & Lloyd, 1997; Hourcade, Pilotte, West, & Parette, 2004; von Tetzchner & Jensen, 1996). Many individuals who grow up with manual communication boards are introduced to electronic devices quite late in their language development careers.

This chapter describes the histories of two aided communicators that in quite different ways illustrate the diverse processes related to a shift from using a manual board to using an electronic device. The first history is about Cara, a young woman who transitioned from using a manual board with Blissymbols (Bliss, 1965) to an electronic communication aid with a communication system called "Language, Learning and Living" (LLL, (Jones, 1997)) and voice output at the age of seven. The second history is about Niall, a young man with cerebral palsy who was introduced to a voice output device after almost two decades of using manual boards with Blissymbols. Their histories highlight the importance of identifying the expectations of voice output use, and the role individual, environmental and cultural factors may have in facilitating and hindering the transition from manual boards to electronic aided communication. Cara's history demonstrates the need for increased support and intervention during the transition to voice output technology, as well as the need for perseverance in order to integrate speech technology in everyday communication. In many respects, Niall's history documents a failed transition, if increased use of synthetic speech output is the measure of success. Although Niall was successful in some activities over the course of a year of targeted intervention, his voice output device never became an integrated part of his communicative means. The chapter focuses on the ancillary factors that may be crucial in determining the extent to which a voice output device is integrated into the daily communication of an aided communicator.

The International Classification of Functioning, Disability and Health (ICF; World Health Organization, 2001) emphasizes participation in social and societal activities, and may be used as a general framework for evaluating the effectiveness of particular interventions, including interventions for individuals developing aided communication (Raghavendra, Bornman, Granlund, & Bjorck-Akesson, 2007). This chapter therefore also discusses the implications of being an aided communicator within the context of community and social inclusion and the challenges faced by aided communicators who may be perceived by others as being involved *in* their communities but who may yet be perceived as far from being part *of* these communities.

BACKGROUND

Aided Communication in a Multi-Modal Context

Augmentative and alternative communication forms are commonly categorized as aided or unaided. *Aided* communication "includes all forms of communication in which the linguistic expression exists in a physical form external to the user" (von Tetzchner & Martinsen, 1992, p.7), including picture communication boards, voice output devices and computers. By contrast *unaided* forms are produced by the 'speaker' with no external props. Gestures, eye gaze and vocalizations are all examples of unaided communication forms. One of the most robust findings in relation to individuals with severe speech impairments is their reliance on multiple modes of communication, including both aided and non-aided forms (Basil, 1992; Brekke & von Tetzchner, 2003; Collins, 1996; Falkman, Dahlgren Sandberg, & Hjelmquist, 2002; Iacono, Mirenda, & Beukelman, 1993; Kraat, 1987; Light, Collier, & Parnes, 1985; Paul, 1998; von Tetzchner & Grove, 2003). Thus, a *communication system* comprises all the forms of communication used for both comprehension and for expression. However, within any multimodal communication system, it is assumed that certain kinds of messages may be more effectively negotiated with particular modes of communication. In other words, modes of communication may not be equal when it comes to solving specific communication problems. In particular, where there is little contextual support, referential communication with specific content may be reliant on access to a large and varied vocabulary. In communication aids, symbols for this vocabulary may be represented in a number of different ways, not all of which rely on electronic technology.

Simple and Complex Electronic Aided Communication

Communication devices vary significantly in their technological sophistication. Simple, "low-tech" or "no-tech" devices require no integrated circuitry (Wasson, Arvidson, & Lloyd, 1997). Communication boards displaying graphic symbols, words or letters and single message voice-output devices are examples of widely used low-tech devices. High-tech devices incorporate an integrated circuit, most commonly in the form of mainstream computers or palm devices with specific software to support communication, or dedicated speech output devices. There are many advantages to low-tech communication devices, including their reliability, low cost, durability and portability (Murphy, 2004; Smith & Connolly, 2008; Wasson et al., 1997). However, such systems often have a restricted vocabulary base, rely on partner co-construction of the message with associated risks of misinterpretation or over-interpretation, and may not be useful for distance communication. High-tech devices with voice output technology can address some of the above limitations. Other advantages of speech output devices are presumed to lie in their potential for more independent communication (Dickerson, Stone, Panchura, & Usiak, 2002; Rackensperger, Krezman, McNaughton, Williams, & D'Silva, 2005), obviating or reducing the need for partner interpretation and formulation of messages. Access to voice output also allows for distance communication, for pre-storing of specific content to enhance speed in interactions and increased potential assertiveness (Clarke, McConachie, Price, & Wood, 2001).

The form of communication may also influence potential communication partners. Attitudes of naturally speaking peers have been found to be more positive towards individuals using voice output over manual and low-tech communication devices, and expectations of successful communication are also higher for sophisticated devices (Gorenflo & Gorenflo, 1991; Lilienfeld & Alant, 2001). The aesthetic appeal of a device may be critical for the willingness of communication partners to engage in dialogue and thus impact greatly on opportunities to participate in communication interactions (Bunning & Horton, 2007; Campbell, Gilmore & Cuskelly, 2003; Milner & Kelly, 2009).

However, there remain features that are common to both low-tech and hi-tech aided communication, including the unique role of communication partners in facilitating successful communication, the relatively slow rate of communication, even with sophisticated speech output devices, and the potential of naturally speaking communication partners to influence the direction, duration and success of communication interactions (Light, 1988; von Tetzchner & Martinsen, 1996).

Aided Communication Competence

The communicative competence of aided communicators may be described in four related dimensions (Light, 1989; Light, Beukelman, & Reichle, 2003). *Operational competence* relates to skills in the technical production and operation of communication aids, including the motor and perceptual skills implicit in use of electronic communication systems. *Linguistic competence* refers to the ability to both understand and use the linguistic code of the community, as well as the linguistic code of the aided communication system in use. *Social competence* comprises the ability to determine the conventions or "rules" of interaction within specific contexts and with specific partners, and to apply those rules effectively. This dimension includes pragmatic knowledge as well as judgment and skills related to relational and interpersonal aspects of communication. Finally, individuals who use communication aids must have *strategic competence*, that is, the ability to use aided communication strategies that allow them to minimize the impact of limitations in the linguistic, operational and/or social dimensions. In addition to these forms of knowledge, judgment and skills, motivation, confidence and attitude towards the use of aided communication may also contribute to their attainment of communicative competence (Light, 2003). These factors combine with the operational, linguistic, social and strategic knowledge to represent the resources brought by the individual using aided communication to the development and demonstration of communication competence.

Communication competence does not reside within the individual however. Language may be considered a cultural tool that children learn and internalize through interaction with more competent members of society (Lock, 1980; Tomasello, 1999; Vygotsky, 1962). Early language is co-constructed within dyads, and for children developing aided language it emerges from the interaction with naturally speaking partners, as communication between aided communicators is quite rare (cf., von Tetzchner and Grove, 2003). Johnson, Baumgart, Helmstetter, and Curry (1996) characterize this co-construction in a filter model, within which they contextualize the skills and abilities of aided communicators and their communication partners, and the extrinsic influence of social and cultural contexts of interactions (cf., also the ecological model of Bronfenbrenner (1979). Environmental factors are related to social and societal *communicative accessibility* and may include the demands and constraints of a given situation, including the cultural expectations to certain social roles, as well as the attitudes, knowledge and skills of possible communication partners and society at large (von Tetzchner & Martinsen, 2000). In this respect, the emergence of aided communicative competence may be vulnerable to environmental influences to a greater extent than spoken communication competence (Murray & Goldbart, 2009). The two histories presented in this chapter reflect this collaborative interdependence between individuals using aided communication and their speaking communication partners in the construction of aided communicative competence. They highlight the significant role that devices with speech synthesis can play in demonstrating the competence of the user, as well as the barriers that need to be considered if communicative competence is to be successfully constructed and used across a range of social and cultural contexts.

CARA

The description of Cara combines evidence and information from a range of sources including parents, inter-professional interviews, intervention notes and discussions with Cara herself. From the age of 3 years Cara attended a school for children with physical disabilities. Immediately, she presented as a happy, energetic child who liked nothing better than playing and communicating with her peers and the adults around her. She did not develop speech but seemed to have good comprehension of spoken language. Cara lived at home with both parents who took a very active role in her personal, educational and communication development. From initial school assessment data, Cara was known to be bright and capable. She had a medical diagnosis of spastic cerebral palsy and a speech and language diagnosis of severe dysarthria. Cara was introduced to Blissymbols at 2 years of age and was still using Blissymbols when, some five years later, she was introduced to a communication device with speech output. Cara was able to move around using either a wheelchair or a rollator during her early school years. As she reached age seven, she primarily used her wheelchair – which by this time was a powered chair.

Blissymbols is a conceptually driven and stylized graphic system (see Figure 1). It has a finite number of elements that are combined to construct words and convey concepts (Bliss, 1965). It is a creative and flexible system that can support the generation of complex communication (McNaughton, 1993; McNaughton & Lindsay, 1995). Although it was one of the first symbol systems to be introduced to support children and adults with severe speech and physical impairments, in many countries it is no longer used extensively. Throughout the UK and Ireland it has largely been replaced by more picture-based symbol systems in combination with voice output devices. Although Blissymbols were used in some early electronic devices with speech output (Hunnicutt, 1984; Moffat & Jolleff, 1987), in the UK and Ireland this graphic system has almost without exception been used with manual communication boards. Cara's new voice-output device therefore came with a new graphic system (see below).

Having started very early with Blissymbols, by the age of seven Cara had already gained expertise in using a communication book with 500 Blissymbols, which were organized taxonomically. She was able to access the symbols directly by pointing using her right index finger. She could

Figure 1. Examples of Blissymbols. Adaptedfrom von Tetzchner and Martinsen, (2000, p.8)), with permission

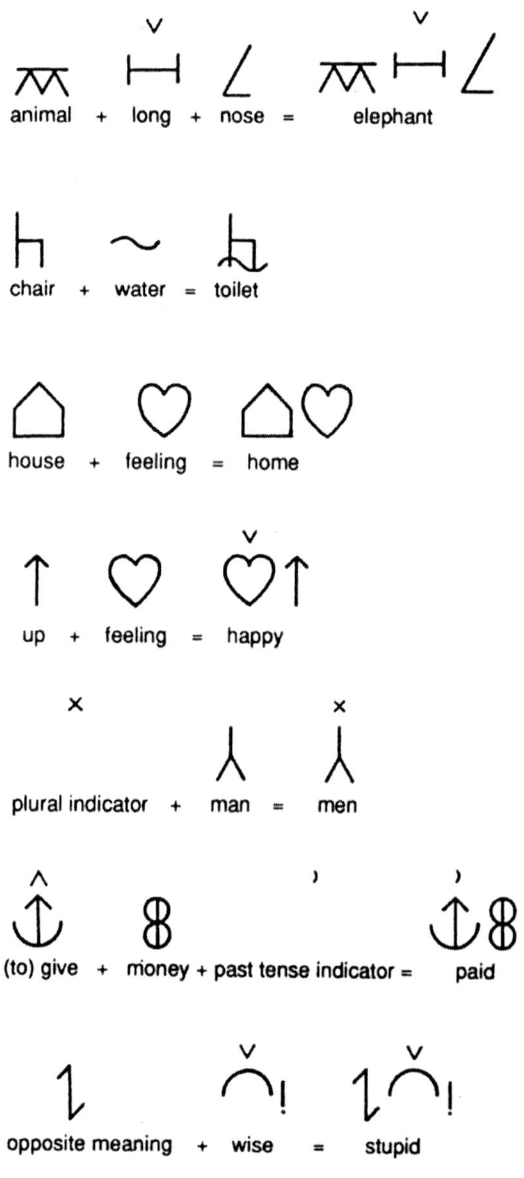

accurately point to squares that were 2cm x 2cm in size. She was also able to turn the pages of her book, although this was effortful, and could be somewhat inaccurate, so she preferred to access themes from the menu page and have her communication partner go to the section selected. The partner then went through each page in the section by asking Cara 'is it on this page' and so on until she could select the specific symbol. She presented herself as a confident, motivated and persistent communicator who was able to generate simple to complex communication messages as appropriate to the conversational context. Like many aided communicators, she needed active involvement from the communication partners to formulate her messages on the basis of her Blissymbol utterances and meaning negotiation. Changes in available communication aid technologies resulted in Cara being introduced to a device with voice output when she was seven years old. Cara and her family were particularly delighted by the prospect of using a voice output communication aid. The aid brought with it great excitement and anticipation that Cara would soon be a more independent communicator, entirely in charge of her own voice. Cara was the first child in the school to change to such a sophisticated system, and parents and professionals had great expectations and were eager to encourage her development. Although none of the people in her environment had previous knowledge of the technology, many of them viewed the new system as easier to use, primarily because the method of message transmission (voice output) was perceived as more normal and typical communication. No one was familiar with the differing demands of technology-mediated conversations. The staff anticipated that these non-optimal conditions might affect Cara's motivation to use the new communication aid, as well as other people's perception of her communication abilities, but there was an overwhelming sense in the environment that Cara's persistence and resilience would enable success.

Changing Language System

Cara's new communication device did not only imply the use of a new message form (speech rather than graphic symbols), but also a new graphic system, "Language, Learning and Living" (LLL; Jones, 1997). LLL is based on "semantic compaction" which is influenced by the multi-meaning Egyptian hieroglyphs (Baker, 1989). The meanings of the icons of the system are altered according to the icons associated with them, in any given sequence. In LLL, each icon or symbol on a display has multiple possible meanings. The specific meaning accessed depends on the choice of layer or "meaning frame" for interpretation of the icon. Each target selection requires specification of the semantic or syntactic class of the target, followed by specification of the specific exemplar within that class. For example, for the target utterance *'cat'* the classifier is the first icon chosen ('animal' [zebra icon]) and the specifier is the second icon chosen, 'cat' [tiger icon], yielding a two-icon sequence, [zebra + tiger]. Similarly for the target utterance *'meat'*, the classifier icon is 'food' [apple icon] and the specifier icon is 'meat' [zebra icon]. The user has to learn the categories associated with each icon and then learn to sequence icons to generate particular words and phrases. Cara moved from using approximately 500 Blissymbols, which she had learned over many years and could combine to construct many more words, to a system with 128 icons with multiple layers of meaning. With LLL, a word was typically produced by sequencing two icons and Cara's device had a potential vocabulary of 10,000 words. Cara's conceptual, semantic and grammatical construction of messages was thus affected by both the change in language representation system (from Blissymbols to LLL) and the mode of message transmission in the communication device. The LLL system implied new demands on Cara's cognitive skills, specifically visual and auditory attention and memory (cf., Carlesimo, Vicari, Albertoni, Turriziani, & Caltagirone, 2000).

Once the new communication aid arrived there was a period of transition from Blissymbols to LLL. Cara continued to use Blissymbols in most of her communications whilst being taught the locations of the different symbols in the device and the words that could be expressed with the new symbol system. Because artificial speech was thought to be easy for Cara to express, within two months the staff had physically replaced the Blissymbols with LLL, even if Cara had not yet learned the equivalent vocabulary items on her new system and was not entirely familiar with key operational components of the technology. This rapid introduction brought some tension into the relationship between the parents, professionals and Cara, who had varying expectations of how quickly and smoothly the transition could and should occur.

Learning to Operate the Electronic Device

When Cara used her manual board, the Blissymbols were "read" and interpreted by the communication partners. It was thus the partners who formulated Cara's utterances. One important reason for choosing an electronic communication system was that Cara should gain independent control of the device by direct access to both the language system and the programming features. In addition, the mounting and positioning of the device were important in terms of the potential impact on her use of her powered wheelchair controls. The communication device she was introduced to, a Deltatalker, offered Cara a range of features in addition to voice output, including infrared environmental controls, computer keyboard emulation, and separate programming features. Cara used all 128 locations on the Deltatalker keyboard, but this challenged her independent mobility because it interfered with access to the wheelchair controls. Cara had difficulty maintaining an upright posture at the same time as making effective movements with her arms and hands. She accessed her powered chair joystick that was positioned on her right armrest, but to additionally re-position her trunk to access the 128 locations on her communication aid reduced the accuracy and speed of her independent communication efforts. These dual demands had implications for her conversations, as communication partners needed to become aware that Cara sometimes needed additional time to get into an effective communication position.

The new communication aid came with one wheelchair mounting system but Cara typically used a manual and powered chair during the school day and a different easy chair at home. In two of these three chairs she had no means of placing her communication aid in an accessible position. It was the knowledge, enthusiasm and persistence of Cara's parents that resulted in her getting an additional mounting system that could be attached to her manual chair. This increased her communication opportunities even if it did not entirely solve the problem of not being able to communicate in every context.

Cara soon learned how to control basic operational features, e.g., switch on/off, speech on/off, volume control, and to select a spelling mode or a symbol communication mode on the device. What remained challenging for her was remembering all the symbol sequences and combinations that were needed to support effective communication. This resulted in frequent 'false starts' during symbol sequences and accidental word productions, which were perceived by people in the environment as Cara 'messing' and holding people up in conversations, or that she was not as linguistically able as they had originally thought. In fact, these early hiccups reflected Cara's efforts in learning to use the new system effectively. However, because the system was perceived by people in the environment as easy to learn, as noted recurrently in team meetings, their attitudes and perceptions of Cara's communication and cognition changed and this negative interpretation proved to be difficult to counteract.

Changes in Perceptions and Interaction Patterns

When Cara got her electronic communication aid, she was perceived as a skilled communicator, using facial expression, vocalization, gesture and body posture to support conversational turns. Aided communication without speech output tends to be unobtrusive because the aided communicator typically must obtain the attention of the communication partner before starting to formulate messages. Many aided communicators depend on others for initiating communication and have limited experience with both initiating and terminating conversations (Kraat, 1987; Light, Arnold & Clarke, 2003). It was not easy for Cara to "take the floor", and she had difficulties knowing how and when to join in a conversation. As she got older it became more apparent that her awareness of the rules of beginning and ending, or of breaking into an on-going conversation, was unclear. She was beginning to be perceived as rather egocentric and insensitive in her interactions. The introduction of voice output did not seem to change her pattern of social engagement. In fact, the new technology brought additional challenges. Accessing LLL in the communication aid was slower than with her Blissymbol communication system; Cara had to look longer at the device whilst constructing her message, thereby reducing her access to non-verbal cues. Moreover, interaction with Blissymbols maintained the attention of the partner, while the new system did not require the partner to co-construct. In fact, partners had to wait longer and often moved the conversation on while Cara was still constructing a message.

The operation of the new system implied a very different message construction process. Cara now had sole responsibility for message generation but it took time to change her long-established construction patterns. For example, although she knew the symbol sequences of simple sentences like *'my turn now'*, she found it difficult to produce these three words without verbal acknowledgement from her communication partner following every word. She would often stop and look up at the partner after each word. The staff interpreted this use of an old strategy as an indication that she was not as able as previously thought. They expressed concern that she was unable to construct typical spoken utterances and may not have a grasp of English word order, rather than noting the fact that message construction naturally would reflect language experience. In effect, Cara was continuing to use the message co-construction pattern that she had used so effectively with Blissymbols.

The introduction of the electronic device with speech output meant that Cara was perceived and reacted to differently by her communication partners. Whilst using Blissymbols, she was perceived as an able communicator. The conflation between the linguistic and operational competences required for the two differing communication systems took some time for those working with Cara to recognize, and this delay had negative consequences for Cara. She recognized the staff's frustration with her, but did not understand the source of their frustration, as she was only using strategies that had previously worked. Cara became more socially isolated and frustrated as messages were no longer timely and were perceived by others as slowing up the conversation. The communication partners became focused on her use of the device, as the synthesized speech output was the most salient of her expressive modes. In the beginning her use of the communication device was certainly not always the most effective or efficient means of communication, so, there was significant differences between the partners' expectations of her communication with synthesized voice and her actual competence in using the device effectively. However, Cara may have been more communicatively strategic at this time than she was often given credit for by people in her environment. She continued to use her full repertoire of communication modes (e.g., vocalizations and gestures) and seemed to choose the mode that was most effective for her in specific situations. For example, when she knew that she had not learned, or did not know where to find a vocabulary item on her device, she would turn the machine off and rather effectively maneuver her conversational partner into a routine with yes/no questions. As her Blissboard had been taken away from her, this strategy was a rather successful alternative for her. However, this particular strategy caused a degree of consternation amongst staff who were concerned that the device had cost a considerable amount of money and that Cara seemed to be indicating that she did not want to use it. Both Cara and her parents reported that they found the pressure to perform and to succeed with the new device quite stressful. It also negatively influenced Cara's interest in others and her eagerness to communicate.

Intervention Needs

Any change of graphic system and communication device represents a huge effort for the user and hence should naturally be accompanied with major intervention measures. Cara received one intervention session per week to support her in aided communication. This allocation of time was typical of service provision at this time. However, a review of the possible influences on Cara's communication development effected a dramatic change in intervention. Cara said that she found the change from Blissymbols to voice output personally challenging. She moved from someone who communicated competently using a system that instantly established close interaction between her and her conversational partner, to someone who had sole control of her voice output system. She found the increased pressure on her to communicate with a less familiar language system socially isolating.

Due to a timely collaboration with a local university, the school was able to provide Cara with more dedicated intervention sessions. Two days every week a speech and language therapist with competence in aided communication offered her sessions related to vocabulary learning, conversations, and system operation. The therapist also gave her some classroom support and guided the staff and the parents in aided conversation strategies. Changes and developments were mapped and recorded in an accessible way, resulting in clearer understanding of the transition process. It soon became clear to everyone that both Cara and the staff needed time and instruction support. There was a positive change in attitudes and expectations, both in Cara and the staff. Cara became more enthusiastic about communication again and staff had realistic expectations of her interactions. She was once again in a position to make her own choice of communication strategies and priorities. She achieved the original goal of becoming a more independent communicator, able to produce sophisticated utterances. Speed of conversational turn was good for an electronic communication aid user but it remained slow and difficult for some of her communication partners to accept.

Further Development

Three years after initial introduction of the device, Cara and her parents were asked to consider a transfer to mainstream education. Cara was the first communication aid user in this education authority to be offered this option. She moved into a mainstream primary school over the following year, moving to full time attendance during the spring term. This was soon followed by a successful transition to a secondary high school. The inclusion team, based in the special school, continued to support the teaching staff in the new schools, including help with Cara's communication device. When Cara completed her high school examinations, she used her device as a keyboard emulator. At the time that this is written, Cara has commenced her second year of college. The speech output device, even if slow, is important for her study activities and social interaction with other students. She continues to find it physically and cognitively demanding to use the electronic device and therefore prefers multi-modal communication. She uses her communication device, a Liberator 14 with LLL, at college and mostly vocalization and gesture at home. The choices Cara has made regarding when and how she uses her different communication modes suggest she views them as equally important.

NIALL

Niall was severely motor disabled from birth but showed good cognitive abilities and comprehension of spoken language. He did not produce speech himself and his first experiences with aided communication were when he was provided with a board with Blissymbols at the age of five. He quickly progressed from a small array of symbols to using a standard chart initially with 100 symbols and then by the age of eight to a chart of 250 symbols, which he accessed using finger pointing. By the time he was a teenager, he used a 400-symbol chart to communicate and was recognized by all communication partners as being an unusually persistent aided communicator and he demonstrated many meta-communicative insights. He was independently mobile in a powered wheelchair operated with joystick controls and accessed a computer using an expanded keyboard with key guard for his schoolwork. Similar to many aided communicators, Niall's academic progress was constrained by his very slow progress in developing reading and spelling skills, and as he progressed across adolescence he became increasingly frustrated with the limitations this placed on him. Although he acquired a small sight vocabulary and developed some initial sound recognition skills, he rarely successfully incorporated these skills to support communication. Within the school context, he was considered to present with specific learning difficulties, and there was a general sense that he did not realize his potential academically. He did not complete any State examinations, although he acquired functional numeracy skills and became independent in many aspects of daily living. Niall's adolescence in the late 1980s coincided with a very significant global shift in technological developments across all domains, but particularly in computer technology and speech synthesis, and by association, electronic communication devices. Across his teenage years, he had several trial periods with electronic devices with speech output, but none of them was found to enhance his communication. As other aided communicators within his school setting acquired voice output devices, the pressure on him to achieve in this domain increased. Culturally, the importance of being an effective user of technology increased and so, although Niall's manual communication board had served him well for many years, its status gradually diminished relative to the emerging high-technology devices. Furthermore, there was a general sense among teachers and professionals that the power of technology was such that if it were not possible to find a device that could be used by a particular individual, somehow that represented a failure on the part of the individual rather than the technology. Thus, his failure to find a useful electronic communication aid increased the impact of his academic problems in school.

After leaving school as a young adult, Niall entered a residential setting for adults with physical disabilities. A new speech and language therapist joined the organization when Niall had lived there several years and she turned her attention to investigating the communication options that technology might have for Niall. He was not employed at that time and although there were some structured recreational activity options available to him, he expressed a desire to engage in more meaningful and rewarding activities. He was independently mobile, using a very old powered chair still with a joystick control and had a keen interest in getting out and about to immerse in the social world around him. He also had a manual chair with a seating insert as a back-up seating option, but he rarely used this chair, as it removed his independence in navigating his environment. At around the same time, Niall started to develop a keen interest in music composition and formed a close working relationship with a musician interested in computer applications for music. He accessed his computer using two switches, accessed with both hands. This newfound interest in technology reinvigorated his desire to gain voice output. A team assessment led to a recommendation and acquisition of a Tellus, an electronic device using MindExpress software, which enabled him to continue using Blissymbols to produce synthetic speech output. However, very little support in learning how to use the device was made available to him. Approximately three years after this device had been purchased, Niall had only minimal experience using it in very structured context-dependent situations, and so he was referred to a university speech and language therapy clinic to get additional support for 'introduction' of his device. Over the course of the following year, Niall attended the university clinic one hour a week to gain skills in using his device. He also participated in a number of interviews about his attitudes to and experiences of aided communication. Excerpts from some of these interviews are interspersed in the discussion below. Around the same time as he started to attend the university clinic, he was seen for a review of his seating at a specialist centre. A new powered chair, still with joystick controls was recommended. One of the advantages of the new powered chair was that it had the potential for mounting his voice output device directly, a factor that was seen to be of crucial importance.

Niall's Use of Manual and Electronic Communication Aids

When first seen in the university clinic, Niall impressed as a very competent Blissymbol communicator. He was still using the same 400-symbol board that he had left school with, even though many of the symbols were difficult to identify, due to the many years' of use. He pointed with his fingers to the 2cm x 2cm symbols, accessing the full display of 400 symbols. Niall could express a wide range of communicative functions and was a very active contributor in conversations, belying the frequent descriptions of conversational passivity of aided communicators (e.g., Basil, 1992; Harris, 1982; Hjelmquist & Dahlgren Sandberg, 1996; Iacono, 2003). He monitored communication partners' comprehension of his symbol use, and readily recognized and repaired communication breakdown. However, he found it difficult to communicate specific information, such as his address, destination or personal names, talking about these tasks as *HARD, TOO MUCH DIFFICULT.*[1] Although his vocalizations were limited to vowel-like utterances, with no intelligible words, he was extremely effective at using these vocalizations and sweeping gestures of his arms to gain attention from potential communication partners. Once attention was established, he formulated his message on the communication board, often embellishing these utterances with facial expression and vocalization to modulate the emotional tone of the utterance. He drew heavily on the strategies intrinsic to his graphic system, for example expanding his available vocabulary by using Blisssymbols such as *SIMILAR-MEANING, OPPOSITE-MEANING* and *COMBINE-MEANING* though rarely using letter cues.

Niall had a strong knowledge of the Blissymbol system and his understanding of spoken language was adequate to support all types of conversations. He produced quite long symbol utterances to express himself, with a word order that usually reflected aided production processes and hence differed from the word order of the spoken language. The following history, produced as a sequence of symbols without partner interruption, is typical of his utterances:

ONE DAY I HE I WAS GO DOWN TRAIN PLACE

PERSON NOT KNOW WHAT I GO ON WHAT TRY TO SAY

I WAS LUCKY NUMBER TELEPHONE TO STICK ON PAGE ON

WHEELCHAIR

THEY DID MAKE BIG THING

THEY NOT KNOW WHAT NUMBER TELEPHONE

MOTHER WAS ANGRY ME.

The story is about a time he had gone to the train station to get a train home and had been unable to communicate his desired destination to the ticket master. Fortunately, his home telephone number was on the arm of his wheelchair and so the ticket master phoned to check what station he needed. Because of his skills in producing narratives such as this example, Niall was regarded as a sophisticated and competent aided communicator, and his language competence was seen as one of his key assets. This competence had strongly influenced the choice of electronic device, as it was seen as essential to maintain the same symbol system in order to minimize the new learning needed, thus focusing new skill development in the domain of operational competence.

Aided communication places challenges not only on the aided communicator, but also requires different skills of the conversational partners than natural speech communication. In the interviews, Niall demonstrated an insight into the situation of his partners. He empathized with the challenges aided communication posed for them, saying *IF I HAVE NOT WORD IT PAIN FOR THEM ME FEEL SORRY FOR THEM.* He especially mentioned the strain of the slow rate of communication, saying *DIFFICULT FOR THEM I FEEL THEY PUT OUT.* Niall appeared to be acutely aware of the image he projected of himself when using the communication board. During conversations, he often mentioned the limitations of graphic symbols without voice output. For example, when explaining the difficulties of using his board, Niall acknowledged its value by saying: *I NEED GET TELL THINGS,* but added *CAN BE DIFFICULT TIMES.* He commented that in shopping centers in particular, staff did not have time for him at the till: *THEY CAN NOT STOP. ME COME UP DESK. THEY QUICK. I NEED QUICK.* Niall frequently referenced his need to have access to speech, for example communicating *I NEED MAKE* "speech" (gestures to mouth). When asked why he wanted voice output, Niall responded *QUICK, SAY QUICK*, indicating a belief that voice output would reduce the time pressure that was typical of his aided interactions. He also recognized the potential of voice output for distance communication and for interacting with those who could not read his symbols: *IF PERSON CAN NOT COME UP FOR READ.* On the other hand, he could identify many activities and interactions where his board was effective, including familiar, communicative predictable situations such as going to a tea-shop where he was known, chatting with friends, and communicating with his mother.

Being able to convey competence to people, particularly people who did not know him, appeared to be very important to him. In his view, using a communication aid with voice output would help people to see that he was a competent individual *BECAUSE THEY CAN SEE PERSON IN BODY.* He expected that having voice output would reveal an image of him as someone who could contribute: *MACHINE MAKE MORE PEOPLE LEARN FROM ME YES BUT NOT THINK THINK ABOUT WHEELCHAIR.* He was anxious to have an opportunity to enter conversations from a position of equality and even authority, and not always as someone who needed help, or who was intimidating. He said his communication board made him less approachable to unfamiliar people *BECAUSE THEY AFRAID TO WHEELCHAIR.*

Thus, what Niall really wanted was conversation in all possible forms. However, he had few conversational opportunities and so tended to make the most of any opportunities that came his way. In common with many individuals who use aided communication, his social networks were small, his opportunities for meaningful and satisfying interactions limited, and his opportunities to develop relationships were constrained. In conversations, he tended to dominate, focusing on topics driven by his own interests and needs, tending to show little interest in what others wanted to say. His strong motivation to express himself was reflected in the demands he placed on students and staff working with him in the university clinic. For a period he had a weekly appointment of one hour working with students and a supervisor, but he frequently arrived up to 90 minutes early for sessions, telling the students that he wanted to start work. The questions of time-keeping and the commitments of all involved in the intervention were discussed extensively by the supervisor and the students with Niall, and he was provided with different types of schedule reminders, alarms and time prompts to help him plan his time-keeping more effectively, but with only limited success. Clearly, his motivation to participate in the intervention outweighed the inconvenience of waiting for long periods of time on a weekly basis. Niall also resisted terminating discussions, so that sessions often over-ran by up to an hour as the students and the supervisor tried to gently guide him towards the exit. While they recognized his need for support, they also had to make him aware of the need to keep time and respect partner signals in relation to conversation termination. At times, the only effective solution seemed to them to be to close his communication board or turn off the device, a strategy that was clearly not acceptable.

However, the result of Niall's communicative motivation and persistence was not more conversation time, but rather that many potential communication partners avoided interacting with him, or limited their interactions to conversations 'on the fly'. Niall complained that the staff where he lived *HEAR WHAT I NEED SAY BUT THEY PLAY PLAY UP ON ME.* Their reactions frustrated him: *I GET ANGRY BECAUSE THEY NOT TALK*, although he also recognized: *THEY NOT STOP BECAUSE THEY HAVE NOT TIME.* His awareness of the time it took for him to say something and the strain this put on the conversational partners seemed to drive his conviction that access to a voice output device would resolve many of his difficulties in conversations. He struggled to understand the tensions his conversational style created for speaking partners, and showed little insight into the fact that increasing his rate of communication would not alone be sufficient in resolving these difficulties. His understanding of time pressure also reflected his experiences and the attitudes, perceptions and understanding of staff in relation to Niall's communication needs.

The Challenges of the New Device

Despite the retention of Blissymbols in Niall's new device, access to the symbols differed significantly from his communication board and the device was also more difficult to manage physically. Niall accessed his Blissboard using finger pointing. His could quickly locate symbols and give the listener his full attention during communication interactions. His pointing was often ambiguous, as he was not always able to isolate one finger, but he readily perceived and corrected the partners' misinterpretations. His old and rather battered Blissboard was stored either under the seat or at the side of his power chair, and he could extract it independently or indicate to the other person that he needed it. With the board placed on the arms of his chair, he could access the full board, although he relied on his communication partner to stabilize it as he selected symbols. Thus, he used his manual communication aid with great skill.

The use of the electronic communication aid required new skills and abilities. Niall was used to a board where all his 400 Blissymbols were visible and in well-known positions, while the screen of the electronic device could display a maximum of 64 symbols and the symbols therefore had to be distributed over several pages. Niall thus had to switch from a static board to a dynamic vocabulary organization. He had to learn page navigation techniques and to remember the locations of "hidden" Blissymbols. The cognitive efforts involved in symbol memory and search seemed to leave fewer cognitive resources for message formulation and dialogue monitoring and participation (cf., Oxley, 2003).

Physical access to the device was also more problematic and effortful. While his finger pointing was adequate when using the manual board, his difficulties in isolating one finger for key pressing meant that associated movements of the other fingers often led to non-target symbol selections or multiple repetitions of the target symbol on the device. A key guard had been attached to the device display, but the guard did not fully match any of the grids available in the software and the alignment of spaces and symbols within the grid was not optimal. Even with timing adjustment and the key guard, Niall found it very difficult to directly access only one symbol on the display. Moreover, when he used the communication board, the communication partner could see the Blissymbols and Niall's movements and filter out potential ambiguities arising from his failure to isolate a single finger, while partner support for 'disambiguation' was not as easy with the electronic device. Both Niall and the partners were frequently frustrated and distracted by the intrusion of non-target symbols. Niall's physical abilities had not changed, but the demands and requirements of the new technology highlighted his difficulties, drawing attention to difficulties that had been less apparent when he used the manual communication board, and making him appear more disabled. Some of the people who knew him well perceived him as less competent than before and became concerned his abilities might have been over-estimated. Given these physical access difficulties, the option of using switches instead of direct selection with the electronic device was considered. When first assessed for an electronic aid, Niall had rejected switch access and there had been no follow-up to explore whether or not access had improved.

Part of the team's delay in reviewing switch access as an option arose from their uncertainty about his seating. When Niall first came to the university clinic, his preferred wheelchair was an old powered chair with joystick controls, but his electronic communication aid could not be mounted onto this chair. It could only be mounted on his manual chair. Having the device mounted in an optimal position increased Niall's accuracy in symbol selection, effectively making it necessary for him to choose between relatively adequate direct access to voice output and independent mobility. Although he had had the device for almost three years when first seen in the university clinic, he had not yet been provided with a communication aid mount that was compatible with his old powered chair, or given a new chair. Decisions about whether or not switch access would be more effective were postponed until after he received his new powered chair, as the new chair offered greater postural control and hence improved his hand function. Partly as a consequence of delays in resolving the seating and access issues, the voice output device had not become an integrated part of his communication. Niall used it mainly during intervention sessions in the university clinic or when the staff working with him brought it to him for a specific purpose. Thus, Niall's high level of aided communication competence when using his manual board contrasted sharply with the many difficulties he faced with the voice output device.

Situational Variation

One way for Niall to make the best of his different communication aids would have been to determine the most effective mode of aided communication for specific situations. In discussions about where he might use either his manual communication board or his electronic device, Niall did not identify any situation where his board might be more effective, despite his very limited experience of successful use of his voice output device compared with his many successful interactions using his board. His expectations were clearly that success in learning to use the electronic device would overcome the limitations he experienced in communication using his manual board. While his motivation and persistence were key factors in his success as an aided communicator, they also appeared to represent vulnerability. His motivation to succeed in using voice output was partly based on unrealistic expectations that having access to speech would solve the communicative challenges he faced with the manual board, despite the fact that in three years he had achieved very little success with the speech technology. His expectation was still that the voice output device would *HELP BIG FUTURE*, suggesting a remarkable persistence in his belief in technology, but also a limited insight into the nature of challenges to be overcome.

Awareness of Grammatical Construction

When Niall used his manual board, he constructed Blissymbol utterances that his partner then interpreted in dialogue with him. Having voice output created a very different conversational structure and made him more aware of the difference between his own productions and natural speech. This contrast became apparent when he prepared a presentation for a meeting of the Irish Chapter of the International Society for Augmentative and Alternative Communication. For this event, he was determined to use his voice output, to speak for himself and have his own voice heard. In this respect, the electronic device provided a new dimension to his communication – an audible voice to tell his story. For the purpose of this presentation, he stored phrases and sentences under single symbols. Niall used his Blissboard to compose the speech, which was then programmed into the device by a helper. During these interactions, Niall selected sequences of symbols whose glosses were written down and entered into the device by the helper. However, when Niall heard the stored utterance that replicated his symbol output, he frequently indicated dissatisfaction with it and requested that it be changed to a more conventional spoken word order and grammar. The structure of his own collaborative language production only seemed to become apparent to him when he started using his voice output device. Being able to review and edit his utterances opened new opportunities for Niall to explicitly evaluate how his communication style and choice of language might impact on others' perceptions of his competence. While utterances with a different grammatical structure were natural in interactions where he used a manual board and the communication partner glossed his message, the opportunity to present his story in (synthetic) spoken utterances without any co-construction turns seemed to raise his awareness of aspects of form that were inconsequential in less formal situations.

Support and Intervention

One of the challenges for adults in Ireland who live in residential settings is the lack of access to services and supports. Many decisions about Niall's device access, mounting, transport and opportunities to practice using the electronic communication aid were reliant on the voluntary support of others. The lack of structured services resulted in significant delays in many aspects of his development and significantly constrained Niall's progress in integrating voice output into his everyday communication. There was no key worker consistently available to advocate for him, and he had to address multiple service agencies to get attention to his different communication and mobility needs. There was little coordination across service agencies and often Niall had to co-ordinate the work across the agencies. These were barriers over which Niall had no effective control, despite the many resources he brought to the task. Another significant influence on Niall's development was his limited communicative access in his environment. There were few communication partners available to support his development of conversational skills. In interviews, Niall spoke of the significant time pressures on staff and others in his social world: *THEY NOT STOP BECAUSE THEY HAVE NOT TIME.* Even his close friends could not always take the time needed to talk with him: *TOO MUCH DO WORK.* His need simply to chat even took up most of the available intervention time, leaving little time for focusing on skills that might make him able to make greater use of the device.

Finally, major decisions about moving to more independent living accommodation came onto the agenda. Niall got the opportunity to move to a small house, several miles from his present residential setting. This move offered him far greater independence and autonomy, but also removed him further from even the limited structural communication supports available to him, including the university clinic. At the time of writing, Niall continues to use his manual board and has not yet integrated the electronic device and speech output into his communication. He has moved into independent living, the speech and language therapist working in the residential setting has left the service and has not been replaced, and Niall is no longer able to access the university clinic because of transport distance and costs. Not surprisingly, his motivation to persist in the face of such adversity appears to be waning, although he has recently expressed interest in attending the university clinic again, because he has received his new powered chair and it might be possible to mount the device directly onto this chair.

FUTURE DIRECTIONS

It seems to be a basic premise implied in much of the literature on aided communication that electronic devices are more flexible, easier to operate and give the user more communicative autonomy and power than manual boards which depend more on active collaboration from the conversational partner. The histories of Cara and Niall presented here illustrate the complexity of the processes involved in transitions from manual communication boards to electronic devices with speech output. Both individuals were extremely motivated to use synthetic speech and both showed significant difficulties in acquiring the skills and strategies required by the electronic devices. For Cara the success of voice output was obvious and direct, although neither immediate nor pervasive. She slowly came to utilize the power of electronic navigation and synthetic speech, but still tended to use them only in more "formal" everyday situations, continuing to use the manual board with people she knew well. Niall used the voice output device to present a pre-prepared talk at a conference, but he never integrated the use of synthetic speech in his everyday communication.

It generally takes longer to produce an aided than a spoken utterance, sometimes several minutes to produce a single aided utterance (Kraat, 1987), contrasting with rates of articulated speech exceeding 100 words per minute (Kent, 1997). A manual board requires sustained attention and collaboration from the communication partner when the user is constructing messages. It is a characteristic of visual communication (such as graphic symbol use) that the conversational situation or joint engagement has to be established before communication is functional. Electronic devices may imply more assertive power for the user, new (synthetic) vocal means for taking the floor and more independence in constructing messages.

However, the partners had a more passive role when Cara and Niall were using electronic devices, and this shift seemed to make them more distant and less involved. Having less active engagement in the interaction also appeared to make them more aware of the slowness of aided communication. This change affected the closeness of the interaction, as experienced by both Cara and Niall. Access to speech synthesis thus brought with it new pressures for them both. People's expectations of what they should be able to achieve and what kinds of support they might need shifted. They were regarded as very competent communicators and therefore not in need of any language or social learning when they got the electronic device, only some initial help with the operational skills. While Blissymbols usually are regarded as 'difficult' and needing to be taught and scaffolded, learning to use a device with speech output is typically perceived as 'easy' by natural speakers (Smith, 2008). Significant people in Cara's environment expected her to immediately communicate more quickly and effectively with the electronic device than with her manual board, even though she was less familiar with all aspects of her new system. Her pioneering status in relation to voice output technology in her setting seemingly made people in the environment place a heavy burden of expectation on her, showing little awareness of the complexity of the task she was undertaking. The changes in interaction style arising from her access to a voice challenged the expectations of her communication partners often with uncomfortable results, while at the same time new expectations of how she should interact were not explicitly explored. For Niall, the struggle to become an effective device user led to a less favorable impression of his abilities for people who knew him well. He never reached a sufficient stage of competence with the electronic device to challenge these perceptions of his interaction style. It was clear that his own expectations of the voice output device also were very high, and likely unrealistic. However, these high expectations no doubt contributed to his motivation and persistence over a prolonged period of time, in the face of considerable barriers to success.

It is a common finding that the provision of new electronic devices does not always come with the understanding that is necessary for successful implementation and realization of the power of the technology. As pointed out by another aided speaker: "Technology is awesome, but it doesn't solve everything" (Lund, 2001, p. 108). The experiences of Cara and Niall disclose a very real reason for concern that failure of technology to solve all the problems of an aided communicator and make his or her communication more normal may be attributed to the user instead of the technological development and implementation – both by parents and professionals, and by the users themselves.

Electronic devices sometimes have to be bulky and heavy in order to function properly, often impacting on the user's access both to the communication device and to other devices. Both Niall and Cara faced challenges in marrying mobility and communication access. Cara was fortunate in facing these challenges in a context where she received help with seating, mounting and access. For Niall, the challenges were far greater because support became limited once he left pediatric services. Niall's experiences are not unique and several studies have reported similar findings (Forster & Iacono, 2007; Hamm & Mirenda, 2006; Murphy, Marková, Collins, & Moodie, 1996; Smith & Connolly, 2008). These reports highlight the need for services that span the lifetime of individuals who use aided communication. Even for Cara, however, the challenges were significant. People who use a number of different wheelchairs are often faced with difficult choices about mounting systems and limited resources and funding agency constraints may force users to make decisions that essentially revolve about where communication is most likely to be a priority over independent mobility, choices that are never a source of concern for natural speakers.

The field of aided communication has to a large extent been driven by technological optimism and an idolization of what technology can achieve in overcoming physical and cognitive impairments (Vanderheiden, 2002). Although communication boards and manual signs had been used with people with impairments of speech, language and cognition for many years, research in aided communication only emerged in the middle of the 1980s when personal computers and electronic communication devices became commercially available (Kiernan, Reid, & Jones, 1982; von Tetzchner & Jensen, 1996). Given the technological advances in the last 20 years, it should seem that it has never been easier for individuals with severe speech impairments to become equal partners in their community. Technology is seen as enabling community participation fitting a general increasing emphasis on the inclusion of people with disability in everyday experiences. However, the histories of Cara and Niall show that communication partners may have unrealistic expectations about how technology may provide participation possibilities, seemingly reflecting a naïve location-focused view of participation and a confounding of physical access with communicative access. Greater physical independence in utterance construction will not always alter the quality of the contribution of people using aided communication within their communities.

For both Cara and Niall, access to voice output brought new opportunities to assert and develop independence. The transition towards greater independence involved a complex evolutionary process for Cara, from a familiar interdependent style of interaction where she was both comfortable and confident, towards a more autonomous but also more unfamiliar role. Initial assumptions were that her speech synthesis would allow her to progress from interdependence to independence in her interactions, whereas in reality, what she needed initially at least was a different type of inter-dependence, one that scaffolded her communication attempts with the same level of supports as were available to her when she used her manual board. The initial delay by professionals in initiating these scaffolds had the effect of increasing her isolation, rather than fostering independence.

Niall expressed independence in all aspects of daily life as a key personal goal. Although he did not achieve this independence directly through significant success in using voice output, engaging in the process of attempting to become more competent using his device still seemed to promote a perception of him as an independent adult. He appeared keenly aware of his isolation and lack of opportunities for communication, including everyday small talk. In reality he changed his focus from trying to achieve more communicative access to trying to increase his autonomy, so that he could independently tackle that isolation. The role of his speech synthesis in that process was largely indirect, but powerful nonetheless. The extent to which Niall's newfound independence will yield genuine participation rather than a new form of isolation within a new community remains to be seen. In the interviews, he often mentioned his desire to be seen as an active agent and a contributing and valuable member of society, rather than as an object of help. Niall clearly viewed the ability to express himself with own voice as central to presenting his independence in such a way as to allow him to assume a role of contributor rather than recipient of support. Attitudes and expectations can thus act as both facilitators and barriers to effective integration of electronic devices into an individual's everyday communication.

In studies, many aided communicators have reported a sense of being an outsider, looking in on their community, while aspiring to authentic roles within and of the communities in which they resided. In interviews they have spoken of their experiences of physical access and presence, but not always communicative access and inclusion; it was not *where,* but *how* they participated that mattered (e.g., Milner & Kelly, 2009). Only through rewarding social interactions between disabled and non-disabled individuals can there be a genuine change in acceptance and involvement in a community (Bunning & Horton, 2007).

The ultimate feeling of *belonging* to a community is complex and for people using communication aids this authentic inclusion may require much professional time and support, over a more extended period of time than has been generally acknowledged. A significant difference between disabled and non-disabled people seems to lie in the different possibilities they are given for developing new skills in response to technological development at an adult age. For most adults without physical disabilities, technological innovations within the workplace that imply new skills automatically lead to new training opportunities, help and support at work, and/or the provision of publicly accessible skill development courses. For many people with disabilities, new technological developments may in fact be decisive for their everyday life. However, the new technologies are expected to give people with disabilities immediate benefits, while as demonstrated by Cara and Niall, keeping up with technology may be a life-span struggle.

Finally, the histories outlined highlight the importance of the resources individuals who use aided communication bring to the challenge of incorporating voice output systems into their communication repertoire. Cara and Niall's own resilience, motivation, persistence and willingness to take risks were extremely important in fostering communicative success. By themselves however, these resources are insufficient, if there are significant barriers to be overcome. One of the core differences between Niall's and Cara's situation was the lack of a key communication support partner for Niall, to support his development towards competence using a voice output device.

CONCLUSION

The histories of Cara and Niall demonstrate that transitioning to competent use of a voice output device may be a bumpy road to an uncertain destination. The journey is often lonely in spite of the fact that users are likely to traverse unknown territory and engage in new forms of communicative interaction. Sometimes the journey and what the user and significant people in the environment learn along the way is more important than arriving somewhere. However, it is also clear that if an aided communicator undertakes the journey alone, with few supports and little understanding of key communication partners of the journey, then the aided communicator is likely to arrive at the same place he or she started, possibly facing both the old and new challenges and barriers. For both Cara and Niall, the theme of time emerged as a core concern – time to simply chat, to fulfill all the common goals of communication.

In both of their stories, people in the environment placed great emphasis and expectation upon equipment, and for both Cara and Niall this emphasis resulted in an unhelpful and superficial focus. They wanted to be valuable and valued members of their talking, listening and acting communities, but their technology was initially a barrier to that fundamental urge towards social identity and belonging. There is a real danger that until professionals utilize what is best about technology by recognizing that it can create as well as break down barriers to participation, they will become surprised again and again when competent aided communicators using manual boards become disempowered by their technology and the expectations of the community. Real community inclusion requires far more than more or less advanced technological solutions. Speech synthesis technology cannot, of itself, generate a new social identity or ensure reciprocity in communication and relationships for people who develop aided communication. Nonetheless, it is important to recognize the positive role that technology can play in allowing individuals to take advantage of new opportunities to participate, to develop their social identity and to experience being valued in a community. In spite of the fact that participation in conversations is the explicit goal of the provision of electronic communication aids to people with speech and language impairments, there is still a great need for research that can provide practitioners with the knowledge they need for scaffolding the development of aided communication with electronic means.

REFERENCES

Arvidson, H. H., & Lloyd, L. L. (1997). History of AAC. In L. L. Lloyd, D. R. Fuller, & H. H. Arvidson (Eds.), *Augmentative and alternative communication: A handbook of principles and practices* (pp. 18-25). Boston: Allyn & Bacon.

Baker, B. (1989). Perspectives: Semantic Compaction Systems. *Communicating Together*, *7*(4), 8–9.

Basil, C. (1992). Social interaction and learned helplessness in severely disabled children. *Augmentative and Alternative Communication*, *8*, 188–199. doi:10.1080/07434619212331276183

Bliss, C. (1965). *Semantography (Blissymbolics)*. Sydney: Semantography Publications.

Brekke, K. M., & von Tetzchner, S. (2003). Co-construction in graphic language development. In S. von Tetzchner & N. Grove (Eds.), *Augmentative and Alternative Communication: Developmental Issues* (pp. 176–210). London: Whurr/Wiley.

Bronfenbrenner, U. (1979). *The ecology of human development: experiments by nature and design*. London: Harvard University Press.

Bunning, K., & Horton, S. (2007). "Border crossing" as a route to inclusion: A shared cause with people with a learning disability? *Aphasiology*, *21*, 9–22. doi:10.1080/02687030600798162

Campbell, J., Gilmore, L., & Cuskelly, M. (2003). Changing student teachers' attitudes towards disability and inclusion. *Journal of Intellectual & Developmental Disability*, *28*, 369–379. doi:10.1080/1366825031000161640

Carlesimo, G., Vicari, S., Albertoni, A., Turriziani, P., & Caltagirone, C. (2000). Developmental dissociation between visual and auditory repetition priming: The role of input lexicons. *Cortex*, *36*, 181–193. doi:10.1016/S0010-9452(08)70523-9

Clarke, M., McConachie, H., Price, K., & Wood, P. (2001). Views of young people using augmentative and alternative communication systems. *International Journal of Language & Communication Disorders*, *36*, 107–115. doi:10.1080/13682820150217590

Collins, S. (1996). Referring expression in conversations between aided and natural speakers. In S. von Tetzchner & M. Jensen (Eds.), *Augmentative and alternative communication: European perspectives* (pp. 89-100). London: Whurr/Wiley.

Dickerson, S. S., Stone, V. I., Panchura, C., & Usiak, D. J. (2002). The meaning of communication: experiences with augmentative communication devices. *Rehabilitation Nursing*, *27*, 215–220.

Falkman, K., Dahlgren Sandberg, A., & Hjelmquist, E. (2002). Preferred communication modes: Pre-linguistic and linguistic communication in non-speaking children with cerebral palsy. *International Journal of Language & Communication Disorders*, *37*, 59–68. doi:10.1080/13682820110096661

Forster, S., & Iacono, T. A. (2007). Perceptions of communication before and after a speech pathology intervention for an adult with intellectual disability. *Journal of Intellectual & Developmental Disability*, *32*, 302–314. doi:10.1080/13668250701654425

Gorenflo, D. W., & Gorenflo, C. W. (1991). The effects of information and augmentative communication technique on attitudes towards nonspeaking individuals. *Journal of Speech and Hearing Research*, *34*, 19–34.

Hamm, B., & Mirenda, P. (2006). Post-school Quality of Life for individuals with developmental disabilities who use AAC. *Augmentative and Alternative Communication*, *22*, 134–147. doi:10.1080/07434610500395493

Harris, D. (1982). Communicative interaction processes involving nonvocal physically handicapped children. *Topics in Language Disorders*, *2*, 21–37.

Hjelmquist, E., & Dahlgren Sandberg, A. (1996). Sounds and silence: Interaction in aided language use. In S. von Tetzchner & M. Jensen (Eds.), *Augmentative and Alternative Communication: European perspectives* (pp. 137–152). London: Whurr/Wiley.

Hourcade, J., Pilotte, J. P., West, E., & Parette, P. (2004). A history of augmentative and alternative communication for individuals with severe and profound disabilities. *Focus on Autism and Other Developmental Disabilities*, *19*, 235–244. doi:10.1177/10883576040190040501

Hunnicutt, S. (1984). Bliss symbol-to-speech conversion: "Bliss-talk". *Stockholm Technical University . Quarterly Progress and Status Report*, *25*, 58–77.

Iacono, T. A. (2003). Pragmatic development in individuals with developmental disabilities who use AAC. In J. Light, D. Beukelman & J. Reichle (Eds.), *Communicative competence for individuals who use AAC: From research to effective practice* (pp. 323–360). London: Paul H Brookes.

Iacono, T. A., Mirenda, P., & Beukelman, D. (1993). Comparison of unimodal and multimodal AAC techniques for children with intellectual disabilities. *Augmentative and Alternative Communication*, *9*, 83–94. doi:10.1080/07434619312331276471

Johnson, J., Baumgart, D., Helmstetter, E., & Curry, C. (1996). *Augmenting basic communication in natural contexts*. Baltimore: Paul H Brookes.

Jones, A. P. (1997). How do you make a dynamic display dynamic? Make it static! Semantic root theory and language structure on dynamic screens. *Communication Matters*, *11*(1), 21–26.

Kent, R. (1997). *Speech sciences*. San Diego: Singular.

Kiernan, C., Reid, B., & Jones, L. (1982). *Signs and symbols: Use of non-vocal communication systems*. London: Heinemann Educational.

Kraat, A. (1987). *Communication interaction between aided and natural speakers: An IPCAS study report* (2nd ed.). Madison, WI: Univ. of Wisconsin-Madison, Trace Research & Development Centre.

Light, J. (1988). Interaction involving individuals using augmentative and alternative communication: State of the art and future directions. *Augmentative and Alternative Communication*, *4*, 66–82. doi:10.1080/07434618812331274657

Light, J. (1989). Toward a definition of communicative competence for individuals using augmentative and alternative communication. *Augmentative and Alternative Communication*, *5*, 137–143. doi:10.1080/07434618912331275126

Light, J. (2003). Shattering the silence: Development of communicative competence by individuals who use AAC. In J. Light, D. Beukelman & J. Reichle (Eds.), *Communicative competence for individuals who use AAC: From research to effective practice* (pp. 3–40). London: Paul H Brookes.

Light, J., Beukelman, D., & Reichle, J. (Eds.). (2003). *Communicative competence for individuals who use AAC: From research to effective practice*. Baltimore: Paul H Brookes.

Light, J., Collier, B., & Parnes, P. (1985). Communicative interaction between young nonspeaking physically disabled children and their primary caregivers: Modes of communication. *Augmentative and Alternative Communication*, *1*, 125–133. doi:10.1080/07434618512331273621

Lilienfeld, M., & Alant, E. (2001). Attitudes of children towards augmentative and alternative communication systems. *The South African Journal of Communication Disorders*, *48*, 45–54.

Lock, A. (1980). *The guided reinvention of language.* London: Academic Press.

Lund, S. (2001). *Fifteen years later: Long-term outcomes for individuals who use augmentative and alternative communication.* Unpublished PhD, Pennsylvania State University.

McNaughton, S. (1993). Graphic representational systems and literacy learning. *Topics in Language Disorders, 13*(2), 58–75.

McNaughton, S., & Lindsay, P. (1995). Approaching literacy with AAC graphics. *Augmentative and Alternative Communication, 11*, 212–228. doi:10.1080/07434619512331277349

Milner, P., & Kelly, B. (2009). Community participation and inclusion: people with disabilities defining their place. *Disability & Society, 24*, 47–62. doi:10.1080/09687590802535410

Moffat, V., & Jolleff, N. (1987). Special needs of physically handicapped severely speech impaired children when considering a communication aid. In P. Enderby (Ed.), *Assistive communication aids for the speech impaired.* London: Churchill Livingstone.

Murphy, J. (2004). "I prefer contact this close": Perceptions of AAC by people with Motor Neuron Disease and their communication partners. *Augmentative and Alternative Communication, 20*, 259–271. doi:10.1080/07434610400005663

Murphy, J., Marková, I., Collins, S., & Moodie, E. (1996). AAC systems: obstacles to effective use. *European Journal of Disorders of Communication, 31*, 31–44. doi:10.3109/13682829609033150

Murray, J., & Goldbart, J. (2009). Cognitive and language acquisition in typical and aided language learning: A review of recent evidence from an aided communication perspective. *Child Language Teaching and Therapy, 25*, 7–34. doi:10.1177/0265659008098660

Oxley, J. (2003). Memory and strategic demands of electronic speech-output communication aids. In S. von Tetzchner & N. Grove (Eds.), *Augmentative and Alternative Communication: Developmental Issues* (pp. 38-66). London: Whurr/Wiley.

Paul, R. (1998). Communicative development in augmented modalities: Language without speech? In R. Paul (Ed.), *Exploring the speech-language connection* (pp. 139–162). Baltimore: Paul H. Brookes.

Rackensperger, T., Krezman, C., McNaughton, D., Williams, M. B., & D'Silva, K. (2005). "When I first got it, I wanted to throw it off a cliff": The challenges and benefits of learning AAC technologies as described by adults who use AAC. *Augmentative and Alternative Communication, 21*, 165–186. doi:10.1080/07434610500140360

Raghavendra, P., Bornman, J., Granlund, M., & Bjorck-Akesson, E. (2007). The World Health Organization's International Classification of Functioning, Disability and Health: implications for clinical and research practice in the field of augmentative and alternative communication. *Augmentative and Alternative Communication, 23*, 349–361. doi:10.1080/07434610701650928

Smith, M. M. (2008). Looking back to look forward: Perspectives on AAC research. *Augmentative and Alternative Communication, 24*, 187–189.

Smith, M. M., & Connolly, I. (2008). Roles of aided communication: perspectives of adults who use AAC. *Disability and Rehabilitation. Assistive Technology, 3*, 260–273. doi:10.1080/17483100802338499

Tomasello, M. (1999). *The cultural origins of human cognition.* London: Harvard University Press.

Vanderheiden, G. C. (2002). A journey through early augmentative communication and computer access. *Journal of Rehabilitation Research and Development, 39*, 39–53.

von Tetzchner, S., & Grove, N. (2003). The development of alternative language forms. In S. von Tetzchner & N. Grove (Eds.), *Augmentative and Alternative Communication: Developmental Issues* (pp. 1–27). London: Whurr/Wiley.

von Tetzchner, S., & Jensen, M. H. (1996). Introduction. In S. von Tetzchner & M. Jensen (Eds.), *Augmentative and alternative communication: European perspectives* (pp. 1–18). London: Whurr/Wiley.

von Tetzchner, S., & Martinsen, H. (1996). Words and strategies: Communicating with young children who use aided language. In S. von Tetzchner & M. Jensen (Eds.), *Augmentative and alternative communication: European perspectives* (pp. 65–88). London: Whurr/Wiley.

von Tetzchner, S., & Martinsen, H. (2000). *Introduction to augmentative and alternative communication* (2nd ed.). London: Whurr/Wiley.

Vygotsky, L. (1962). *Thought and language.* Cambridge, MA: MIT Press.

Wasson, C., Arvidson, H., & Lloyd, L. (1997). Low technology. In L. Lloyd, D. Fuller & H. Arvidson (Eds.), *Augmentative and alternative communication: A handbook of principles and practices* (pp. 127–136.). Boston: Allyn and Bacon.

Williams, M. B., Krezman, C., & McNaughton, D. (2008). "Reach for the stars": Five principles for the next 25 years of AAC. *Augmentative and Alternative Communication, 24*, 194–206. doi:10.1080/08990220802387851

World Health Organization. (2001). *International classification of functioning, disability and health.* Geneva: World Health Organization.

KEY TERMS AND DEFINITIONS

Aided Communication: Communication in which the expression of the intended message relies in part at least, on some physical form external to the communicator, such as a communication aid, a graphic symbol, a picture, or an object.

Blissymbols: A conceptually driven stylized graphic symbol system. Symbols are morphologically based, so that all symbol components carry meaning and new symbols can be generated through application of systematic principles intrinsic to the system.

Communication Aid: Any physical object or device used to represent communication forms, ranging from simple object or picture sets to computer based technology incorporating synthetic speech output.

Communicative Competence: The set of knowledge and skills that allow individuals to convey and interpret messages and negotiate meaning in interpersonal interactions across a range of contexts.

Communication Access: The opportunity, skills and knowledge to engage meaningfully in interpersonal interactions across a range of contexts.

Communication Partner: Refers in this chapter to a naturally speaking partner within a conversational context.

Intervention: A set of principles and procedures applied systematically in the pursuit of a specific (in this context, communication) goal implying a change (and development) in knowledge and/or skills on the part of those involved in the intervention process, directly or indirectly.

ENDNOTE

1 In line with current notation, graphic utterances are written in capital italicized letters (see von Tetzchner & Martinsen, 2000).

Chapter 16
Tossed in the Deep End: Now What?!

Jeff Chaffee
Easter Seals Society, Ohio, USA

ABSTRACT

The purpose of this chapter is to minimize the shock and stigma of adding device users to a caseload in a school, medical, or rehabilitation setting. To this end, the author gives four strategic rules for adapting the device to the therapy setting as well as four additional strategies for improving carryover into activities of daily living, the classroom, and other settings with caregivers and loved ones. To illustrate each of these strategies, the case of Corey, an adult AAC device user, is presented. His case highlights the need for clinicians and support staff to work together towards the common goal of improving communication through the use of the computerized speech output device.

INTRODUCTION

One of the more daunting challenges to any therapist is the "NEW CLIENT." It is already a stressful enough situation in all parts of the therapy world--adding a computerized speech device to the mix seems to make it worse. When that word "DEVICE" enters the mix, the rush of questions can be dizzying: Will I know how and be able to teach others how to program? What happens if I run into problems? Will the client know more than me about using the device? Will the client *want* to use the device?

DOI: 10.4018/978-1-61520-725-1.ch016

BACKGROUND

To address all of these questions (and more), I submit the case of Corey. Corey is a 40-year-old male, diagnosed with cerebral palsy and a lifetime nonverbal communicator. He was referred to my outpatient rehabilitation facility in early 2007. The referral paperwork in hand, my supervisor sat the department down and explained: "We've gotten a referral for an adult AAC user." As you might expect, everyone was somewhat worried. Corey had already been through the referral, evaluation and acquisition process for his device and he was to be using The Great Talking Box Company's E-Talk

8400. Because of this, the ordeal of choosing a device and seeking funding was already done—as such that aspect of device use/ownership will not be included in this case study.

Corey had previously been evaluated by a physical therapist also working at our center. During this evaluation, the physical therapist recognized the beginnings of good candidacy for a device with Corey, as he was able to use basic picture symbols. These were similar to the icons used in the Picture Exchange Communication System (also known as PECS) and the therapist used them with Corey to indicate pain, to indicate its intensity and to relate basic messages during the physical therapy evaluation process. On the strength of these early trials, his caregivers had taken the proactive step of having Corey formally evaluated by another speech therapist before his time with me. This fact aside, he came to me a blank slate—he had no "low-tech" or "medium tech" trials, there were no failed attempts on previous devices…in fact, at 40 the man had not received speech therapy services, nor had had any kind of AAC system in place to this point.

THE FOUR RULES FOR TREATMENT

Corey's situation was somewhat unique. There would be approximately 1 month before he was to start coming for speech therapy—time enough for even the most terrified and technologically-backward therapist to "learn" the basics of a device and its particular ins-and-outs. In this pre-therapy time, I got to know the E-Talk well, taking it home with me, referring to online and paper manuals, and quickly bending it to my will (instead of the opposite). This taught me **THERAPY RULE #1: "PREPARE!"**

While "Prepare!" might seem a simple and almost pedantic first rule of thumb, there is no single better piece of advice I can give a therapist approaching "that 'talking computer' kid" or "the device client." The month of preparation time I got is a rarity (some might even say a luxury), and it is certainly nothing I can tell all therapists to insist on. The practical reality is that you will receive your device-user's case file or referral information on Monday. By their first session, it's up to you to be a professional with the device. Preparing your sessions will take on different aspects at all points in your client's journey with their device.

In situations where you do not have the device first, it is the therapist's responsibility to contact the user's family or caregiver(s). Ask them which device they are using, how many pictures are on a page, and if there have been issues with use of the touch screen, joysticks, button selection, etc. While this will not allow you to make a button saying "Good Morning, Mr. Jeff" before that first session, it does allow for preparation of your therapy space. It may also show you other areas of device usage that you may need to learn the basics of prior to that session (e.g. programming basics, linking pages, selecting icons, importing photos/pictures, etc.). With this information about the device in hand, I turn immediately to the maker's websites. Be the device a Prentke-Romich *Vantage*, an *E-Talk 8400* like Corey's, a Dynavox *VMax*, or any other system, contacting the maker of the device via email or phone call should answer most introductory questions about the basics of use.

The internet is a fantastic pre-session resource, as many devices now feature "emulator" software which allows parents/caregivers, therapists, or teachers to program the device on their personal computer, using the full QWERTY keyboard, arrow keys, and mouse. This immediately takes away the stigma of hunching over the device, terrified that your ham-fisted attempts at programming will inevitably break the screen, wipe out the memory, and leave your loved one/client voiceless. These emulators are also a boon for therapists, who can use their planning time to program new vocabulary quickly and easily without need for the client to surrender their device for extended periods while new content is added. And lastly, using these emulators has been the single best way for me to learn the foibles of specific devices quickly...and how to overcome them.

The information that comes from the internet and phone calls should be collected and put into a "cheat sheet" for you and the user's support system, so that it can be used as an easy troubleshooting guide should questions arise.

Armed with my rudimentary knowledge of programming buttons and pages, and with a device now set up with a series of 2x5[1] arrays featuring buttons for emotions, greetings, etc., I was as ready as I thought I could be for Corey. I decided to use a "category>specific" layout with the specific targets loaded with whole phrases. Here, and elsewhere in the chapter, the use of "Word 1> Word 2" shorthand indicates that "Word 2" is a change of page; thus the pages move from a broad category on the first page to choices of specific vocabulary on the second. This was a layout that made sense to me and seemed the least labor intensive for Corey. In addition, it did not require him to do much with regard to syntactical layout and sidestepped literacy problems which may have existed by eliminating the use of the E-Talk's text window.

It is here that the role of client/clinician begins to blur for Corey and I, a blurring which has tended to repeat itself with the majority of my AAC clients. I certainly knew Corey's device much better than he or his caregivers, making me the "teacher" of sorts. But Corey knew **Corey** better than his caregivers or I did, making him just as valid a teacher.

I learned in our first session that finger isolation—in this case, extending *only* the index finger to activate, versus a more gross motor movement such as patting or slapping—was tough for Corey, and as a result, he very frequently "mis-hit" the device, sending us all over the place instead of formulating messages. While this was sometimes a true error (e.g. touching an incorrect target), he also struggled with keeping his other fingers out of the way, and they would often times brush the screen causing many problems with purposeful activation. Corey was also a very fun-loving client in sessions, and as many users will do from time to time, he found a particular "favorite" button which he would activate *all the time*, making structured practice a challenge at times. Developing the rapport that Corey and I shared was important to overcoming these issues in the initial sessions which had nothing to do with the device itself. The device, it seemed, had its own agenda!

As our first month closed, I managed to learn how much a single device can go from perfectly-ordered to complete chaos in the six days between sessions. Technical issues popped up: odd "write" commands (ones not programmed to the buttons); 10 identical icons on a page that had been programmed as 2x3 and had featured six unique choices; all buttons being invisible, or keeping only the icons invisible, or "no speech;" even the time a fully-charged battery was reading as dead and refused to turn the device on.

Those weeks' sessions that made me reflect on **THERAPY RULE #2: ANTICIPATE THE FOUL-UPS.** The device is going to get messed up at some point, and usually more frequently than you would expect, hope, or want it to! This rule has served me well and is as invaluable as the "Prepare" rule is. Corey's device can have a very severe "attitude problem," in as much as a computer can have one. But adhering to the first rule allows users to prepare themselves for every possible outcome. Knowing the device—at least the basics—and continuing to learn its commands will undo the vast majority of system errors that arise.

How can you anticipate what will happen? Taking a moment between sessions, or during your programming time with the device or its emulator, look for potential issues such as similar or confusing icon choices, problems with links, etc. Also, taking a moment to speak with family members or caregivers (or reviewing your notes from speaking with them before) can help you get a feel for the client's daily activities and communication needs. This allows you to plan for things like transportation of the device, other people who may be encountering the device, etc. The safest bet is to assume that the device will be put through a rigorous test each time it leaves your session from both a technological (i.e. system errors) and non-technological standpoint (dropping the device). It then becomes your job to include needed education on things like safe transportation, general care, and integration of the device into daily use.

The technology and non-technology issues above allow me to spring right into **RULE #3: BACK UP, BACK UP, BACK UP!** Whether you are using a series of memory cards, a dedicated computer that runs only your device's emulation/synchronizing software, or even paper print-outs, it is imperative to make sure that your device is backed up after EVERY change to the programming, whether that reflects changes after your session or those made outside the session. In fact, I have taken to making my AAC sessions 60 minutes instead of our center's usual 30 to allow for pre-therapy and post-therapy back-up synchronizing.

It seems intuitive, I am certain, to most computer users that saving your work often is of the *utmost* importance. But many times this "conventional wisdom" seems to be forgotten on devices, a failing I was guilty of during the early days of Corey's treatment. This made the sessions when his E-Talk would come in with scores of programming errors all the more nightmarish as I was sent back to the beginning—or at least my last "saved" point, which sometimes was nowhere near Corey's current level.

Corey's progress during those first four months was not as slow as the problems I have spoken about might suggest. And to be fair, I was not sure just what to expect after four months, so all the gains we made were pleasantly surprising. While he was not able--or expected— to use his device for complex sentences at conversational speed, he was not relying on hand-over-hand cuing—where the client's "choice" is directed by the physical manipulation of their hand by their communication partner— either. Corey's issues with mis-hits continued, so the use of "dead spaces" was used. This meant that since he had difficulty in removing his hand after a dynamic button would change the page, the same space in the next page would be left without of programming and black (Figure 1). In addition to these "dead spots" the device was set up to show a red selection box around Corey's choice, to make a click sound indicating that a screen touch had been made, and changing settings that waited for Corey to *let go* of the button he wanted before activating (versus activating on the touch of the button) all helped to overcome the issues with mis-hits as we continued in treatment.

These strategies seemed to help Corey without the need for the clear Lucite die-cut overlay pieces that the E-Talk uses to limit finger drag. I chose to go this direction over the overlay direction simply because I felt that Corey could continue to benefit from increasing his available locations and vocabulary—meaning that for each new layout, he would need either a new plastic overlay or one that could handle several styles at one time (e.g. a 2x4 overlay supporting 16, 32, or 48 locations by having the cut-out slots on the overlay have several buttons on the screen itself). On top of the problems of cost and effort that such a selection of overlays would create, I saw that as we progressed, Corey was better able to limit his "press and hold" behaviors and improve finger isolation.

With the touch selection issues resolved in a functional way, it was time to start challenging Corey. In our first months together, I started with 10 icons in a 2x5 layout. But as sessions continued and Corey continued to make progress, 2x5 became an array that limited Corey more than it helped him. Initially, each page I created stopped once the selection was made and the dynamic page change occurred. The pages did not reset to the home page. In addition, adding the dead space to a page reduced my number of choices to

Figure 1. The Family button is selected on the left, causing the screen to change. On the right side, the choices for "family" are shown, and the same location of the original touched button, the "dead space" is a button which is turned off to prevent mis-hits. This "dead space is noted in black; the other blank spaces are simply those without programmed messages in them.

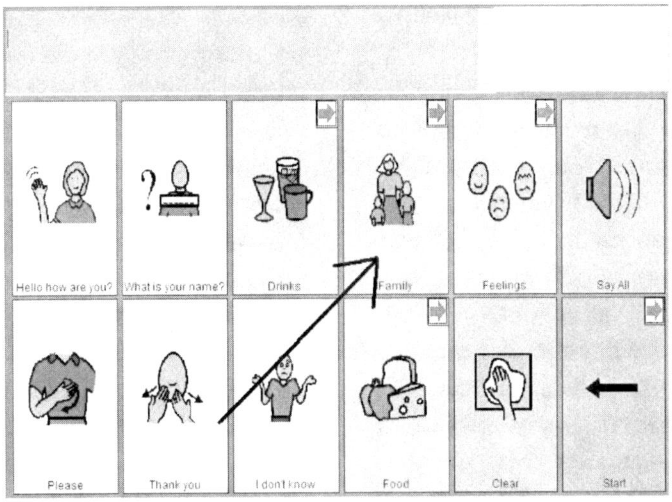

(a)

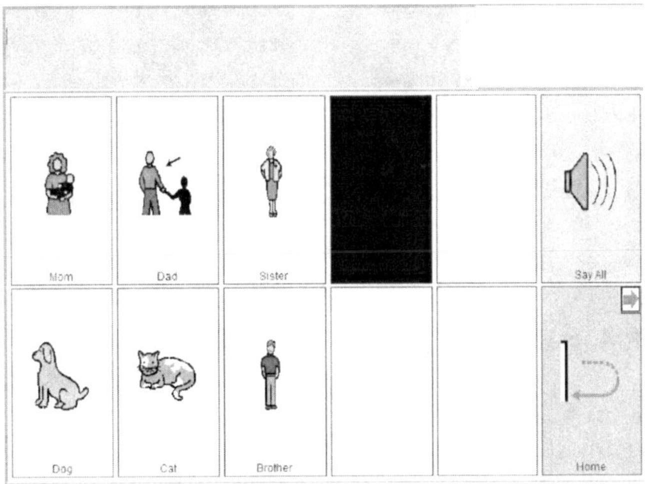

(b)

a maximum of nine. The need for a "home" icon to reset the pages then cut the usable buttons to eight. On pages where more choices were offered beyond the first group, there was need for "more choices" buttons (leaving seven slots) and a "step back" button (cutting it to six slots). I was initially reluctant to make the buttons too much smaller than the 2x5 grid created. Corey already had difficulty with finger isolation and resting the hand on the screen—it seemed that shrinking the button size and complicating what he saw on-screen would be too much change too quickly.

All of these issues, fixes, and considerations led me to **THERAPY RULE #4: BE FLEXIBLE**. Working together with the other rules to this point, keeping your expectations flexible is the "oil" making the machine of your sessions run smoothly today, tomorrow, and in the long term. Staying flexible and keeping the client and his caregivers calm throughout any technical glitch, outright system failure, or other setback in treatment will allow each person involved in treatment to view each challenge as the unique opportunity for learning that it is.

Other instances of the need for flexibility include the need for redesigning—sometimes from the ground up—the device's contents to meet improving or declining function. Corey began, as noted, with a 2x5 layout. The constraints of this layout and his excellent grasp of the use of the icons made it necessary to add additional choices. He moved from 2x5 to the more challenging 2x6 first, then 3x5. That layout served him very well until recently when therapy trials showed that 6x6 would work very well for Corey. There are other considerations as well. It may become apparent that a new selection technique is needed (joysticks, switches, pointers, eye scanners, etc.). The client may have been issued a "lemon" of a device—and the therapist/support staff may need to seek out extensive repairs or even a new/replacement device. And, depending on progress, funding sources and many other things, it may come time for a new, updated device. Keeping all options on the table, adapting and adjusting as needed to the everyday challenges of device use—keeping a *flexible* mindset—will make these challenges simpler to deal with.

While you may be trained more in the speech-language area than parents or caregivers, or you may have more experience with computerized speech devices (or computers in general), your knowledge, patience and everything else will be tested more than once by the device. Allowing your set-up to be changed quickly making it easier or more challenging as needed or setting up the device so that buttons can be added or taken away quickly is absolutely central to successful device use. That successful use is not meant for you—it is for the *user*.

Ultimately, all of what you are doing— the preparing, anticipating breakdowns, backing your work up, and being flexible—is being done not so that you can show off your prowess as a programmer or a speech therapist. It is done to give a voice to the person without one, to put into words their emotions. That may seem a lofty and high aspiration, but it is the simple truth of what it is you are attempting to do with that device. Keeping all of this in mind and reflecting on Corey's progress from the early days until now, it was all of those rules working together that have allowed him to move from the simplicity of basic use on a 2x5 grid loaded with full sentences to his current 6x6 grid which uses multiple selections of phrases and words to formulate longer messages.

But ending your planning here gives you only *half* of the picture. It is at this juncture in the treatment period that many therapists and caregivers—myself included—fail to make adequate plans for transitioning the client and his device out of the therapy room. Your session once a week will never be enough to ensure that the device is well cared-for, that the user's support system knows how to program, and that the proper steps are taken to make certain that your device is not treated as an $8000 video game.

THE FOUR RULES FOR SUCCESSFUL CARRYOVER AND HOME USAGE

Taking the next step and ensuring that your device user and his device are released from therapy into a supporting and willing environment will be the most difficult thing for any therapist. This is just as challenging as seeing conversational mastery of a new speech sound or language concept. Keep in mind that as you are establishing a home program the client's family, loved ones and caregivers likely feel the exact same panic that passed through your mind when you first started planning your treatment sessions. It has been my experience that whether it is Corey and his staff of home health aides or a child with parents and teachers, the single biggest concern is "I just do not know what to do with this...thing." To this end, I will offer four new rules for developing the nurturing environment you will need to help your device user continue to grow in their mastery of the device.

When planning home carryover, the first thing you must do is actually an extension of your therapy Rule #1 (Prepare!). **CARRYOVER RULE #1: ASSESS THE ENVIRONMENT**. This need not necessarily include a full home evaluation in the same way that discharge from a skilled nursing facility might, but it does involve finding out details about what happens to your client and his device after they leave your session. The nice part about this environmental assessment is that you are likely to get a good thumbnail sketch of the home, school, or work environment your client is likely to be placed in on a daily basis in the session. Then, simply flesh this basic outline out with hobbies, specialties and limitations, as well as other secondary information. Not only will this allow you to customize the device to make it unique to the user, it allows you to see potential roadblocks in the non-therapy setting that you and the caregivers will need to plan for.

For example, here is an environmental assessment on Corey. He lives in an assisted-living apartment community with his roommate Ralph. He and Ralph have a common living room area with a TV and stereo and a collection of videos and music. Both Corey and Ralph like to play *Connect 4*. During the day, Corey goes to a special needs workshop where he receives physical and occupational therapy in addition to doing some basic manufacturing tasks. Corey is continent of bowel and bladder and is able to use the toilet with moderate physical assist for transfers. He has around-the-clock care provided by health aides. There is frequent turnover of the aides, as the parent company tries to keep the aides flexible by limiting how attached they get to any specific client. These aides have a basic understanding of some computer technology, but are not experienced users of home/office computing, let alone being experienced with AAC devices (I will explain more about how I found this out in a moment).

About six months into Corey's treatment, when his progress in the sessions started to warrant planning for discharge (or reduction of therapy), it became VITAL to keep the staff in the loop with regard to his device.

I came up with a basic questionnaire for them to gauge where the various staff members felt more- and less-comfortable with computers in general and with Corey's device in specific. What I saw surprised me—most of the people knew next to nothing about Corey's device, having used it very little in the home environment. Additionally, many members of the staff were extremely uncomfortable with computers, even things that I had assumed (incorrectly) that most people would be familiar with, including basic operations, saving files, and search functions. It was at this point that I learned **CARRYOVER RULE #2: TEACH THE PEOPLE. THEN TEACH AGAIN UNTIL IT CLICKS**.

This information in hand, I planned a series of inservice meetings to introduce the care staff to the E-Talk, run though basic maintenance, and discuss the "basic basics" of programming. The teaching sessions included people from all aspects of Corey's day: the supervisors of the care company, three of his aides, and also staff and therapists from his workshop. I ended each of the sessions with free discussion time, allowing each "delegation" the opportunity to suggest vocabulary for Corey, to vent their frustrations, and discuss his case in general and specific terms. The sessions went very well; I was very pleased with the interest in Corey and his device.

A very strange thing happened, however, in the weeks after the first training days. Corey started to get *worse*. There was not a medical status change that I was informed of or that I found out about. There had not been any major changes at his house, with the staff, or in his daily activities in the workshop. It was as though Corey simply unlearned all the excellent progress on his device.

For example, our sessions used hypothetical questions, a task that Corey usually did a very good job with. In this exercise, I would ask a hypothetical question: "Corey, if you had a bad stomachache, how could you tell me?" The correct sequence was Main Page> Pain> Stomachache (with the programmed message "I have a stomach ache"). While the occasional mis-hit might give me "I have a headache" (which was next to "stomachache") or the toolbox menu (since it was near the "Pain" menu), Corey typically excelled at this exercise.

Corey's activations in both free-reply (where he was given no specific cues and allowed to touch any button he preferred) and questions in more structured tasks became increasingly scattered and random. His energy level in sessions varied wildly, with some struggles to keep Corey awake and some frantic flurries of redirection to keep him oriented to simple activation tasks.

Phone calls to his staff eventually led to a meeting with his caseworker through the local Mental Health/Mental Handicap office, who I will call Frances. In ten minutes, I discovered that the root cause for Corey's abrupt turn-around was not due to some drastic medical emergency. In my estimation, I had given the aides ample suggestions for homework or new programming during the sessions. Where I had failed, however, was in putting these recommendations in writing on the paperwork Corey brought with him each week, instead relying on the aides to pass word about these assignments among themselves. This failure had not translated—at all—into a working action plan for the staff to integrate Corey's E-Talk into his daily life. No wonder he was acting as though he had never seen the device—30-60 minutes once a week with me were his *only* exposure to the E-Talk! This leads to **CARRYOVER RULE #3: COMMUNICATE...ALWAYS AND OFTEN!**

This communication takes on many forms. You need to let the family or caregivers know what is happening with the device. This means that you are informing them of changes to layout, to array size, or even to colors and icons. There is also a need to define and communicate clear roles for the use of the device outside the therapy setting—who is doing what to the computer where and when. You will find yourself talking to parents, writing notes to teachers, calling employers, and liaising with caseworkers. Your communication with them is what allows them to chart the course to success for their loved one or client after that user has left therapy.

Frances worked closely with the staff to make a functional care plan for the home while I went to work on my next teaching experience. The focus this time was not so much to alleviate computer angst or to focus heavily on programming for the daily aides, but to include strategies for integrating the device, its vocabulary, and (by extension) Corey's voice into the day to day activities. These strategies focused on pairing activities with demonstrations of activation (e.g. when toileting, a demonstration of "bathroom" button), moving to hand-over-hand activations of the same (e.g. rather than showing Corey how to hit "bathroom," a hand-over-hand cue is given), and so on through the steps of learning until use of the button is independent. As these types of pairings and their cueing hierarchies are mastered, less structured activities take their place; things like listening and replying with "yes/no/I don't know", turn taking for a game (which was a great one for Corey and his love of *Connect 4*), or "tell me what you want" interactions with staff and family, where the user is in complete control and has free reign to activate any buttons he likes.

With another round of teaching done (remember: *teach the people, then teach them again until it clicks*) and a series of meetings with Corey's caregivers later, a full plan for his continued use of the E-Talk outside of the session was ready to go. With my role clear, and the roles of the caregivers equally clear, an amazing rebound took place with Corey. While he was still, at times, the loveable goof that Corey could be (and that sense of humor could derail the most carefully-planned sessions), his progress showed he was ready for additional vocabulary and additional challenges.

New arrays were introduced (the 3x5 and 6x6 sizes alluded to previously) and with them plenty of open communication with the care staff. Corey continued to do well. Once again, the question of decreasing his reliance on me to do basic vocabulary upgrades was brought up. Frances was more involved in the discussion this time, and she was on board so long as the communication was still good with the home staff's agency. It was time now, nearly 15 months from his first session, for what I had thought would be the final teaching session, the big one, the one most likely to confuse everyone: programming the E-Talk.

To begin this process I took a moment and rewrote the questionnaire from the first trial. The revised questionnaire looked in more detail at the staff's comfort level with computers in general, as well as with Corey's device in specific: what things the various users had used computers for across any kind of use day-to-day? Had they used a word processor like Word or WordPerfect? Had they used the internet, and could they find their way around if I needed them to use Great Talking Box's website? Had they ever contacted technical support for their computer, for a gadget at home, or for another kind of AAC device?

The response to the questionnaires was mixed. I had a group with highly varying computer experience and comfort. To make sure that everyone was on the same level, I made the programming seminar *very* basic. E-Talk has a PC-based software package that runs all the same functions as the device itself, meaning you can do your programming on your desktop computer, and then synchronize it with the device's memory card. For this session, I had our clinic's computer department get together a handful of our older computers that could run the software, so that the teaching session would be very hands-on. Everyone could have a chance to be programming in the same way (or roughly the same way) that they would be doing it on the E-Talk without needing to pass only Corey's single device around the room. This ensured the session moved at a good pace, minimizing the lag time, and keeping people on the task at hand without a lot of opportunity for idle chit-chat.

It was the day of the teaching session. The room was set up; I had a projector hooked to my laptop so I could be demonstrating while the aides were experimenting for themselves. My notes were ready. 8:30—the starting time—came and went and nobody had shown up. The same thing happened as the clock hit 9:00 A.M. By 9:15, *one* out of the four aides scheduled to come was in the building. As luck might have it, it was the only aide who had had the experience of seeing Corey use his device in person, had done some rudimentary programming in sessions, and was reasonably comfortable with the day-to-day usage of the E-Talk. We waited for a little longer, but no one else came. The short version of what came next involves rescheduling the session, making certain to note how important this information was, and a faxed apology from Corey's care agency about the problems with attendance.

The sessions that elapsed between the cancelled training session and the rescheduled one were largely unremarkable, except for one important thing. I noticed that the "homework" I was giving to the aide who brought him, whom I will call Terri, consistently was not completed. This involved simple additions to existing pages, a concept she had indicated enough comfort with in sessions. I felt this was the easiest possible route towards downgrading Corey towards once-a-month "tech check" sessions, where we made sure the device was in a good working condition.

When I asked Terri what the problem seemed to be, she told me "We're not allowed to program. The bosses told all the aides of people who use computers like this that we're not supposed to mess with them. If we think the computer needs to have changes to it, we have to let the bosses or the therapists do it."

It is here that I would love to tell you that I had a moment of clarity, saw that I was straying from my own "rules" in my sessions and that

I took charge of the situation changing all the things that needed changing starting with my shortcomings. The reality of it, however, was that I had finally had just about all I could take with the way this device was being handled. After a 25-minute call, one that at times was very tense, to Frances and Corey's caregivers later, we came up with an action plan that everyone was happy with and in agreement.

First off, all practice with the E-Talk would be logged in a book so that Frances could audit how much time was being spent with Corey on structured tasks and free-form communication, as well as what issues were experienced, new vocabulary requests, etc. This was a hold-over from the initial "no formal home plan" problems we had had previously. Secondly, the paranoia related to changing the programming was done away with—the daytime aides who worked with Corey the most would have access to the programming menus, password, etc. This allowed for an optimal amount of "on the fly" types of customization and flexibility, where the E-Talk could quickly be converted to meet the changing needs that daily life would present to Corey.

A rescheduled session, again with the four primary daytime-aides that Corey had the most contact with, was put into place. It was light and fun, this session, and all four aides indicated by the end that they were more comfortable with programming.

I started the session with a joke for the group. I took a second to program a hidden button where it showed a blank screen with only a button that said "push here." When this happened, the screen turned black, with the words "All Data Erased: Critical Error" and an explosion noise sounded at the device's current loudness level. It broke the ice and got everyone laughing; I clarified that I was not making fun of their bosses or their policies, but rather getting them to overcome that fear—the E-Talk, like all computers, should NEVER do anything you as the user have not specifically programmed it to do (at least under the normal daily run of things). I would, if I were reading this chapter instead of writing it, copy that last sentence down in big black block letters and hang it somewhere everyone could see it.

After the session, I asked everyone to program their own button on Corey's current array which would allow Corey to greet them when he saw them, tell them goodbye when they left, and, I added with optimism, eventually allow him to create custom requests like "Emily, I need bathroom" or similar. Every time they entered the room, before anything else, they were to have Corey greet them with "Hello (Name)" as a two-button, two-page task. The usual cuing hierarchy of demonstration, then hand-over-hand activation, verbal prompting, and independent activation was to apply here as well. It was a task, I assured the aides, that I would be doing myself with both my own button and one for the receptionist.

In addition, I asked each aide to, on a sticky-note or similar, to come up with four or five important words. These would be ones that Corey would be using every day, or at least more than simply for a holiday. These notes were to be sent with Corey over the next few weeks during his weekly sessions. It was for words like these—or even the situations which would require the buttons—that they were in the unique position to do important "on the fly" programming to enable Corey to request or comment on the things IMMEDIATELY near him at any given time.

Both of these tasks might seem trivial to take the time to explicitly point out to healthcare professional. They might even seem to be my form of talking down to the staff, but I stand by them, as they frame **CARRYOVER RULE #4: MAKE THE HOMEWORK REASONABLE AND FREQUENT**.

To step away from speech devices for just a second, I want to talk about the maturation process I went through as a clinician. When I was on my graduate school externships, both with my adult clients in a rehabilitation hospital and with my pediatric clients at a clinic not-so-dissimilar to where Corey and I worked together, I had a *bear* of a time with homework assignments. Not with my own assignment, that is, (as that would have certainly complicated my final semesters of graduate school) but rather those assigned to my clients. At times, I gave none. Some days would see me giving a little bit to target one goal, and a little targeting a separate goal. And there were times where I was practically having the client not only reinvent the wheel but write a step-by-step book on their method. As I came to my time with Corey, however, I had struck a pretty good balance between homework and no-homework. The problem was that I had never had a speech device client like Corey before. Most of my previous device users were far under him, using lower-tech systems with minimal room for further growth or the need for a $6000 talking computer. So I had to take those lessons from externships, my clinical fellowship time, and my licensed-therapist days and retool them for this situation.

You, as the therapist, will find that this is the case when planning the home program for your own clients. You will have prepared, anticipated the possible issues, backed up the programming, kept yourself flexible, assessed the non-clinical environment, kept lines of communication open, and taught just as often as you need, so you have the tools and information you need to make homework reasonable. There should be *no* session where at least some homework is not assigned, even a session where your device user was *unable to use the device with you during your time*. How can this happen?

It seems that just after the "explosion noise" training session, one of the aides (I still never found out which one) took it upon themselves to use a blue ball-point pen to complete one of their programming assignments. No, they did not use the pen to write the assignment down, or to organize their thoughts on a separate page. Rather, they used it to tap the screen while programming. When the device came to the session, Corey was still groggy, as they had been late in arriving since he had overslept. Owing to the late arrival, I waived the usual "Hello" task at the front desk, and took him right back to the treatment room. The screen was so covered in tiny blue flecks that it was making the touch screen behave badly, and by the time a reset of the device, a recalibration and cleaning of the screen, and a synchronization with my office computer were all finished, we had no time to complete any therapeutic trials that day. The assignment? Sixty minutes each day for the next week of unstructured and structured tasks with a minimum of 45 activations, logged meticulously in the home practice book. These sixty minutes a day did NOT include any other "free form" activations, however, a point explicitly mentioned in the homework. I asked simply for 60 minutes of intense data-keeping; other uses in context were expected and were intended as more—and better—independent practice as far as I was concerned. The last part of this particular home assignment, a brush-up of responsible use of the device by the aides, was accomplished with letter to the aides (forwarded to Frances as well), which required signatures from each of them.

This was not done to be punitive or to throw my weight around as "THE THERAPIST." Simply stated, that 60 minutes of time—which was only a single hour out of their shift/Corey's day—included all the time from the session I had to take to clean the device, which was time *not* spent on furthering Corey's understanding of the E-Talk. It also included some "continuing education" for the staff as to what their role as custodian of the E-Talk was when I was not working with Corey. The note, while admittedly curt compared to the majority of my communications with the staff, got across in no uncertain terms what was acceptable and what was not with regard to use and programming, as well as teaching them the basics of caring for other devices they may encounter in their treatment times.

CONCLUSION

While I have spent a great amount of time cataloging the pitfalls (and some pratfalls as well) of the course of Corey's treatment, I can say with some certainty that as this chapter was being written, Corey was again mentioned for reduction of services and eventual discharge from formal therapy. The good news was that his care company decided that it might be a possibility, but that they were not ready to do so just yet. His timeline, it seems, will continue on with me for at least another six months to a year. The aides—still in flux from resident to resident— have said that they continue to be uncomfortable with the E-Talk. There are concerns that the lack of my "every week" presence will reduce the use of the device, turning it into what Frances referred to as "another toy, a video game." So it seems that Corey, his staff, and I will continue to apply the Four Rules for Carryover. I will keep teaching, keep evaluating the situation, keep leaving the lines of communication open, and keep sending reasonable homework.

As I compiled this chapter, I spoke with my current co-workers on their own experiences with devices, clients who use them and families/caregivers. Their experiences, amazingly, were startlingly similar to my own. Even the families that our department considers "the GOOD families" seem to balk at giving their loved ones a voice at some point in the process. It is a natural tendency, I suppose, to get angry at these folks for dropping the ball. "How could I make it simpler?" the frustrated therapist finds himself asking. "This is basic stuff here!"

It is here that I recalled a bit of theorizing my mother put forth to me a long time ago. I was frustrated with something or other, and this particular problem was not going away on its own accord and certainly was not following *my* schedule for it to be resolved by itself. "Jeff," she told me, "We all go through the five stages of grief every day." And while the problem then—as now with speech devices—is not grieving the loss of someone or something, the thinking is the same.

There is the denial of a proud, but still worried, parent. "MY child does not need a device. You just need to work harder with them" (there may even be even a little bit of anger in there as well). There is the denial of an overworked care staff administrator: "I do not have the time to teach my employees, and they are never going to go for it anyway." The anger follows, as in the parental scenario above, and even "You're telling me that this $8000 device is going to take you a *month* to learn how to program?!" Bargaining here is not the typical kind of plea you might hear in other situations, but rather it is more "You've just *got* to teach him how to use something other than 'want cookie!' He's driving me nuts!" Depression follows on, usually apathetic in tone: "Yeah, I guess we practice with it. It is hard because we have X, Y, and Z going on, so…"

This creates the ideal climate for a system failure—not of the device, but of the therapy session, the home plan, and possibly the relationship between the client, his loved ones, and you the therapist. Powering through this, though, brings you to that final stage of the grief cycle: *acceptance*! Here, the device has been integrated into daily life in ways that may not immediately seem flawless, but are no less functional. The family/loved ones have understanding of the working of the device and of how to include the user in conversation—and make use of that understanding to decrease their reliance on the therapist to do everything for them. The torch is passed: the planned sessions for device updates are reduced to consults once a month (or even less frequently) for overall system checks, as the therapist becomes, in a word, obsolete to the process.

Using these rules of mine is no specific guarantee of getting a specific client to a specific level of mastery. Nor does it ensure that the client's support system will embrace every aspect of their device usage. What they **do**, however, is give the therapist and family a framework on which to build stronger sessions both in and outside the clinical setting. That word "session" might not seem like it belongs next to "outside the clinical setting," but consider the home practice that is structured time—"We're going to spend forty-five minutes on requesting different toys." This to me is no different than the same kind of trials conducted at an outpatient therapy facility. The proctor of this trial is different, but the aim is the same: trials targeting a specific activation skill set to increase overall mastery of the device.

ENDNOTE

1 A note on my use of array dimensions here: I use the shorthand which puts rows before columns, thus "2x5" means "two rows of five columns." This style will be used the same way throughout the chapter.

Compilation of References

Abbeduto, L., & Nuccio, J. B. (1991). Relation between receptive language and cognitive maturity in persons with intellectual disabilities. *American Journal of Intellectual Disabilities*, *96*, 143–149.

Abbeduto, L., & Rosenberg, S. (1992). Linguistic communication in persons with mental retardation. In S. Warren & J. Reichle (Eds.), *Causes and effects in communication and language intervention* (pp. 331-359). Maryland: Paul H. Brookes.

Abbeduto, L., Evans, J., & Dolan, T. (2001). Theoretical perspectives on language and communication problems in mental retardation and developmental disabilities. *Mental Retardation and Developmental Disabilities Research Reviews*, *7*, 45–55. doi:10.1002/1098-2779(200102)7:1<45::AID-MRDD1007>3.0.CO;2-H

Abbeduto, L., Furman, L., & Davies, B. (1989). Relation between the receptive language and mental age of persons with mental retardation. *American Journal of Mental Retardation*, *93*, 535–543.

Aboutabit, N. A., Beautemps, D., & Besacier, L. (Accepted). Lips and hand modeling for recognition of the cued speech gestures: The French vowel case. *Speech Communication.*

Aboutabit, N., Beautemps, D., Clarke, J., & Besacier, L. (2007). A HMM recognition of consonant-vowel syllables from lip contours: the cued speech case. Paper presented at the Interspeech, Antwerp, Belgium.

Abrams, D., Jackson, D., & St. Claire, L. (1990). Social identity and the handicapping functions of stereotypes: Children's understanding of mental and physical handicap. *Human Relations*, *43*, 1085–1098. doi:10.1177/001872679004301103

Abrams, J. J. (Director). (2009). *Star Trek* [Motion picture]. United States: Paramount Pictures.

Abry, C., Badin, P., & Scully, C. (1994). Sound-to-gesture inversion in speech: the Speech Maps approach. In K. Varghese & S. Pfleger & J. P. Lefèvre (Eds.), Advanced speech applications (pp. 182-196). Berlin: Springer Verlag.

Acoustical Society of America. (2009). *Meetings of the Acoustical Society of America.* Retrieved from http://asa.aip.org/meetings.html.

Actroid. (n.d.). Retrieved July 2, 2009, from Wikipedia: http://en.wikipedia.org/wiki/Actroid

Adamlab. (1988). *WOLF manual.* Wayne, MI.

Adams, F.-R., Crepy, H., Jameson, D., & Thatcher, J. (1989). *IBM products for persons with disabilities.* Paper presented at the Global Telecommunications Conference (GLOBECOM'89), Dallas, TX, USA.

Adamson, L. B., Romski, M. A., Deffebach, K., & Sevcik, R. A. (1992). Symbol vocabulary and the focus of conversations: Augmenting language development for youth with mental retardation. *Journal of Speech and Hearing Research*, *35*, 1333–1343.

Adaptive Communication Systems (n.d.). *AllTalk.* Clinton, PA: AllTalk.

Ai Squared. (2009). *Corporate homepage.* Retrieved from http://aisquared.com/

Alcatel-Lucent. (2009). *Bell Labs Historical Timeline*. Retrieved from http://www.alcatel-lucent.com/wps/portal/!ut/p/kcxml/Vc5LDoIwGATgs3CCvxKKuqxI-JBIeCkhh00BaFW0LwQfh9sLCGHeTb5LJQAkFlLp-6N5fq2bS6kkChtBlhlu3P1RxNF0PxZ4iRnwReq8T-kxXICvPMhBYosltxQt08zHCQ8j7nbheO49k-pg8Jtf-dgMncYvKuWY52VUazs7Kynqux3xSjoPhwTmtWX-EgCP4EM-fvuN5LzQXPXQqo8Ni5SliGB_8NT1f/delta/base64xml/L3dJdyEvd0ZNQUFzQUsvNElVRS82X-zlfSVA!

Alencar, M. S., & da Rocha, V. C., Jr. (2005). *Communication systems*. New York: Springer US.

Allauzen, C., Mohri, M., & Riley, M. (2004). Statistical modeling for unit selection in speech synthesis. In *Proceedings of the 42nd Annual Meeting of the Association for Computational Linguistics (ACL'2004)*, (pp. 55-62).

Allen, J. (2005). Designing desirability in an augmentative and alternative communication device. *Universal Access in the Information Society*, *4*, 135–145. doi:10.1007/s10209-005-0117-2

Allen, J., Hunnicutt, S., & Klatt, D. (1987). *From text to speech: The MITalk system*. Cambridge, UK. Cambridge University Press. Bangalore, S., Hakkani-Tür, D., & Tur, G. (2006). Introduction to the special issue on spoken language understanding in conversational systems. *Speech Communication*, *48*(3-4), 233–238.

Allport, G. W. (1958). *The nature of prejudice*. Garden City, NY: Doubleday.

American Psychiatric Association. (2000). *Diagnostic and statistical manual of mental disorders* (4th ed., Text revision). Washington, DC.

American Speech and Hearing Association (ASHA). Retrieved September 14, 2009, http://www.asha.org/public/speech/disorders/AAC.htm

American Speech-Language-Hearing Association. (2005). *Roles and Responsibilities of Speech-Language Pathologists With Respect to Augmentative and Alternative Communication: Position Statement*. Available from www.asha.org/policy.

Anderson, R. J., & Antonak, R. F. (1992). The influence of attitudes and contact on reactions to persons with physical and speech disabilities. *Rehabilitation Counseling Bulletin*, *35*, 240–247.

Angelo, D. H., Kokosa, S. M., & Jones, S. D. (1996). Family perspective on augmentative and alternative communication: families of adolescents and young adults. *Augmentative and Alternative Communication*, *12*(1), 13–20. doi:10.1080/07434619612331277438

Apple Inc. (2009a). *Accessibility-VoiceOver in Depth*. Retrieved from http://www.apple.com/accessibility/voiceover/

Apple Inc. (2009b). *iPhone-Accessibility*. Retrieved from http://www.apple.com/iphone/iphone-3gs/accessibility.html

Aron, M., Berger, M.-O., & Kerrien, E. (2008). Multimodal fusion of electromagnetic, ultrasound and MRI data for building an articulatory model. Paper presented at the International Seminar on Speech Production, Strasbourg, France.

Arvidson, H. H., & Lloyd, L. L. (1997). History of AAC. In L. L. Lloyd, D. R. Fuller, & H. H. Arvidson (Eds.), *Augmentative and alternative communication: A handbook of principles and practices* (pp. 18-25). Boston: Allyn & Bacon.

Ashman, A. F., & Suttie, J. (1996). The medical and health status of older people with mental retardation in Australia. *Journal of Applied Gerontology*, *15*, 57–72. doi:10.1177/073346489601500104

Atal, B. S., & Hanauer, S. L. (1971). Speech analysis and synthesis by linear prediction of Speech Wave. *The Journal of the Acoustical Society of America*, *50*(2b), 637–655. doi:10.1121/1.1912679

Atwell, E., Howarth, P., & Souter, C. (2003). The ISLE Corpus: Italian and German Spoken Learners' English. *ICAME JOURNAL - Computers in English Linguistics*, *27*, 5-18.

Axmear, E., Reichle, J., Alamsaputra, M., Kohnert, K., Drager, K., & Sellnow, K. (2005). Synthesized speech intelligibility in sentences: A comparison of monolingual English speaking and bilingual children. *Language, Speech, and Hearing Services in Schools, 36*, 244–250. doi:10.1044/0161-1461(2005/024)

Badin, P., Elisei, F., Bailly, G., & Tarabalka, Y. (2008). An audiovisual talking head for augmented speech generation: Models and animations based on a real speaker's articulatory data. Paper presented at the Conference on Articulated Motion and Deformable Objects, Mallorca, Spain.

Badin, P., Tarabalka, Y., Elisei, F., & Bailly, G. (2008). Can you "read tongue movements"? Paper presented at the Interspeech, Brisbane, Australia.

Baggia, P., Badino, L., Bonardo, D., & Massimino, P. (2006). *Achieving Perfect TTS Intelligibility.* Paper presented at the AVIOS Technology Symposium, Speech-TEK West 2006, San Francisco, CA, USA.

Bailly, G., Fang, Y., Elisei, F., & Beautemps, D. (2008). Retargeting cued speech hand gestures for different talking heads and speakers. Paper presented at the Auditory-Visual Speech Processing Workshop (AVSP), Tangalooma, Australia.

Baker, B. (1989). Perspectives: Semantic Compaction Systems. *Communicating Together*, 7(4), 8–9.

Balandin, S., & Morgan, J. (2001). Preparing for the future: Aging and alternative and augmentative communication. *Augmentative and Alternative Communication, 17*, 99–108.

Basil, C. (1992). Social interaction and learned helplessness in severely disabled children. *Augmentative and Alternative Communication, 8*, 188–199. doi:10.1080/07434619212331276183

Beautemps, D., Girin, L., Aboutabit, N., Bailly, G., Besacier, L., Breton, G., et al. (2007). TELMA: telephony for the hearing-impaired people. From models to user tests. Toulouse, France.

Beck, A. R., & Fritz, H. (1998). Can people who have aphasia learn iconic codes? *Augmentative and Alternative Communication, 14*, 184–196. doi:10.1080/07434619812331278356

Beck, A. R., & Fritz-Verticchio, H. (2003). The influence of information and role-playing experiences on children's attitudes toward peers who use AAC. *American Journal of Speech-Language Pathology, 12*, 51–60. doi:10.1044/1058-0360(2003/052)

Beck, A., & Dennis, M. (1996). Attitudes of children toward a similar-aged child who uses augmentative communication. *Augmentative and Alternative Communication, 12*, 78–87. doi:10.1080/07434619612331277528

Becker, L. A. (1999). *Effect size calculators.* Retrieved on July 21, 2008, from http://web.uccs.edu/lbecker/Psy590/escalc3.htm

Bedrosian, J. L. (2003). On the subject of subject selection in AAC: Implications for planning and interpreting efficacy research. In R. W. Schlosser (Ed.), *The efficacy of augmentative and alternative communication: Toward evidence-based practice* (pp. 57-83). Boston: Academic Press.

Bell Telephone Laboratories, Inc. (1981). *Impact: A compilation of Bell System innovations in science and engineering that have led to the creation of new products and industries, while improving worldwide telecommunications* (2nd ed.), (L.K. Lustig, Ed.). Murray Hill, NJ: Bell Laboratories.

Bellugi, U., & Klima, E. S. (1976). Two faces of sign: Iconic and abstract. *Annals of the New York Academy of Sciences, 280*, 514–538. doi:10.1111/j.1749-6632.1976.tb25514.x

Benesty, J., Makino, M., & Chen, J. (2005). *Speech enhancement.* New York: Springer.

Bennett, C. L. (2005). Large scale evaluation of corpus-based synthesizers: results and lessons from the Blizzard challenge 2005. In *Proceedings of the 9th European Conference on Speech Communication and Technology (Interspeech-2005/Eurospeech)* (pp. 105–108), Lisbon, Portugal.

Bennett, W., & Runyah, C. (1982). Educator's perceptions of the effects of communication disorders upon educational performance. *Language, Speech, and Hearing Services in Schools, 13*, 260–263.

Benoît, C., Grice, M., & Hazan, V. (1996). The SUS test: A method for the assessment of text-to-speech synthesis intelligibility using Semantically Unpredictable Sentences. *Speech Communication*, *18*(4), 381–392. doi:10.1016/0167-6393(96)00026-X

Berry, B. P. (1972). Comprehension of possessive and present continuous sentences by nonretarded, mildly retarded, and severely retarded children. *American Journal of Mental Deficiency*, *76*, 540–544.

Beukelman, D. R. (1991). Magic and cost of communicative competence. *Augmentative and Alternative Communication*, *7*, 2–10. doi:10.1080/07434619112331275633

Beukelman, D. R., & Mirenda, P. (2005). *Augmentative & alternative communication: Supporting children & adults with complex communication needs* (3rd ed.). Baltimore: Paul H. Brookes Publishing Company.

Beukelman, D. R., Yorkston, K. M., & Reichle, J. (2000). *Augmentative and alternative communication for adults with acquired neurological disorders*. Baltimore, MD: Paul H. Brooks Publishing.

Beukelman, D., & Ansel, B. (1995). Research priorities in augmentative and alternative communication. *Augmentative and Alternative Communication*, *11*, 131–134. doi:10.1080/07434619512331277229

Beukelman, D., Fager, S., Ball, L., & Dietz, A. (2007). AAC for adults with acquired neurological conditions: A review. *Augmentative and Alternative Communication*, *23*, 230–242. doi:10.1080/07434610701553668

Beutnagel, M., Conkie, A., & Syrdal, A. K. (1998). Diphone synthesis using unit selection, In *Proceedings of the 3rd ESCA/COCOSDA International Workshop on Speech Synthesis*, (pp. 185-190).

Beutnagel, M., Conkie, A., Schroeter, J., Stylianou, Y., & Syrdal, A. (1999). *The AT&T Next-Gen TTS System*. Presented at the Joint Meeting of ASA, EAA, and DAGA, Berlin, Germany.

Bigorgne, D., Boeffard, O., Cherbonnel, B., Emerard, F., Larreur, D., Le Saint-Milon, J. L., et al. (1993). Multilingual PSOLA text-to-speech system. In *IEEE International Conference on Acoustics, Speech, and Signal Processing, ICASSP-93*, (Vol.2, pp.187-190).

Binger, C., & Light, J. (2006). Demographics of preschoolers who require augmentative and alternative communication. *Language, Speech, and Hearing Services in Schools*, *37*, 200–208. doi:10.1044/0161-1461(2006/022)

Bishop, D. V. M. (1992). The underlying nature of specific language impairment. *Journal of Child Psychology and Psychiatry, and Allied Disciplines*, *33*, 3–66. doi:10.1111/j.1469-7610.1992.tb00858.x

Black, A. W., & Lenzo, K. A. (2007). *Building synthetic voices*. Retrieved February 2, 2007, from http://festvox.org/festvox/festvox_toc.html

Black, A., & Tokuda, K. (2005). The Blizzard Challenge - 2005: Evaluating corpus-based speech synthesis on common datasets. *INTERSPEECH-2005*, 77-80.

Black, M., Tepperman, J., Kazemzadeh, A., Lee, S., & Narayanan, S. (2008). *Pronunciation Verification of English Letter-Sounds in Preliterate Children*. Paper presented at the 10th International Conference on Spoken Language Processing (ICSLP - Interspeech), Brisbane, Australia.

Blackstone, S., & Hunt-Berg, M. (2004). *Social networks: A communication inventory for individuals with complex communication needs and their communication partners*. Verona, WI: Attainment Company.

Blackstone, S., & Wilkins, D. P. (2009). Exploring the Importance of emotional competence in children with complex communication needs. *Perspectives on Augmentative and Alternative Communication*, *18*, 78–87. doi:10.1044/aac18.3.78

Blau, A. F. (1986). Communication in the back-channel: social structural analyses of nonspeech/speech conversations (augmentative communication, discourse analysis). Ph.D. dissertation, City University of New York, New York. Retrieved August 10, 2009, from Dissertations & Theses: Full Text.(Publication No. AAT 8629674).

Blischak, D. M., & Lloyd, L. L. (1996). Multimodal augmentative and alternative communication: Case study. *Augmentative and Alternative Communication*, *12*, 37–46. doi:10.1080/07434619612331277468

Bliss, C. (1965). *Semantography (Blissymbolics)*. Sydney: Semantography Publications.

Bloch, S., & Wilkinson, R. (2004). The understandability of AAC: a conversation analysis study of acquired dysarthria. *Augmentative and Alternative Communication*, *20*(4), 272–282. doi:10.1080/07434610400005614

Bloch, S., & Wilkinson, R. (2007). The understandability of AAC: A conversation analysis study of acquired dysarthria. *Augmentative and Alternative Communication*, *20*, 272–282. doi:10.1080/07434610400005614

Blockberger, S., Armstrong, R., O'Connor, A., & Freeman, R. (1993). Children's attitudes toward a nonspeaking child using various augmentative and alternative communication techniques. *Augmentative and Alternative Communication*, *9*, 243–250. doi:10.1080/07434619312331276661

Borland, J. (2006, January 26). *Sony puts Aibo to sleep*. Retrieved from http://news.cnet.com/Sony-puts-Aibo-to-sleep/2100-1041_3-6031649.html?tag=mncol

Brady, N. C., & Halle, J. W. (2002). Breakdowns and repairs in conversations between beginning AAC users and their partners. In J. Reichle, D. R. Beukelman, & J. C. Light (Eds.), *Exemplary practices for beginning communicators: Implications for AAC* (pp. 323-351). Baltimore: Paul H. Brookes Publishing Co.

Brady, N. C., McLean, J. E., McLean, L. K., & Johnston, S. (1995). Initiation and repair of intentional communicative acts by adults with severe to profound cognitive disabilities. *Journal of Speech and Hearing Research*, *38*, 1334–1348.

Brain-computer interfaces. (n.d.) Retrieved July 1, 2009, from The Psychology Wiki http://psychology.wikia.com/wiki/Brain-computer_interfaces

Brandenburg, K. (1999). *MP3 and AAC explained*. Paper presented at the AES 17th International Conference on High Quality Audio Coding. Retrieved February 23, 2009 from http://iphome.hhi.de/smolic/MMK/mp3_and_aac_brandenburg.pdf

Brekke, K. M., & von Tetzchner, S. (2003). Co-construction in graphic language development. In S. von Tetzchner & N. Grove (Eds.), *Augmentative and Alternative Communication: Developmental Issues* (pp. 176–210). London: Whurr/Wiley.

Bridges Freeman, S. (1990). Children's attitudes toward synthesized speech varying in quality. (Doctoral dissertation, Michigan State University, 1990). *Dissertation Abstracts International*, *52*(06), 3020B. (UMI No. 9117814)

Bronfenbrenner, U. (1979). *The ecology of human development: experiments by nature and design*. London: Harvard University Press.

Brown, R. (1978). Why are signed languages easier to learn than spoken languages? (Part Two). *Bulletin - American Academy of Arts and Sciences. American Academy of Arts and Sciences*, *32*, 25–44. doi:10.2307/3823113

Bu, N., Tsuji, T., Arita, J., & Ohga, M. (2005). Phoneme classification for speech synthesiser using differential EMG signals between muscles. Paper presented at the IEEE Conference on Engineering in Medicine and Biology, Shanghai, China

Bunnell, H. T., & Lilley, J. (2008). Schwa variants in American English. *Proceedings: Interspeech*, *2008*, 1159–1162.

Bunnell, H. T., Hoskins, S. R., & Yarrington, D. M. (1998). A biphone constrained concatenation method for diphone synthesis. *SSW3-1998*, 171-176.

Bunnell, H. T., Pennington, C., Yarrington, D., & Gray, J. (2005). Automatic personal synthetic voice construction. *INTERSPEECH-2005*, 89-92.

Bunning, K., & Horton, S. (2007). "Border crossing" as a route to inclusion: A shared cause with people with a learning disability? *Aphasiology*, *21*, 9–22. doi:10.1080/02687030600798162

Buzolich, M. J., & Wiemann, J. W. (1988). Turn taking in atypical conversations: The case of the speaker/augmented-communicator dyad. *Journal of Speech and Hearing Research*, *31*, 3–18.

Cameron, J. (Director). (1984). *The Terminator* [Motion picture]. United States: Helmdale Film.

Campbell, J. P. Jr. (1997). Speaker recognition: A tutorial. *Proceedings of the IEEE*, *85*(9), 1437–1462. doi:10.1109/5.628714

Campbell, J., Gilmore, L., & Cuskelly, M. (2003). Changing student teachers' attitudes towards disability and inclusion. *Journal of Intellectual & Developmental Disability*, *28*, 369–379. doi:10.1080/13668250310001616407

Carlesimo, G., Vicari, S., Albertoni, A., Turriziani, P., & Caltagirone, C. (2000). Developmental dissociation between visual and auditory repetition priming: The role of input lexicons. *Cortex*, *36*, 181–193. doi:10.1016/S0010-9452(08)70523-9

Carnegie Mellon University. (2009). *Festvox—Blizzard Challenge*. Retrieved from http://festvox.org/blizzard/

Carr, A., & O'Reilly, G. (2007). Diagnosis, classification and epidemiology. In A. Carr, G. O'Reilly, P. Noonan Walsh, & J. McEvoy (Eds.), *The handbook of intellectual disability and clinical psychology practice* (pp. 3-49). London: Routledge.

Carson, C. (1994). *Star Trek: Generations* [Motion picture]. United States: Paramount Pictures.

Carter, M., & Iacono, T. (2002). Professional judgments of the intentionality of communicative acts. *Augmentative and Alternative Communication*, *18*, 177–191. doi:10.1080/07434610212331281261

Caruso, D. J. (Director). (2008). *Eagle Eye* [Motion picture]. United States: DreamWorks SKG.

Carver, C. S., Glass, D. C., & Katz, I. (1978). Favorable evaluations of blacks and the handicapped: Positive prejudice, unconscious denial, or social desirability. *Journal of Applied Social Psychology*, *8*, 97–106. doi:10.1111/j.1559-1816.1978.tb00768.x

Case, R. (1985). *Intellectual development: Birth to adulthood.* Toronto, ON: Academic Press, Inc.

Cater, J. (1983). *Electronically Speaking: Computer Speech Generation*. Indianapolis: Howard W. Sams & Co., Inc.

Cetta, D.S. (Producer). (2008, November 4). Brain Power [segment]. *60 Minutes* [Television series]. New York: CBS News.

Chambers, J. K. (1995). *Sociolinguistic theory.* Oxford: Blackwell.

Cheslock, M. A., Barton-Hulsey, A., Romski, M. A., & Sevcik, R. A. (2008). Using a speech-generating device to enhance communicative abilities for an adult with moderate intellectual disability. *Intellectual and Developmental Disabilities*, *46*, 376–386. doi:10.1352/2008.46:376-386

Chou, F.-C. (2005). *Ya-Ya Language Box - A Portable Device for English Pronunciation Training with Speech Recognition Technologies.* Paper presented at the 9th European Conference on Speech Communication and Technology (Eurospeech-Interspeech), Lisbon, Portugal.

Choudhury, M. (2003). *Rule-based grapheme to phoneme mapping for Hindi speech synthesis.* A paper presented at the 90th Indian Science Congress of the International Speech Communication Association (ISCA), Bangalore, India.

Church, G., & Glennen, S. (1992). *The handbook of assistive technology.* San Diego: Singular Publishing Co.

Clark, H. H. (1996). *Using language*. Cambridge, UK: Cambridge University Press.

Clark, H. H., & Brennan, S. E. (1991). Grounding in communication. In *Perspectives on socially shared cognition* (pp. 127-149). Washington, DC: American Psychological Association.

Clark, H., Horn, L. R., & Ward, G. (2004). Pragmatics of language performance. In *Handbook of Pragmatics* (pp. 365-382). Oxford: Blackwell.

Clark, R. A., Richmond, K., & King, S. (2004). Festival 2 – build your own general purpose unit selection speech synthesizer. In *Proceedings of the 5th International Speech Communication Association Speech Synthesis Workshop (SSW5)* (pp. 173–178), Pittsburgh, PA.

Clarke, M., & Wilkinson, R. (2007). Interaction between children with cerebral palsy and their peers 1:

Organizing and understanding VOCA use. *Augmentative and Alternative Communication, 23*, 336–348. doi:10.1080/07434610701390350

Clarke, M., & Wilkinson, R. (2008). Interaction between children with cerebral palsy and their peers 2: Understanding initiated VOCA-mediated turns. *Augmentative and Alternative Communication, 24*, 3–15. doi:10.1080/07434610701390400

Clarke, M., McConachie, H., Price, K., & Wood, P. (2001). Views of young people using augmentative and alternative communication systems. *International Journal of Language & Communication Disorders, 36*, 107–115. doi:10.1080/13682820150217590

Cleuren, L., Duchateau, J., Sips, A., Ghesquiere, P., & Van Hamme, H. (2006). *Developing an Automatic Assessment Tool for Children's Oral Reading.* Paper presented at the 9th International Conference on Spoken Language Processing (ICSLP - Interspeech), Pittsburgh, PA, USA.

Cohen, J. (1988). *Statistical power analysis for the behavioral sciences* (2nd ed). Hillsdale, NJ: Lawrence Erlbaum Associates.

Cohen, J. (1992). A power primer. *Psychological Bulletin, 112*, 15–159.

Coker, C. H. (1985). A dictionary-intensive letter-to-sound program. *Journal of the Acoustical Society of America., suppl. 1, 78*(S1), S7.

Coker, C. H., Denes, P. B., & Pinson, E. N. (1963). *Speech Synthesis: An Experiment in Electronic Speech Production.* Baltimore: Waverly Press.

Cole, R., Halpern, A., Ramig, L., van Vuuren, S., Ngampatipatpong, N., & Yan, J. (2007). A Virtual Speech Therapist for Individuals with Parkinson Disease. *Journal of Education Technology, 47*(1), 51–55.

Colella, A., & Varma, A. (1999). Disability-job fit stereotypes and the evaluation of persons with disabilities at work. *Journal of Occupational Rehabilitation, 9*, 79–95. doi:10.1023/A:1021362019948

Collins, S. (1996). Referring expression in conversations between aided and natural speakers. In S. von Tetzchner & M. Jensen (Eds.), *Augmentative and alternative communication: European perspectives* (pp. 89-100). London: Whurr/Wiley.

Comer, R. J., & Piliavin, J. A. (1972). The Effects of Physical Deviance upon Face-to Face Interaction: The Other Side. *Journal of Personality and Social Psychology, 23*, 33–39. doi:10.1037/h0032922

Conkie, A., & Isard, S. (1994). Optimal coupling of diphones. *SSW2-1994*, 119-122.

Connor, S. (2009). The strains of the voice. In K. Izdebski (ed.), *Emotions in the human voice, volume 3: Culture and perception* (1st ed.), (pp. 297-306). San Diego, CA: Plural Publishing Inc.

Cook, S. W., & Selltiz, C. (1964). A multiple-indicator approach to attitude measurement. *Psychological Bulletin, 62*, 36–55. doi:10.1037/h0040289

Cooper, H. M., & Hedges, L. V. (Eds.). (1994). Research synthesis as a scientific enterprise. In *The handbook of research synthesis* (pp. 3-14). New York: Russell Sage Foundation.

Cornett, R. O. (1967). Cued speech. *American Annals of the Deaf, 112*, 3–13.

Coulston, R., Oviatt, S., & Darves, C. (2002). Amplitude convergence in children's conversational speech with animated personas. In *Proceedings of the 7th International Conference on Spoken Language Processing* (pp. 2689–2692), Boulder, CO.

Cowley, C. K., & Jones, D. M. (1992). Synthesized or digitized? A guide to the use of computer speech. *Applied Ergonomics, 23*(3), 172–176. doi:10.1016/0003-6870(92)90220-P

Cox, R. M., Alexander, G. C., & Gilmore, C. (1987). Intelligibility of average talkers in typical listening environments. *The Journal of the Acoustical Society of America, 81*(5), 1598–1608. doi:10.1121/1.394512

Crabtree, M., Mirenda, P., & Beukelman, D. R. (1990). Age and gender preferences for synthetic and natural speech. *Augmentative and Alternative Communication, 6*(4), 256–261. doi:10.1080/07434619012331275544

Crandall, C. S., & Eshleman, A. (2003). A justification-expression model of the expression and experience of prejudice. *Psychological Bulletin, 119*, 414–446. doi:10.1037/0033-2909.129.3.414

Crawford, D., & Ostrove, J. M. (2003). Representations of Disability and the Interpersonal Relationships of Women with Disabilities. *Women & Therapy, 26*, 179–194. doi:10.1300/J015v26n03_01

Creech, R. (1996) *Extemporaneous speaking: Pragmatic principles*. Paper Presented at the 4th. Annual Pittsburgh Employment Conference, Pittsburgh, PA.

Creehan, D. (2003). *Artificial Intelligence for ASIMO*. Retrieved from http://popularrobotics.com/asimo_ai.htm
de Kermadec, F. J. (2004). *Are You Talking to Me? Speech on Mac OS X*. Retrieved from http://www.macdevcenter.com/pub/a/mac/2004/03/17/speech.html

Creer, S. M., Cunningham, S. P., Green, P. D., & Fatema, K. (in press). Personalizing synthetic voices for people with progressive speech disorders: judging voice similarity. In *Proceedings of Interspeech2009.*

Cruice, M., Worrall, L., & Hickson, L. (2006). Quantifying aphasic people's social lives in the context of non-aphasic peers. *Aphasiology, 20*, 1210–1225. doi:10.1080/02687030600790136

Cucchiarini, C., Lembrechts, D., & Strik, H. (2008). *HLT and communicative disabilities: The need for co-operation between government, industry and academia.* Paper presented at the LangTech2008, Rome, Italy.

Darves, C., & Oviatt, S. (2002). Adaptation of users' spoken dialogue patterns in a conversational interface. In *Proceedings of the 7th International Conference on Spoken Language Processing* (pp. 561–564), Boulder, CO.

Dattilo, J., & Camarata, S. (1991). Facilitating conversation through self-initiated augmentative communication treatment. *Journal of Applied Behavior Analysis, 24*, 369–378. doi:10.1901/jaba.1991.24-369

DeHouwer, J., & Moors, A. (2007). How to define and examine the implicitness of implicit measures. In B. Wittenbrink & N. Schwarz (eds.) *Implicit measures of attitudes: Procedures and controversies*. New York: Guilford Press (pp. 179-194).

Demasco, P. (1994). Human factors considerations in the design of language interfaces in AAC. *Assistive Technology, 6*, 10–25.

Dempster, F. N. (1981). Memory span: Sources of individual and developmental differences. *Psychological Bulletin, 89*, 63–100. doi:10.1037/0033-2909.89.1.63

Dickerson, S. S., Stone, V. I., Panchura, C., & Usiak, D. J. (2002). The meaning of communication: experiences with augmentative communication devices. *Rehabilitation Nursing, 27*, 215–220.

Dowden, P. (1997). Augmentative and alternative communication decision making for children with severely unintelligible speech. *Augmentative and Alternative Communication, 13*, 48–59. doi:10.1080/07434619712331277838

Drager, K. D. R., & Reichle, J. E. (2001a). Effects of age and divided attention on listeners' comprehension of synthesized speech. *Augmentative and Alternative Communication, 17*, 109–119.

Drager, K. D. R., & Reichle, J. E. (2001b). Effects of discourse context on the intelligibility of synthesized speech for young adult and older adult listeners: Applications for AAC. *Journal of Speech, Language, and Hearing Research: JSLHR, 44*, 1052–1057. doi:10.1044/1092-4388(2001/083)

Drager, K. D. R., Anderson, J. L., DeBarros, J., Hayes, E., Liebman, J., & Panek, E. (2007). Speech synthesis in background noise: Effects of message formulation and visual information on the intelligibility of American English DECtalk. *Augmentative and Alternative Communication, 23*, 177–186. doi:10.1080/07434610601159368

Drager, K. D. R., Clark-Serpentine, E. A., Johnson, K. E., & Roeser, J. L. (2006). Accuracy of repetition of digitized and synthesized speech for young children in background noise. *American Journal of Speech-Language Pathology, 15*(2), 155–164. doi:10.1044/1058-0360(2006/015)

Drager, K. D. R., Postal, V. J., Carrolus, L., Castellano, M., Gagliano, C., & Glynn, J. (2006). The effect of aided language modeling on symbol comprehension and production in two preschoolers with autism. *American Journal of Speech-Language Pathology, 15*, 112–125. doi:10.1044/1058-0360(2006/012)

Drager, K., Ende, E., Harper, E., Iapalucci, M., & Rentschler, K. (2004). *Digitized Speech Output for Young Children Who Require AAC.* Poster presented at the annual convention of the American Speech-Language-Hearing Association, Philadelphia, PA.

Drager, K., Finke, E., Gordon, M., Holland, K., Lacey, L., Nellis, J., et al. (2008, August). *Effects of Practice on the Intelligibility of Synthesized Speech for Young Children.* Poster presented at the biennial conference of the International Society for Augmentative and Alternative Communication, Montréal, Québec, Canada.

Duchateau, J., Cleuren, L., Van Hamme, H., & Ghesquiere, P. (2007). *Automatic Assessment of Children's Reading Level.* Paper presented at the 10th European Conference on Speech Communication and Technology (Eurospeech-Interspeech), Antwerp, Belgium.

Duffy, J. (2005). *Motor speech disorders: substrates, differential diagnosis and management* (2nd ed.). St Louis, MO: Elsevier Mosby.

Duffy, S. A., & Pisoni, D. B. (1992). Comprehension of synthetic speech produced by rule: A review and theoretical interpretation. *Language and Speech, 35*, 351–389.

Duker, P. C., van Driel, S., & van de Bracken, J. (2002). Communication profiles of individuals with Down's syndrome, Angelman syndrome, and pervasive developmental disorders. *Journal of Intellectual Disability Research, 46*, 35–40. doi:10.1046/j.1365-2788.2002.00355.x

Dunn, H. K., & White, S. D. (1940). Statistical measurements on conversational speech. *The Journal of the Acoustical Society of America, 11*(3), 278–288. doi:10.1121/1.1916034

Dutoit, T. (1997). High-quality text-to-speech synthesis: An overview. *Electrical and electronics . Engineers Australia, 17*(1), 25–36.

Dutoit, T., & Leich, H. (1993). MBR-PSOLA: Text-to-speech synthesis based on an MBE re-synthesis of the segments database. *Speech Communication, 13*(3-4), 435–440. doi:10.1016/0167-6393(93)90042-J

Dynavox Technologies (n.d.). *Dynavox MT4.* Pittsburgh, PA.

EAR Studio, Inc. (n.d.). *Listening Post Homepage.* Retrieved July 1, 2009 from http://www.earstudio.com/projects/listeningpost.html.

EAR Studio, Inc. (Producer). (2002, December). *Listening Post – Part 1.* Video posted to http://video.google.com/videoplay?docid=-1219120608081240028

Ebert. (2009). *Finding my own voice.* Retrieved September 14, 2009 from http://blogs.suntimes.com/ebert/2009/08/finding_my_own_voice.html

Elliot, T., & Frank, R. (1990). Social and interpersonal reactions to depression and disability. *Rehabilitation Psychology, 35*, 135–147.

Enabling Devices (n.d.). *7-Level Communicator.* Hastings on Hudson, NY.

Engwall, O., & Bälter, O. (2007). Pronunciation feedback from real and virtual language teachers. *Journal of Computer Assisted Language Learning, 20*(3), 235–262. doi:10.1080/09588220701489507

Engwall, O., & Wik, P. (2009). *Are real tongue movements easier to speech read than synthesized?* Paper presented at the 11th European Conference on Speech Communication and Technology (Eurospeech-Interspeech), Brighton, UK.

Eriksson, E., Bälter, O., Engwall, O., & Öster, A.-M. (2005). *Design Recommendations for a Computer-Based Speech Training System Based on End-User Interviews.* Paper presented at the 10th International Conference Speech and Computer (SPECOM), Patras, Greece.

Evans, J. L., Viele, K., Kass, R. E., & Tang, F. (2002). Grammatical morphology and perception of synthetic and natural speech in children with specific language impairments. *Journal of Speech, Language, and Hearing Research: JSLHR, 45*, 494–504. doi:10.1044/1092-4388(2002/039)

Falkman, K., Dahlgren Sandberg, A., & Hjelmquist, E. (2002). Preferred communication modes: Pre-linguistic and linguistic communication in non-speaking children with cerebral palsy. *International Journal of Language & Communication Disorders, 37*, 59–68. doi:10.1080/13682820110096661

Fant, C. G. M. (1960). *Acoustic theory of speech production*. The Hague, The Netherlands: Mouton.

Fant, G. (1960). *Acoustic theory of speech production*. The Hague, The Netherlands: Mouton & Co.

Fant, G. (Ed.). (1960). *Acoustic theory of speech production*. The Hague, Netherlands: Mouton.

Fichten, C. S., & Amsel, R. (1986). Trait Attributions about College Students with a Physical Disability: Circumplex Analyses and Methodological Issues. *Journal of Applied Social Psychology, 16*, 410–427. doi:10.1111/j.1559-1816.1986.tb01149.x

Fichten, C. S., & Bourdon, C. V. (1986). Social Skill Deficit or Response Inhibition: Interaction between Disabled and Nondisabled College Students. *Journal of College Student Personnel, 27*, 326–333.

Fichten, C. S., Robillard, K., Judd, D., & Amsel, R. (1989). College students with physical disabilities: Myths and realities. *Rehabilitation Psychology, 34*, 243–257.

Findler, L., Vilchinsky, N., & Werner, S. (2007). The multidimensional attitudes scale toward persons with disabilities (MAS): Construction and validation. *Rehabilitation Counseling Bulletin, 50*, 166–176. doi:10.1177/00343552070500030401

Fine, M., & Asch, A. (1988). *Women with disabilities: Essays in psychology, culture, and politics*. Temple University Press: Philadelphia.

Fiske, S. T. (2005). Social cognition and the normality of prejudgment. In J. F. Dovidio, P. Glick, & L. A. Rudman (Eds.), *Reflecting on "The Nature of Prejudice,"* (pp. 36-53). Malden, MA: Blackwell.

Fiske, S. T., Cuddy, A. J. C., Glick, P., & Xu, J. (2002). A model of (often mixed) stereotype content: Competence and warmth respectively follow from status and competition. *Journal of Personality and Social Psychology, 82*, 878–902. doi:10.1037/0022-3514.82.6.878

Fitzpatrick, T. (2006) *Teenager moves video icons just by imagination*. Retrieved from http://news-info.wustl.edu/news/page/normal/7800.html

Flanagan, J. L. (1957). Note on the design of terminal analog speech synthesizers. *The Journal of the Acoustical Society of America, 29*(2), 306–310. doi:10.1121/1.1908864

Forster, S., & Iacono, T. A. (2007). Perceptions of communication before and after a speech pathology intervention for an adult with intellectual disability. *Journal of Intellectual & Developmental Disability, 32*, 302–314. doi:10.1080/13668250701654425

Fowler, C. A. (1980). Coarticulation and theories of extrinsic timing. *Journal of Phonetics, 8*, 113–133.

FreedomScientific. (2009). *Products page*. Retrieved from http://www.freedomscientific.com/product-portal.asp

Fucci, D., Reynolds, M. E., Bettagere, R., & Gonzales, M. D. (1995). Synthetic speech intelligibility under several experimental conditions. *Augmentative and Alternative Communication, 11*, 113–117. doi:10.1080/07434619512331277209

Fujiki, M., Brinton, B., Isaacson, T., & Summers, C. (2001). Social behaviors of children with language impairments on the playground: A pilot study. *Language, Speech, and Hearing Services in Schools, 32*, 101–113. doi:10.1044/0161-1461(2001/008)

Fukada, T., Tokuda, K., Kobayashi, T., & Imai, S. (1992). An adaptive algorithm for mel-cepstral analysis of speech. In *Proceedings of IEEE International Conference on Acoustics, Speech, and Signal Processing* (pp. 137–140), San Francisco, CA.

Furnham, A., & Thompson, R. (1994). Actual and perceived attitudes of wheelchair users. *Counselling Psychology Quarterly, 7*, 35. doi:10.1080/09515079408254133

García-Gómez, R., López-Barquilla, R., Puertas-Tera, J.-I., Parera-Bermúdez, J., Haton, M.-C., Haton, J.-P., et al. (1999). *Speech Training for Deaf and Hearing Impaired*

People: ISAEUS Consortium. Paper presented at the 6th European Conference on Speech Communication and Technology (Eurospeech-Interspeech), Budapest, Hungary.

Garrett, K. L & Kimelman M. D. Z. (2000) AAC and aphasia: Cognitive-linguistic considerations. In: Beukelman D. R, Yorkston K. M & Reichle J (Eds.) *Augmentative and alternative communication for adults with acquired neurologic disorders* (pp.339-374). Baltimore: Paul H. Brookes.

Gerosa, M., & Narayanan, S. (2008). *Investigating Assessment of Reading Comprehension in Young Children.* Paper presented at the International Conference on Acoustics, Speech and Signal Processing (ICASSP), Las Vegas, NV, USA.

Gertner, B., Rice, M., & Hadley, P. (1994). Influence of communicative competence on peer preferences in a preschool classroom. *Journal of Speech and Hearing Research, 37,* 913–923.

Gibert, G., Bailly, G., & Elisei, F. (2006). Evaluating a virtual speech cuer. Paper presented at the InterSpeech, Pittsburgh, PE.

Gibert, G., Bailly, G., Beautemps, D., Elisei, F., & Brun, R. (2005). A analysis and synthesis of the 3D movements of the head, face and hand of a speaker using cued speech. *The Journal of the Acoustical Society of America, 118*(2), 1144–1153. doi:10.1121/1.1944587

Gilbert, D. T., & Hixon, J. G. (1991). The trouble of thinking: Activation of stereotypic beliefs. *Journal of Personality and Social Psychology, 60,* 509–517. doi:10.1037/0022-3514.60.4.509

Glennen, S. L., & Decoste, D. C. (1997). *Handbook of augmentative and alternative communication.* San Diego: Singular Publishing Group.

Goffman, E. (1963). *Stigma: Notes on the management of spoiled identity.* Englewood Cliffs, NJ: Prentice Hall.

Goffman, L., Smith, A., Heisler, L., & Ho, M. (2008). The breadth of coarticulatory units in children and adults. *Journal of Speech, Language, and Hearing Research: JSLHR, 51*(6), 1424–1437. doi:10.1044/1092-4388(2008/07-0020)

Gong, L., & Lai, J. (2003). To mix or not to mix synthetic speech and human speech? Contrasting impact on judge-rated task performance versus self-rated performance and attitudinal responses. *International Journal of Speech Technology, 6,* 123–131. doi:10.1023/A:1022382413579

Gong, L., & Nass, C. (2007). When a talking-face computer agent is half-human and half-humanoid: Human identity and consistency preference. *Human Communication Research, 33,* 163–193.

Gorenflo, C. W., & Gorenflo, D. W. (1991). The effects of information and augmentative communication technique on attitudes toward nonspeaking individuals. *Journal of Speech and Hearing Research, 34,* 19–26.

Gorenflo, C. W., Gorenflo, D. W., & Santer, S. A. (1994). Effects of synthetic voice output on attitudes toward the augmented communicator. *Journal of Speech and Hearing Research, 37,* 64–68.

Gorenflo, D. W., & Gorenflo, C. W. (1997). Effects of synthetic speech, gender, and perceived similarity on attitudes toward the augmented communicator. *Augmentative and Alternative Communication, 13,* 87–91. doi:10.1080/07434619712331277878

Gouvier, W. D., Sytsma-Jordan, S., & Mayville, S. (2003). Patterns of discrimination in hiring job applicants with disabilities: The role of disability type, job complexity, and public contact. *Rehabilitation Psychology, 48,* 175–181. doi:10.1037/0090-5550.48.3.175

Granström, B. (2005). *Speech Technology for Language Training and e-Inclusion.* Paper presented at the 9th European Conference on Speech Communication and Technology (Eurospeech-Interspeech), Lisbon, Portugal.

Green, B. G., Logan, J. S., & Pisoni, D. B. (1986). Perception of synthetic speech produced automatically by rule: Intelligibility of eight text-to-speech systems. *Behavior Research Methods, Instruments, & Computers, 18*(2), 100–107.

Green, S., Davis, C., Karshmer, E., Marsh, P., & Straight, B. (2005). Living stigma: The impact of labeling, stereotyping, separation, status loss, and discrimination in the lives of individuals with disabilities and their families. *Sociological Inquiry*, *75*, 197–215. doi:10.1111/j.1475-682X.2005.00119.x

Greenberg, H. (2001, June 25). Watch It! The Traps Are Set The best investing advice is the most basic: Beware of getting too clever. *Fortune*. Retrieved from http://money.cnn.com/magazines/fortune/fortune_archive/2001/06/25/305449/index.htm

Greene, B. G. (1983). Perception of synthetic speech by children. In *Research on Speech Perception Progress Report No. 9*. Bloomington, IN: Speech Research Laboratory, Indiana University.

Greene, B. G., & Pisoni, D. B. (1982). Perception of synthetic speech by children: A first report. In *Research on Speech Perception Progress Report No. 8*. Bloomington, IN: Speech Research Laboratory, Indiana University.

Greene, B. G., Logan, J. S., & Pisoni, D. B. (1986). Perception of synthetic speech produced automatically by rule: Intelligibility of eight text-to-speech systems. *Behavior Research Methods, Instruments, & Computers*, *18*, 100–107.

Greene, B. G., Manous, L. M., & Pisoni, D. B. (1984). *Perceptual evaluation of DECtalk: A final report on version 1.8* (Progress Report No. 10). Bloomington, IN: Indiana University Speech Research Laboratory.

Greenspan, S. L., Nusbaum, H. C., & Pisoni, D. B. (1988). Perceptual learning of synthetic speech produced by rule. *Journal of Experimental Psychology. Human Perception and Performance*, *14*, 421–433.

Greenwald, A. G., McGhee, D. E., & Schwartz, J. L. K. (1998). Measuring individual differences in implicit cognition: The Implicit Association Test. *Journal of Personality and Social Psychology*, *74*, 1464–1480. doi:10.1037/0022-3514.74.6.1464

Gregory, D. (1998). Reactions to Ballet with Wheelchairs: Reflections of Attitudes toward People with Disabilities. *Journal of Music Therapy*, *35*(4), 274–283.

Grice, H. P. (1975). Logic & conversation. *Syntax & Semantics*, *3*, 41–58.

Guéguin, M., Le Bouquin-Jeannès, R., Gautier-Turbin, V., Faucon, G., & Barriac, V. (2008). On the evaluation of the conversational speech quality in telecommunications. EURASIP Journal on Advances in Signal Processing, Article ID 185248, 185215 pages.

Guenther, F. H., Ghosh, S. S., & Tourville, J. A. (2006). Neural modeling and imaging of the cortical interactions underlying syllable production. *Brain and Language*, *96*(3), 280–301. doi:10.1016/j.bandl.2005.06.001

Guenther, F., & Brumberg, J. (2009, May). *Real-time speech synthesis for neural prosthesis*. Paper presented at the 157th Meeting of the Acoustical Society of America, Portland, OR.

Hamm, B., & Mirenda, P. (2006). Post-school Quality of Life for individuals with developmental disabilities who use AAC. *Augmentative and Alternative Communication*, *22*, 134–147. doi:10.1080/07434610500395493

Hanson, E. K., & Sundheimer, C. (2009). Telephone talk: Effects of timing and use of a floorholder message on telephone conversations using synthesized speech. *Augmentative and Alternative Communication*, *25*, 90–98. doi:10.1080/07434610902739926

Hanson, H. M., & Stevens, K. N. (2002). A quasiarticulatory approach to controlling acoustic source parameters in a Klatt-type formant synthesizer using HLsyn. *The Journal of the Acoustical Society of America*, *112*(3), 1158–1182. doi:10.1121/1.1498851

Harber, K. (1998). Feedback to minorities: Evidence of a positive bias. *Journal of Personality and Social Psychology*, *74*, 622–628. doi:10.1037/0022-3514.74.3.622

Haring, N. G., McCormick, L., & Haring, T. G. (Eds.). (1994). *Exceptional children and youth* (6th ed.). New York: Merrill.

Harper, D. C. (1999). Social psychology of difference: Stigma, spread, and stereotypes in childhood. *Rehabilitation Psychology*, *44*, 131–144. doi:10.1037/0090-5550.44.2.131

Harris, D. (1982). Communicative interaction processes involving nonvocal physically handicapped children. *Topics in Language Disorders, 2*, 21–37.

Harris, M. D., & Reichle, J. (2004). The impact of aided language stimulation on symbol comprehension and production in children with moderate cognitive disabilities. *Am. Journ. of Speech-Language Pathology, 13*, 155–167. doi:10.1044/1058-0360(2004/016)

Harris, Z. S. (1955). From phoneme to morpheme. *Language, 31*(2), 190–222. doi:10.2307/411036

Harrison, A.-M., Lau, W.-Y., Meng, H., & Wang, L. (2008). *Improving mispronunciation detection and diagnosis of learners' speech with context-sensitive phonological rules based on language transfer.* Paper presented at the 10th International Conference on Spoken Language Processing (ICSLP - Interspeech), Brisbane, Australia.

Hart, R. D., & Williams, D. E. (1995). Able-Bodied Instructors and Students with Physical Disabilities: A Relationship Handicapped by Communication. *Communication Education, 44*, 140–154. doi:10.1080/03634529509379005

Haskins Laboratories. (1953). *Haskins Laboratories.* Retrieved from http://www.haskins.yale.edu/history/haskins1953.pdf

Haskins Laboratories. (2008a). *The "Adventure" Film.* Retrieved from http://www.haskins.yale.edu/history/Adventure.html

Haskins Laboratories. (2008b). *Decades of Discovery–1950s.* Retrieved from http://www.haskins.yale.edu/decades/fifties.html

Hatzis, A. (1999). *Optical Logo-Therapy: Computer-Based Audio-Visual Feedback Using Interactive Visual Displays for Speech Training.* Unpublished doctoral dissertation, University of Sheffield, United Kingdom.

Hatzis, A., Green, P., Carmichael, J., Cunningham, S., Palmer, R., Parker, M., & O'Neill, P. (2003). *An Integrated Toolkit Deploying Speech Technology for Computer Based Speech Training with Application to Dysarthric Speakers.* Paper presented at the 8th European Conference on Speech Communication and Technology (Eurospeech-Interspeech), Geneva, Switzerland.

Hatzis, A., Green, P.-D., & Howard, S.-J. (1997). *Optical Logo-Therapy (OLT): A Computer-Based Real Time Visual Feedback Application for Speech Training.* Paper presented at the 5th European Conference on Speech Communication and Technology (Eurospeech-Interspeech), Rhodes, Greece.

Hawking, S. (2009). *Prof. Stephen Hawking's disability advice.* Retrieved September 14, 2009, from http://www.hawking.org.uk/index.php/disability/disabilityadvice

Hawking, S. (n.d.). *Prof. Stephen Hawking's Computer.* Retrieved June 30, 2009, from http://www.hawking.org.uk/index.php/disability/thecomputer

Hebl, M., & Kleck, R. E. (2000). The social consequences of physical disability. In T. F. Heatherton, R. E. Kleck, J. Hull, & M. R. Hebl, J. G. Hull (Eds.), *The social psychology of stigma* (pp. 88-125). New York: Guilford Press.

Hebl, M., Tickle, J., & Heatherton, T. (2000). Awkward moments in interactions between nonstigmatized and stigmatized individuals. In T. F. Heatherton, R. E. Kleck, J. Hull, & M. R. Hebl, J. G. Hull (Eds.), *The social psychology of stigma* (pp. 88-125). New York: Guilford Press.

Heinemann, W. (1990). Meeting the handicapped: A case of affective-cognitive inconsistency. In W. Stroebe & M. Hewstone (Eds.) *European review of social psychology,* (Vol.1, pp. 323-335). London: John Wiley.

Henderson, M., & Naughton, P. (2009, April 21). Prof Stephen Hawking 'comfortable' in hospital after health scare. *TimesOnline.* Retrieved from http://www.timesonline.co.uk/tol/news/uk/science/article6139493.ece

Henton, C. (2002). Challenges and rewards in using parametric or concatenative speech synthesis. *International Journal of Speech Technology, 5*(2), 117–131. doi:10.1023/A:1015416013198

Henton, C. (2003). Taking a look at TTS. *Speech Technology,* (January-February), 27-30.

Hertz, S. R., & Huffman, M. K. (1992). A nucleus-based timing model applied to multi-dialect speech synthesis by rule. *ICSLP-1992*, 1171-1174.

Hesseldahl, A. (2001, January 19). Disaster Of The Day: Lernout & Hauspie. *Forbes*. Retrieved from http://www.forbes.com/2001/01/19/0119disaster.html

Hetzroni, O. E., & Harris, O. L. (1996). Cultural aspects in the development of AAC users. *Augmentative and Alternative Communication*, *12*(1), 52–58. doi:10.1080/07434619612331277488

Higginbotham, D. J., & Baird, E. (1995). Analysis of listeners' summaries of synthesized speech passages. *Augmentative and Alternative Communication*, *11*, 101–112. doi:10.1080/07434619512331277199

Higginbotham, D. J., & Caves, K. (2002). AAC performance and usability issues: the effect of AAC technology on the communicative process. *Assistive Technology*, *14*(1), 45–57.

Higginbotham, D. J., & Wilkins, D. (2009). In-person interaction in AAC: New perspectives on utterances, multimodality, timing and device design. *Perspectives on Augmentative Communication.*

Higginbotham, D. J., & Wilkins, D. P. (1999). Slipping through the timestream: Time and timing issues in augmentative communication. In J. Duchan, D. Kovarsky & M. Maxwell (eds.), *The social construction of language incompetence*, (pp. 49-82). Mahwah, NJ: Lawrence Erlbaum Publishing.

Higginbotham, D. J., Drazek, A. L., Kowarsky, K., Scally, C. A., & Segal, E. (1994). Discourse comprehension of synthetic speech delivered at normal and slow presentation rates. *Augmentative and Alternative Communication*, *10*, 191–202. doi:10.1080/07434619412331276900

Higginbotham, D. J., Kim, K., & Scally, C. (2007). The effect of the communication output method on augmented interaction. *Augmentative and Alternative Communication*, *23*, 140–153. doi:10.1080/07434610601045344

Higginbotham, D. J., Scally, C. A., Lundy, D. C., & Kowarsky, K. (1995). Discourse comprehension of synthetic speech across three augmentative and alternative communication (AAC) output methods. *Journal of Speech, Language, and Hearing Research: JSLHR*, *38*, 889–901.

Higginbotham, D. J., Scally, C., Lundy, D., & Kowarsky, K. (1995). The effect of communication output method on the comprehension of synthesized discourse passages. *Journal of Speech and Hearing Research*, *38*, 889–901.

Higginbotham, D. J., Shane, H., Russell, S., & Caves, K. (2007). Access to AAC: Present, past, and future. *Augmentative and Alternative Communication*, *23*, 243–257. doi:10.1080/07434610701571058

Higginbotham, D.J. (1997). Class Lecture.

Hilari, K., & Northcott, S. (2006). Social support in people with chronic aphasia. *Aphasiology*, *20*, 17–36. doi:10.1080/02687030500279982

Hill, K. J. (2001). *The development of a model for automated performance measurement and the establishment of performance indices for augmented communicators under two sampling conditions.* Ph.D. dissertation, University of Pittsburgh, Pennsylvania. Retrieved August 10, 2009, from Dissertations & Theses: Full Text.(Publication No. AAT 3013368).

Hjelmquist, E., & Dahlgren Sandberg, A. (1996). Sounds and silence: Interaction in aided language use. In S. von Tetzchner & M. Jensen (Eds.), *Augmentative and Alternative Communication: European perspectives* (pp. 137–152). London: Whurr/Wiley.

Hofe, R., & Moore, R. K. (2008). AnTon: an animatronic model of a human tongue and vocal tract. Paper presented at the Interspeech, Brisbane, Australia.

Hollingum, J., & Cassford, G. (1988). *Speech technology at work*. London: IFS Publications.

Holmes, J. N. (1961). Research on Speech Synthesis Carried out during a Visit to the Royal Institute of Technology, Stockholm, from November 1960 to March 1961. *Joint Speech Resear4ch Unit Report JU 11.4, British Post Office, Eastcote, England.*

Holmes, J. N. (1973). The influence of the glottal waveform on the naturalness of speech from a parallel formant synthesizer. *IEEE Trans., AU-21*, 298–305.

Holmes, J., & Holmes, W. (2001). *Speech synthesis and recognition* (2nd Ed.). London: Taylor and Francis.

Honda Motor Company, Ltd. (2009, March 31). *Honda, ATR and Shimadzu Jointly Develop Brain-Machine Interface Technology Enabling Control of a Robot by Human Thought Alone*. Retrieved from http://world.honda.com/news/2009/c090331Brain-Machine-Interface-Technology/

Hoover, J., Reichle, J., Van Tasell, D., & Cole, D. (1987). The intelligibility of synthesized speech: Echo II versus Votrax. *Journal of Speech and Hearing Research, 30*, 425–431.

Hourcade, J., Pilotte, J. P., West, E., & Parette, P. (2004). A history of augmentative and alternative communication for individuals with severe and profound disabilities. *Focus on Autism and Other Developmental Disabilities, 19*, 235–244. doi:10.1177/10883576040190040501

Howland, C. A., & Rintala, D. H. (2001). Dating behaviors of disabled women. *Sexuality and Disability, 19*, 41–70. doi:10.1023/A:1010768804747

Huang, X., Acero, A., Adcock, J., Hon, H.-W., Goldsmith, J., Liu, J., & Plumpe, M. (1996). Whistler: A trainable text-to-speech system. In *Proceedings of the 4th International. Conference on Spoken Language Processing (ICSLP '96)*, (pp. 2387-2390).

Huckvale, M. (2004) *SCRIBE manual version 1.0*. Retrieved January 7, 2009, from http://www.phon.ucl.ac.uk/resource/scribe/scribe-manual.htm

Hueber, T., Chollet, G., Denby, B., Dreyfus, G., & Stone, M. (2007). Continuous-speech phone recognition from ultrasound and optical images of the tongue and lips. Paper presented at the Interspeech, Antwerp, Belgium.

Humes, L. E., Nelson, K. J., & Pisoni, D. B. (1991). Recognition of synthetic speech by hearing-impaired listeners. *Journal of Speech and Hearing Research, 34*, 1180–1184.

Hunnicutt, S. (1984). Bliss symbol-to-speech conversion: "Bliss-talk". *Stockholm Technical University. Quarterly Progress and Status Report, 25*, 58–77.

Hustad, K. C., Kent, R. D., & Beukelman, D. R. (1998). DECtalk and MacinTalk speech synthesizers: Intelligibility differences for three listener groups. *Journal of Speech, Language, and Hearing Research: JSLHR, 41*, 744–752.

Hutt, M. L., & Gibby, R. G. (1979). *The mentally retarded child: Development training and education* (4th ed.). Boston: Allyn and Bacon.

Hyams, P. (Director). (1984). *2010* [Motion picture]. United States: Metro-Goldwyn-Mayer

Iacono, T. A. (2003). Pragmatic development in individuals with developmental disabilities who use AAC. In J. Light, D. Beukelman & J. Reichle (Eds.), *Communicative competence for individuals who use AAC: From research to effective practice* (pp. 323–360). London: Paul H Brookes.

Iacono, T. A., Mirenda, P., & Beukelman, D. (1993). Comparison of unimodal and multimodal AAC techniques for children with intellectual disabilities. *Augmentative and Alternative Communication, 9*, 83–94. doi:10.1080/07434619312331276471

IBM. (2009a). *1971*. Retrieved from http://www-03.ibm.com/ibm/history/history/year_1971.html

IBM. (2009b). *The First 10 Years*. Retrieved from http://www-03.ibm.com/ibm/history/exhibits/pc25/pc25_tenyears.html

IBM. (2009c). *History of IBM*. Retrieved from http://www-03.ibm.com/ibm/history/history/history_intro.html

Iida, A., & Campbell, N. (2003). Speech database for a concatenative text-to-speech synthesis system for individuals with communication disorders. *International Journal of Speech Technology, 6*(4), 379–392. doi:10.1023/A:1025761017833

IMDb. (2009). *Ben Burtt*. Retrieved from http://www.imdb.com/name/nm0123785/

IMDb. (2009). *Filmography by TV series for Majel Barrett.* Retrieved from http://www.imdb.com/name/nm0000854/filmoseries#tt0060028

International Speech Communication Association. (2009). *Interspeech 2009.* Retrieved from http://www.interspeech2009.org/

Jakobson, R. (1960). Linguistics and poetics. In T. A. Sebeok, (Ed.), *Style in language*, (pp. 350-377). Cambridge, MA: MIT Press.

Jayant, N. S., & Noll, P. (1984). *Digital coding of waveforms.* Englewood Cliffs, NJ: Prentice-Hall.

Jenkins, J. J., & Franklin, L. D. (1982). Recall of passages of synthetic speech. *Bulletin of the Psychonomic Society, 20*(4), 203–206.

Jeunet, J. (Director). (1997). *Alien: Resurrection* [Motion picture]. United States: Twentieth Century Fox.

Johnson, J., Baumgart, D., Helmstetter, E., & Curry, C. (1996). *Augmenting basic communication in natural contexts.* Baltimore: Paul H Brookes.

Jokisch, O., & Hoffmann, R. (2008). *Towards an Embedded Language Tutoring System for Children.* Paper presented at the Workshop on Child, Computer and Interaction, Chania, Greece.

Jones, A. P. (1997). How do you make a dynamic display dynamic? Make it static! Semantic root theory and language structure on dynamic screens. *Communication Matters, 11*(1), 21–26.

Jreige, C., Patel, R., & Bunnell, H. T. (2009). VocaliD: Personalizing Text-to-Speech Synthesis for Individuals with Severe Speech Impairment. In *Proceedings of ASSETS 2009.*

Kageyama, Y. (2009, March 11). *Human-like robot smiles, scolds in Japan classroom.* Retrieved from http://www.physorg.com/news155989459.html.

Kail, R. (1992). General slowing of information processing by persons with mental retardation. *American Journal of Mental Retardation, 97*, 333–341.

Kamm, C., Walker, M., & Rabiner, L. (1997). *The role of speech processing in human-computer intelligent communication.* Paper presented at NSF Workshop on human-centered systems: Information, interactivity, and intelligence.

Kangas, K. A., & Allen, G. D. (1990). Intelligibility of synthetic speech for normal-hearing and hearing-impaired listeners. *The Journal of Speech and Hearing Disorders, 55*, 751–755.

Kawahara, H., Masuda-Katsuse, I., & de Cheveigné, A. (1999). Restructuring speech representations using a pitch-adaptive time-frequency smoothing and an instantaneous-frequency-based F0 extraction: possible role of a repetitive structure in sounds. *Speech Communication, 27*, 187–207. doi:10.1016/S0167-6393(98)00085-5

Kaye, A. S. (2005). Gemination in English. *English Today, 21*(2), 43–55. doi:10.1017/S0266078405002063

Kemp, B. (1999). Quality of life while ageing with a disability. *Assistive Technology, 11*, 158–163.

Kennedy, C. H. (2005). *Single-case designs for educational research.* Boston: Allyn and Bacon.

Kent, R. (1997). *Speech sciences.* San Diego: Singular.

Kent, R. D., & Read, W. C. (1992). *The acoustic analysis of speech.* San Diego: Singular Publishing Group.

Kent, R., Weismer, G., Kent, J., & Rosenbek, J. (1989). Toward phonetic intelligibility testing in dysarthria. *The Journal of Speech and Hearing Disorders, 54*, 482–499.

Kiernan, C., Reid, B., & Jones, L. (1982). *Signs and symbols: Use of non-vocal communication systems.* London: Heinemann Educational.

Kim, J., & Davis, C. (2004). Investigating the audio–visual speech detection advantage. *Speech Communication, 44*(1-4), 19–30. doi:10.1016/j.specom.2004.09.008

Kim, K. (2001). *Effect of speech-rate on the comprehension and subjective judgments of synthesized narrative discourse.* University at Buffalo, Communicative Disorders and Sciences.

Kindler, A. (2002). *Survey of the states' limited English proficient students and available educational programs and services, summary report.* Washington, DC: National Clearinghouse for English Language Acquisition & Language Instruction Educational Programs.

Kintsch, W., & van Dijk, T. A. (1978). Towards a model for text comprehension and production. *Psychological Review, 85*, 363–394. doi:10.1037/0033-295X.85.5.363

Kiritani, S. (1986). X-ray microbeam method for measurement of articulatory dynamics: techniques and results. *Speech Communication, 5*(2), 119–140. doi:10.1016/0167-6393(86)90003-8

Klatt, D. H. (1980). Software for a cascade/parallel formant synthesizer. *The Journal of the Acoustical Society of America, 67*(3), 971–995. doi:10.1121/1.383940

Klatt, D. H. (1986). *Audio recordings from the Appendix of D. Klatt, "Review of text-to-speech conversion for English."* Retrieved from http://cslu.cse.ogi.edu/tts/research/history/

Klatt, D. H. (1987). Review of text-to-speech conversion for English. *The Journal of the Acoustical Society of America, 82*(3), 737–793. doi:10.1121/1.395275

Klatt, D. H., & Klatt, L. C. (1990). Analysis, synthesis and perception of voice quality variations among female and male talkers. *The Journal of the Acoustical Society of America, 87*(2), 820–857. doi:10.1121/1.398894

Kleck, R., Ono, H., & Hastorf, A. H. (1966). The Effects of Physical Deviance upon Face-to-Face Interaction. *Human Relations, 19*, 425–436. doi:10.1177/001872676601900406

Koester, H. H., & Levine, S. P. (1997). Keystroke-level models for user performance with word prediction. *Augmentative and Alternative Communication, 13*, 239–257. doi:10.1080/07434619712331278068

Kominek, J., & Black, A. W. (2003). *CMU Arctic databases for speech synthesis.* Retrieved April 20, 2006, from http://festvox.org/cmu arctic/cmu arctic report.pdf

Kornilov, A.-U. (2004). *The Biofeedback Program for Speech Rehabilitation Of Oncological Patients After Full Larynx Removal Surgical Treatment.* Paper presented at the 9th International Conference Speech and Computer (SPECOM), Saint Petersburg, Russia.

Korzeniowski, P. (2008). An Emotional Mess. *SpeechTechMag.com*, Retrieved March 30, 2009. http://www.speechtechmag.com/Articles/Editorial/Cover-Story/An-Emotional-Mess-51042.aspx

Koul, R. (2003). Synthetic speech perception in individuals with and without disabilities. *Augmentative and Alternative Communication, 19*(1), 49–58. doi:10.1080/0743461031000073092

Koul, R. K., & Allen, G. D. (1993). Segmental intelligibility & speech interference thresholds of high-quality synthetic speech in the presence of noise. *Jrnl. of Speech & Hearing Rsrch., 36*, 790–798.

Koul, R. K., & Clapsaddle, K. C. (2006). Effects of repeated listening experiences on the perception of synthetic speech by individuals with mild-to-moderate intellectual disabilities. *Augmentative and Alternative Communication, 22*, 1–11. doi:10.1080/07434610500389116

Koul, R. K., & Corwin, M. (2003). Efficacy of AAC intervention in chronic severe aphasia. In R.W. Schlosser, H.H. Arvidson, & L.L. Lloyd, (Eds.), *The efficacy of augmentative and alternative communication: Toward evidence-based practice* (pp. 449-470). San Diego, CA: Academic Press.

Koul, R. K., & Hanners, J. (1997). Word identification and sentence verification of two synthetic speech systems by individuals with intellectual disabilities. *Augmentative and Alternative Communication, 13*, 99–107. doi:10.1080/07434619712331277898

Koul, R. K., & Hester, K. (2006). Effects of repeated listening experiences on the recognition of synthetic speech by individuals with severe intellectual disabilities. *Journal of Speech, Language, and Hearing Research: JSLHR, 49*, 1–11.

Koul, R. K., & Schlosser, R. W. (2004). Effects of synthetic speech output in the learning of graphic symbols of varied iconicity. *Disability and Rehabilitation, 26*, 1278–1285. doi:10.1080/09638280412331280299

Koul, R., & Clapsaddle, K. C. (2006). Effects of repeated listening experiences on the perception of synthetic speech by individuals with mild-to-moderate disabilities. *Augmentative and Alternative Communication, 22*, 112–122. doi:10.1080/07434610500389116

Koul, R., & Hanners, J. (1997). Word identification and sentence verification of two synthetic speech systems by individuals with mental retardation. *Augmentative and Alternative Communication, 13*, 99–107. doi:10.1080/07434619712331277898

Koul, R., & Harding, R. (1998). Identification and production of graphic symbols by individuals with aphasia: Efficacy of a software application. *Augmentative and Alternative Communication, 14*, 11–24. doi:10.1080/07434619812331278166

Koul, R., & Hester, K. (2006). Effects of listening experiences on the recognition of synthetic speech by individuals with severe intellectual disabilities. *Journal of Speech, Language, and Hearing Research: JSLHR, 49*, 47–57.

Koul, R., & Schlosser, R. W. (2004). Effects of synthesized speech output in the learning of graphic symbols of varied iconicity [Electronic version]. *Disability and Rehabilitation, 26*, 1278–1285. doi:10.1080/09638280412331280299

Koul, R., Corwin, M., & Hayes, S. (2005). Production of graphic symbol sentences by individuals with aphasia: Efficacy of a computer-based augmentative and communication intervention. *Brain and Language, 92*, 58–77. doi:10.1016/j.bandl.2004.05.008

Koul, R., Corwin, M., Nigam, R., & Oetzel, S. (2008). Training individuals with severe Broca's aphasia to produce sentences using graphic symbols: Implications for AAC intervention. *Journal of Assistive Technologies, 2*, 23–34.

Koul, R.-K. (2003). Synthetic Speech Perception in Individuals with and without Disabilities. *Augmentative and Alternative Communication, 19*, 49–58. doi:10.1080/0743461031000073092

Kraat, A. (1987). *Communication interaction between aided and natural speakers: An IPCAS study report* (2nd ed.). Madison, WI: Univ. of Wisconsin-Madison, Trace Research & Development Centre.

Kreiman, J., & Papcun, G. (1991). Comparing discrimination and recognition of unfamiliar voices. *Speech Communication, 10*(3), 265–275. doi:10.1016/0167-6393(91)90016-M

Kröger, B. J., Birkholz, P., Kannampuzha, J., & Neuschaefer-Rube, C. (2006). Modeling sensory-to-motor mappings using neural nets and a 3D articulatory speech synthesizer. Paper presented at the Interspeech, Pittsburgh, PE.

Kubrick, S. (Director). (1968). *2001: A Space Odyssey* [Motion picture]. United Kingdom: Metro- Goldwyn-Mayer.

Kurzweil, R. (1999). *The Age of Spiritual Machines*. New York: Penguin.

LaBerge, D., & Samuels, S. L. (1974). Toward a theory of automatic information processing in reading. *Cognitive Psychology, 6*, 293–323. doi:10.1016/0010-0285(74)90015-2

Lancioni, G. E., Singh, N. N., O'Reilly, M. F., Sigafoos, J., Oliva, D., & Baccani, S. (2006). Teaching 'Yes' and 'No' responses to children with multiple disabilities through a program including microswitches linked to a vocal output device. *Perceptual and Motor Skills, 102*, 51–61. doi:10.2466/PMS.102.1.51-61

Lasker, J., & Beukelman, D. R. (1999). Peers' perceptions of storytelling by an adult with aphasia. *Aphasiology, 12*, 857–869.

Lee, J. (2001, November 29). Buyers of Units Of Lernout Are Disclosed. *New York Times*. Retrieved from http://www.nytimes.com/2001/11/29/business/buyers-of-units-of-lernout-are-disclosed.html?scp=1&sq=Buyers%20of%20Units%20Of%20Lernout%20Are%20Disclosed&st=cse

Lee, J. R., Nass, C., Brave, S. B., Morishima, Y., Nakajima, H., & Yamada, R. (2007). The case for caring colearners:

The effects of a computer-mediated colearner agent on trust and learning. *The Journal of Communication*, *57*, 183–204. doi:10.1111/j.1460-2466.2007.00339.x

Lee, K. M., Liao, K., & Ryu, S. (2007). Children's responses to computer-synthesized speech in educational media: Gender consistency and gender similarity effects. *Human Communication Research*, *33*, 310–329. doi:10.1111/j.1468-2958.2007.00301.x

Lehiste, I., & Shockey, L. (1972). On the perception of coarticulation effects in English VCV syllables. *Journal of Speech and Hearing Research*, *15*(3), 500–506.

Levinson, S. E., Olive, J. P., & Tschirgi, J. S. (1993). Speech synthesis in telecommunications. *IEEE Communications Magazine*, *31*(11), 46–53. doi:10.1109/35.256873

Light, J. (1988). Interaction involving individuals using augmentative and alternative communication systems: state of the art and future directions. *Augmentative and Alternative Communication*, *4*(2), 66–82. doi:10.1080/07434618812331274657

Light, J. (1989). Toward a definition of communicative competence for individuals using augmentative and alternative communication. *Augmentative and Alternative Communication*, *5*, 137–143. doi:10.1080/07434618912331275126

Light, J. (1996). "Communication is the essence of human life": Reflections on communicative competence. *Augmentative and Alternative Communication*, *13*, 61–70. doi:10.1080/07434619712331277848

Light, J. (2003). Shattering the silence: Development of communicative competence by individuals who use AAC. In J. Light, D. Beukelman & J. Reichle (Eds.), *Communicative competence for individuals who use AAC: From research to effective practice* (pp. 3–40). London: Paul H Brookes.

Light, J., & Drager, K. (2007). AAC technologies for young children with complex communication needs: State of the science and future research directions. *Augmentative and Alternative Communication*, *23*, 204–216. doi:10.1080/07434610701553635

Light, J., Beukelman, D., & Reichle, J. (Eds.). (2003). *Communicative competence for individuals who use AAC: From research to effective practice*. Baltimore: Paul H Brookes.

Light, J., Collier, B., & Parnes, P. (1985). Communicative interaction between young nonspeaking physically disabled children and their primary caregivers: Modes of communication. *Augmentative and Alternative Communication*, *1*, 125–133. doi:10.1080/07434618512331273621

Light, J., Page, R., Curran, J., & Pitkin, L. (2007). Children's ideas for the design of AAC assistive technologies for young children with complex communication needs. *Augmentative and Alternative Communication*, *23*(4), 274–287. doi:10.1080/07434610701390475

Lilienfeld, M., & Alant, E. (2001). Attitudes of children towards augmentative and alternative communication systems. *The South African Journal of Communication Disorders*, *48*, 45–54.

Lilienfeld, M., & Alant, E. (2002). Attitudes of children toward an unfamiliar peer using an AAC device with and without voice output. *Augmentative and Alternative Communication*, *18*(2), 91–101. doi:10.1080/07434610212331281191

Lloyd, L. L., & Fuller, D. R. (1990). The role of iconicity in augmentative and alternative communication symbol learning. In W. I. Fraser (Ed.), *Key issues in mental retardation research* (pp. 295-306). London: Routledge.

Lloyd, L. L., Fuller, D. R., & Arvidson, H. (1997). *Augmentative and alternative communication: A handbook of principles and practices*. Needham Heights, MA: Allyn & Bacon.

Lock, A. (1980). *The guided reinvention of language*. London: Academic Press.

Locke, J. L. (1998). Where did all the gossip go?: Casual conversation in the information age. *The Magazine of the American Speech-Language-Hearing Association*, *40*(3), 26–31.

Logan, J. S., Greene, B. G., & Pisoni, D. B. (1989). Segmental intelligibility of synthetic speech produced by rule. *The Journal of the Acoustical Society of America*, *86*, 566–581. doi:10.1121/1.398236

Louvet, E. (2007). Social judgment toward job applicants with disabilities: Perceptions of personal qualities and competencies. *Rehabilitation Psychology*, *52*, 297–303. doi:10.1037/0090-5550.52.3.297

Lucas, G. (Director). (1977). *Star Wars* [Motion picture]. United States: Twentieth Century Fox.

Luce, P. A., Feustel, T. C., & Pisoni, D. B. (1983). Capacity demands in short-term memory for natural and synthetic speech. *Human Factors*, *25*, 17–32.

Luce, P. A., Feustel, T. C., & Pisoni, D. B. (1983). Capacity demands in short-term memory for natural and synthetic speech. *Human Factors*, *25*, 17–32.

Lund, S. (2001). *Fifteen years later: Long-term outcomes for individuals who use augmentative and alternative communication.* Unpublished PhD, Pennsylvania State University.

Luo, F. (2009). *Personal narrative telling by individuals with ALS who use AAC devices.* Ph.D. dissertation, State University of New York at Buffalo, New York. Retrieved August 10, 2009, from Dissertations & Theses: Full Text. (Publication No. AAT 3342143).

Luo, F., Higginbotham, D. J., & Cornish, J. (2008). *Personal Narrative Telling of AAC Users with ALS.* American Speech Language and Hearing Association, Chicago, IL, November 21, 2008.

Maas, A., Castelli, L., & Arcuri, L. (2000). Measuring prejudice: Implicit versus explicit techniques. In D. Capozza & R. Brown (Eds.) *Social identity processes: Trends in theory and research.* London: Sage (pp. 96-116).

MacArthur, C. A. (2000). New tools for writing: Assistive technology for students with writing difficulties. *Topics in Language Disorders*, *20*(4), 85–100.

Mack, M., Tierney, J., & Boyle, M.E.T. (1990). The intelligibility of natural and LPC-coded words and sentences of native and non-native speakers of English. *Massachusetts Institute of Technology Lincoln Laboratory Technical Report, 869.*

Magen, H. S., Kang, A. M., Tiede, M. K., & Whalen, D. H. (2003). Posterior pharyngeal wall position in the production of speech. *Journal of Speech, Language, and Hearing Research: JSLHR*, *46*(1), 241–251. doi:10.1044/1092-4388(2003/019)

Makas, E. (1988). Positive attitudes toward disabled people: Disabled and nondisabled persons' perspectives. *The Journal of Social Issues*, *44*, 49–62.

Makashay, M. J., Wightman, C. W., & Syrdal, A. K. A. K., & Conkie, A. D. (2000). Perceptual *evaluation of automatic segmentation in text-to-speech synthesis.* A paper presented at the ICSLP 2000 Conference, Beijing, China.

Marics, M. A., & Williges, B. H. (1988). The intelligibility of synthesized speech in data inquiry systems. *Human Factors*, *30*, 719–732.

Marques, J. M., Yzerbyt, V. Y., & Leyens, J. P. (1988). The "black sheep effect": Extremity of judgments towards ingroup members as a function of group identification. *European Journal of Social Psychology*, *18*, 1–16. doi:10.1002/ejsp.2420180102

Martin, J. G., & Bunnell, H. T. (1981). Perception of anticipatory coarticulation effects. *The Journal of the Acoustical Society of America*, *69*(2), 559–567. doi:10.1121/1.385484

Martin, J. G., & Bunnell, H. T. (1982). Perception of anticipatory coarticulation effects in vowel-stop consonant-bowel sequences. *Journal of Experimental Psychology. Human Perception and Performance*, *8*(3), 473–488. doi:10.1037/0096-1523.8.3.473

Maslow, A. H. (1943). A theory of human motivation. [Retrieved from: http://www.emotionalliteracyeducation.com/abraham-maslow-theory-human-motivation.shtml]. *Psychological Review*, *50*, 370–396. doi:10.1037/h0054346

Massachusetts Institute of Technology. (2009). *University homepage.* Retrieved from http://mit.edu

Massaro, D. W. (1998). *Perceiving talking faces: From speechperception to a behavioral principle.* Cambridge, MA: MIT Press.

Massaro, D. W. (2004). From multisensory integration to talking heads and language learning. In G. Calvert, C. Spence, & B.E. Stein (Eds.), *Handbook of multisensory processes* (pp. 153-176). Cambridge, MA: MIT Press.

Massaro, D. W. (2006). A computer-animated tutor for language learning: Research and applications. In P. E. Spencer & M. Marshark (Eds.), Advances in the spoken language development of deaf and hard-of-hearing children (pp. 212-243). New York, NY: Oxford University Press.

Massaro, D.-W. (2008). *Just in Time Learning: Implementing Principles of Multimodal Processing and Learning for Education of Children with Special Needs.* Paper presented at the Workshop on Child, Computer and Interaction, Chania, Greece.

Massey, J.-H. (1988). Language-Impaired Children's Comprehension of Synthesized Speech. *Language, Speech, and Hearing Services in Schools, 19*, 401–409.

Masuko, T., Tokuda, K., Kobayashi, T., & Imai, S. (1997). Voice characteristics conversion for HMM-based speech synthesis system. In *Proceedings of ICASSP*, (pp.1611–1614).

Matson, J. L. (Ed.). (2007). *Handbook of assessment in persons with intellectual disability.* San Diego: Academic Press.

McCall, D., Shelton, J. R., Weinrich, M., & Cox, D. (2000). The utility of computerized visual communication for improving natural language in chronic global aphasia: Implications for approaches to treatment in global aphasia. *Aphasiology, 14*, 795–826. doi:10.1080/026870300412214

McCarthy, J., & Light, J. (2005). Attitudes toward individuals who use augmentative and alternative communication: Research review. *Augmentative and Alternative Communication, 21*, 41–55. doi:10.1080/07434610410001699753

McCree, A. V., & Barnwell, T. P. III. (1995). A mixed Excitation LPC vocoder model for low bit rate speech coding. *IEEE Transactions on Speech and Audio Processing, 3*(4), 242–250. doi:10.1109/89.397089

McGregor, G., Young, J., Gerak, J., Thomas, B., & Vogelsberg, R. T. (1992). Increasing functional use of an assistive communication device by a student with severe disabilities. *Augmentative and Alternative Communication, 8*, 243–250. doi:10.1080/07434619212331276233

McKelvey, M. L., Dietz, A. R., Hux, K., Weissling, K., & Beukelman, D. R. (2007). Performance of a person with chronic aphasia using personal and contextual pictures in a visual scene display prototype. *Journal of Medical Speech-Language Pathology, 15*, 305–317.

McNaughton, D., Fallon, D., Tod, J., Weiner, F., & Neisworth, J. (1994). Effects of repeated listening experiences on the intelligibility of synthesized speech. *Augmentative and Alternative Communication, 10*, 161–168. doi:10.1080/07434619412331276870

McNaughton, D., Fallon, K., Tod, J., Weiner, F., & Neisworth, J. (1994). Effect of repeated listening experiences on the intelligibility of synthesized speech. *Augmentative and Alternative Communication, 10*, 161–168. doi:10.1080/07434619412331276870

McNaughton, S. (1993). Graphic representational systems and literacy learning. *Topics in Language Disorders, 13*(2), 58–75.

McNaughton, S., & Lindsay, P. (1995). Approaching literacy with AAC graphics. *Augmentative and Alternative Communication, 11*, 212–228. doi:10.1080/07434619512331277349

Mechling, L. C., & Cronin, B. (2006). Computer-based video instruction to teach the use of augmentative and alternative communication devices for ordering at fast-food restaurants. *The Journal of Special Education, 39*, 234–245. doi:10.1177/00224669060390040401

Mermelstein, P. (1973). Articulatory model for the study of speech production. *The Journal of the Acoustical Society of America, 53*(4), 1070–1082. doi:10.1121/1.1913427

Merrill, E. C., & Jackson, T. S. (1992). Sentence processing by adolescents with and without intellectual disabilities. *American Journal on Intellectual Disabilities, 97*, 342–350.

Microsoft Corporation. (2009a). *Accessibility in Microsoft Products*. Retrieved from http://www.microsoft.com/enable/products/default.aspx

Microsoft Corporation. (2009b). *Microsoft's Commitment to Accessibility*. Retrieved from http://www.microsoft.com/enable/microsoft/default.aspx

Microsoft Corporation. (2009c). *Older Versions of Microsoft Internet Explorer*. Retrieved from http://www.microsoft.com/enable/products/IE.aspx

Microsoft Corporation. (2009d). *Windows 2000 Professional Accessibility Resources*. Retrieved from http://www.microsoft.com/enable/products/windows2000/default.aspx

Millar, D. C., Light, J. C., & Schlosser, R. W. (2006). The impact of augmentative and alternative communication intervention on the speech production of individuals with developmental disabilities: A research review. *Journal of Speech, Language, and Hearing Research: JSLHR, 49*, 248–264.

Miller, J. F., & Paul, R. (1995). *The clinical assessment of language comprehension*. Baltimore: Brookes.

Miller, N., Noble, E., Jones, D., & Burn, D. (2006). Life with communication changes in Parkinson's disease. *Age and Ageing, 35*, 235–239. doi:10.1093/ageing/afj053

Milner, P., & Kelly, B. (2009). Community participation and inclusion: people with disabilities defining their place. *Disability & Society, 24*, 47–62. doi:10.1080/09687590802535410

Mirenda, P. (2003). Toward functional augmentative and alternative communication for students with autism: Manual signs, graphic symbols, and voice output communication aids. *Language, Speech, and Hearing Services in Schools, 34*, 203–216. doi:10.1044/0161-1461(2003/017)

Mirenda, P., & Beukelman, D. (1990). A comparison of intelligibility among natural speech and seven speech synthesizers with listeners from three age groups. *Augmentative and Alternative Communication, 6*, 61–68. doi:10.1080/07434619012331275324

Mirenda, P., & Beukelman, D. R. (1987). A comparison of speech synthesis intelligibility with listeners from three age groups. *Augmentative and Alternative Communication, 3*, 120–128. doi:10.1080/07434618712331274399

Mirenda, P., & Beukelman, D. R. (1987). A comparison of speech synthesis intelligibility with listeners from three age groups. *Augmentative and Alternative Communication, 5*, 84–88.

Mirenda, P., & Beukelman, D. R. (1990). A comparison of intelligibility among natural speech and seven speech synthesizers with listeners from three age groups. *Augmentative and Alternative Communication, 6*(1), 61–68. doi:10.1080/07434619012331275324

Mirenda, P., & Brown, K. E. (2009). A picture is worth a thousand words: Using visual supports for augmented input with individuals with autism spectrum disorders. In P. Miranda & T. Iacono (Eds.), *Autism spectrum disorders and AAC* (pp. 303-332). Baltimore: Paul H. Brookes Publishing Co.

Mirenda, P., & Iacono, T. (Eds.) (2009). *Autism spectrum disorders and AAC*. Baltimore: Paul H. Brookes Publishing Co.

Mirenda, P., Eicher, D., & Beukelman, D. R. (1989). Synthetic and natural speech preferences of male and female listeners in four age groups. *Journal of Speech and Hearing Research, 32*, 175–183.

Mirenda, P., Wilk, D., & Carson, P. (2000). A retrospective analysis of technology use patterns of students with autism over a five-year period. *Journal of Special Education Technology, 15*, 5–6.

Mitchell, P. R., & Atkins, C. P. (1989). A comparison of the single word intelligibility of two voice output communication aids. *Augmentative and Alternative Communication, 5*, 84–88. doi:10.1080/07434618912331275056

Möbius, B. (2003). Rare events and closed domains: Two delicate concepts in speech synthesis . *International Journal of Speech Technology*, *6*(1), 57–71. doi:10.1023/A:1021052023237

Moffat, V., & Jolleff, N. (1987). Special needs of physically handicapped severely speech impaired children when considering a communication aid. In P. Enderby (Ed.), *Assistive communication aids for the speech impaired*. London: Churchill Livingstone.

Monaghan, A. I. C. (1990). A multi-phrase parsing strategy for unrestricted text. In *Proceedings of ESCA workshop on speech synthesis*, (pp. 109-112).

Moon, Y., & Nass, C. (1996). How "real" are computer personalities? Psychological responses to personality types in human-computer interaction. *Communication Research*, *23*, 651–674. doi:10.1177/009365096023006002

Moore, R., & Morris, A. (1992). Experiences collecting genuine spoken enquiries using WOZ techniques. In *Proceedings of DARPA Speech and Natural Language Workshop* (pp. 61–63), New York.

Moray, N. (1967). Where is capacity limited? A survey and a model. *Acta Psychologica*, *27*, 84–92. doi:10.1016/0001-6918(67)90048-0

Moulines, E., & Charpentier, F. (1990). Pitch-synchronous wave-form processing techniques for Text-to-Speech synthesis using diphones. *Speech Communication*, *9*(5-6), 453–467. doi:10.1016/0167-6393(90)90021-Z

Mullennix, J. W., Stern, S. E., Wilson, S. J., & Dyson, C. (2003). Social perception of male and female computer synthesized speech. *Computers in Human Behavior*, *19*, 407–424. doi:10.1016/S0747-5632(02)00081-X

Murphy, J. (2004). 'I prefer contact this close': perceptions of AAC by people with motor neurone disease and their communication partners. *Augmentative and Alternative Communication*, *20*(4), 259–271. doi:10.1080/07434610400005663

Murphy, J., Marková, I., Collins, S., & Moodie, E. (1996). AAC systems: obstacles to effective use. *European Journal of Disorders of Communication*, *31*, 31–44. doi:10.3109/13682829609033150

Murray, J., & Goldbart, J. (2009). Cognitive and language acquisition in typical and aided language learning: A review of recent evidence from an aided communication perspective. *Child Language Teaching and Therapy*, *25*, 7–34. doi:10.1177/0265659008098660

Nabelek, A. K., Czyzewski, Z., Krishnan, L. A., & Krishnan, L. A. (1992). The influence of talker differences on vowel identification by normal-hearing and hearing-impaired Listeners. *The Journal of the Acoustical Society of America*, *92*(3), 1228–1246. doi:10.1121/1.403973

Nakajima, Y., Kashioka, H., Shikano, K., & Campbell, N. (2003). Non-audible murmur recognition Input Interface using stethoscopic microphone attached to the skin. Paper presented at the International Conference on Acoustics, Speech and Signal Processing.

Nakamura, K., Toda, T., Saruwatari, H., & Shikano, K. (2006). Speaking aid system for total laryngectomees using voice conversion of body transmitted artificial speech. Paper presented at the InterSpeech, Pittsburgh, PE.

Nass, C., & Brave, S. (2005). *Wired for speech: How voice activates and advances the human-computer relationship*. Cambridge, MA: MIT Press.

Nass, C., & Lee, K. (2001). Does computer-synthesized speech manifest personality? Experimental tests of recognition, similarity-attraction, and consistency-attraction. *Journal of Experimental Psychology. Applied*, *7*(3), 171–181. doi:10.1037/1076-898X.7.3.171

Nass, C., & Moon, Y. (2000). Machines and mindlessness: Social responses to computers. *The Journal of Social Issues*, *56*, 81–103. doi:10.1111/0022-4537.00153

Nass, C., Fogg, B. J., & Moon, Y. (1996). Can computers be teammates? *International Journal of Human-Computer Studies*, *45*, 669–678. doi:10.1006/ijhc.1996.0073

Nass, C., Moon, Y., & Green, N. (1997). Are machines gender neutral? Gender-stereotypic responses to computers with voices. *Journal of Applied Social Psychology*, *27*, 864–876. doi:10.1111/j.1559-1816.1997.tb00275.x

National Institute of Deafness and Other Communication Disorders. (2001). *About hearing*. Retrieved October 24, 2001 from http://www.nidcd.nih.gov/health

NaturalSoft Limited. (2009). *NaturalReaders homepage*. Retrieved from http://naturalreaders.com/

Nelson, P., Soli, S., & Seitz, A. (2002). *Acoustical barriers to learning.* Melville, NY: Technical Committee on Speech Communication of the Acoustical Society of America.

NeoSpeech. (2009) Corporate homepage. Retrieved from http://neospeech.com/

Neri, A., Cucchiarini, C., & Strik, H. (2006). *Improving Segmental Quality in L2 Dutch by Means of Computer Assisted Pronunciation Training With Automatic Speech Recognition.* Paper presented at the CALL 2006, Antwerp, Belgium.

Nicholas, M., Sinotte, M. P., & Helms-Estabrooks, N. (2005). Using a computer to communicate: Effect of executive function impairments in people with severe aphasia. *Aphasiology, 19*, 1052–1065. doi:10.1080/02687030544000245

Nota, Y., & Honda, K. (2004). Brain regions involved in motor control of speech. *Acoustical Science and Technology, 25*(4), 286–289. doi:10.1250/ast.25.286

Nuance Communications, Inc. (2009). *Nuance Corporate Website*. Retrieved from http://www.nuance.com/

O'Keefe, B, M., & Dattilo, J. (1992). Teaching the response-recode form to adults with mental retardation using AAC systems. *Augmentative and Alternative Communication, 8*, 224–233. doi:10.1080/0743461921 2331276213

O'Keefe, B. M., Brown, L., & Schuller, R. (1998). Identification and rankings of communication aid features by five groups. *Augmentative and Alternative Communication, 14*(1), 37–50. doi:10.1080/07434619812331278186

O'Shaughnessy, D. (1987). *Speech communication: human and machine*. Reading, MA: Addison-Wesley Publishing Company.

O'Shaughnessy, D. (1992). Recognition of hesitations in spontaneous speech. *Proceedings of the IEEE Conference on Acoustics, Speech, and Signal Processing*, 521-524.

O'Shaughnessy, D., Barbeau, L., Bernardi, D., & Archambault, D. (1988). Diphone speech synthesis. *Speech Communication, 7*(1), 55–65. doi:10.1016/0167-6393(88)90021-0

Ochs, E., & Schieffelin, B. (2008). Language socialization: An historical overview. In P. A. Duff & N. H. Hornburger (Eds.), *Encyclopedia of language and education (2nd edition), 8*, 3-15.

Oddcast Inc. (2008). *SitePal homepage*. Retrieved from http://www.sitepal.com/

Öhman, S. E. G. (1966). Coarticulation in VCV Utterances: Spectrographic Measurements. *The Journal of the Acoustical Society of America, 39*(1), 151–168. doi:10.1121/1.1909864

Olive, J. P., Greenwood, A., & Coleman, J. (1993). *Acoustics of American English: A dynamic approach.* New York: Springer-Verlag.

Olive, J., van Santen, J., Möbius, B., & Shih, C. (1998). Synthesis. In R. Sproat (Ed.), *Multilingual text-to-speech synthesis: The Bell Labs approach.* (pp. 191–228). Dordrecht, The Netherlands: Kluwer Academic Publishers.

Olkin, R., & Howson, L. (1994). Attitudes Toward and Images of Physical Disability. *Journal of Social Behavior and Personality, 9*(5), 81–96.

Oshrin, S. E., & Siders, J. A. (1987). The effect of word predictability on the intelligibility of computer synthesized speech. *Journal of Computer-Based Instruction, 14*, 89–90.

Öster, A.-M. (1996). *Clinical Applications of Computer-Based Speech Training for Children with Hearing Impairment.* Paper presented at the 4th International Conf. on Spoken Language Processing (ICSLP-Interspeech), Philadelphia, PA, USA.

Öster, A.-M., House, D., Protopapas, A., & Hatzis, A. (2002). *Presentation of a new EU project for speech therapy: OLP (Ortho-Logo-Paedia).* Paper presented at the XV Swedish Phonetics Conference (Fonetik 2002), Stockholm, Sweden.

Ouni, S., & Laprie, Y. (2005). Modeling the articulatory space using a hypercube codebook for acoustic-to-articulatory inversion. *The Journal of the Acoustical Society of America, 118*(1), 444–460. doi:10.1121/1.1921448

Oxley, J. (2003). Memory and strategic demands of electronic speech-output communication aids. In S. von Tetzchner & N. Grove (Eds.), *Augmentative and Alternative Communication: Developmental Issues* (pp. 38-66). London: Whurr/Wiley.

Parette, P., & Huer, M. B. (2002). Working with Asian American families whose children have augmentative and alternative communication needs. *Journal of Special Education Technology E-Journal, 17*(4). Retrieved January 4, 2009, from http://jset.unlv.edu/17.4T/parette/first.html

Paris, C. R., Gilson, R. D., Thomas, M. H., & Silver, N. C. (1995). Effect of synthetic voice on intelligibility on speech comprehension. *Human Factors, 37*, 335–340. doi:10.1518/001872095779064609

Parsons, T. (1987). *Voice and speech processing.* New York: McGraw-Hill Book Company.

Paul, R. (1998). Communicative development in augmented modalities: Language without speech? In R. Paul (Ed.), *Exploring the speech-language connection* (pp. 139–162). Baltimore: Paul H. Brookes.

Peterson, G., Wang, W., & Siversten, E. (1958). Segmentation techniques in speech synthesis. *The Journal of the Acoustical Society of America, 30*, 739–742. doi:10.1121/1.1909746

Petty, R. E., & Cacioppo, J. T. (1986). *Communication and persuasion.* New York: Springer.

Phillips, M. J. (1985). "Try Harder": The Experience of Disability and the Dilemma of Normalization. *The Social Science Journal, 22*, 45–57.

Pickett, J. M. (1999). *The acoustics of speech communication.* Boston: Allyn and Bacon.

Pisoni, D. B., Manous, L. M., & Dedina, M. J. (1987). Comprehension of natural and synthetic speech: II. Effects of predictability on the verification of sentences controlled for intelligibility. *Computer Speech & Language, 2*, 303–320. doi:10.1016/0885-2308(87)90014-3

Pitrelli, J. F., Bakis, R., Eide, E. M., Fernandez, R., Hamza, W., & Picheny, M. A. (2006). The IBM expressive text-to-speech synthesis system for American English. *IEEE Transactions on Audio Speech and Language Processing, 14*(4), 1099–1108. doi:10.1109/TASL.2006.876123

Popich, E., & Alant, E. (1997). Interaction between a teacher and the non-speaking as well as speaking children in the classroom. *The South African Journal of Communication Disorders, 44*, 31–40.

Portnuff, C. (2006). *Augmentative and Alternative Communication: A Users Perspective.* Lecture delivered at the Oregon Health and Science University, August, 18, 2006. http://aac-rerc.psu.edu/index-8121.php.html

Prentke Romich Company (n.d.). *TouchTalker.* Wooster, OH.

Proyas, A. (Director). (2004). *I, Robot* [Motion picture]. United States: Twentieth Century Fox.

Rabiner, L. R. (1989). A tutorial on hidden Markov models and selected applications in speech recognition. *IEEE Transactions on Audio, Speech, and Language Processing, 77*, 257–286.

Rackensperger, T., Krezman, C., McNaughton, D., Williams, M. B., & D'Silva, K. (2005). "When I first got it, I wanted to throw it off a cliff": The challenges and benefits of learning AAC technologies as described by adults who use AAC. *Augmentative and Alternative Communication, 21*, 165–186. doi:10.1080/07434610500140360

Raghavendra, P., Bornman, J., Granlund, M., & Bjorck-Akesson, E. (2007). The World Health Organization's International Classification of Functioning, Disability and Health: implications for clinical and research practice in the field of augmentative and alternative communication. *Augmentative and Alternative Communication, 23*, 349–361. doi:10.1080/07434610701650928

Ralston, J. V., Pisoni, D. B., & Mullennix, J. W. (1995). Perception and comprehension of speech. In A. Syrdal, R. Bennet, & S. Greenspan (Eds.), *Applied speech technology* (pp. 233-288). Boca Raton, FL: CRC Press.

Ralston, J. V., Pisoni, D. B., & Mullennix, J. W. (1995). Perception and comprehension of speech. In A. Syrdal, R. Bennet, & S. Greenspan (Eds.), *Applied speech technology* (pp. 233-288). Boca Raton, FL: CRC Press.

Ralston, J. V., Pisoni, D. B., Lively, S. E., Greene, B. G., & Mullennix, J. W. (1991). Comprehension of synthetic speech produced by rule: Word monitoring and sentence-by-sentence listening times. *Human Factors*, *33*, 471–491.

Ratcliff, A., Coughlin, S., & Lehman, M. (2002). Factors influencing ratings of speech naturalness in augmentative and alternative communication. *AAC: Augmentative and Alternative Communication*, *18*(1), 11–19.

Recasens, D. (2002). An EMA study of VCV coarticulatory direction. *The Journal of the Acoustical Society of America*, *111*(6), 2828–2840. doi:10.1121/1.1479146

Reeves, B., & Nass, C. (1996). *The media equation: How people treat computers, television, and new media like real people and places.* New York: Cambridge University Press/CSLI.

Reichle, J., York, J., & Sigafoos, J. (1991). *Implementing augmentative and alternative communication: Strategies for learners with severe disabilities.* Baltimore: Paul H. Brookes Publishing Co.

Reynolds, M. E. D., Bond, Z. S., & Fucci, D. (1996). Synthetic speech intelligibility: Comparison of native and non-native speakers of English. *Augmentative and Alternative Communication*, *12*(1), 32. doi:10.1080/07434619612331277458

Reynolds, M. E., & Fucci, D. (1998). Synthetic speech comprehension: A comparison of children with normal and impaired language skills. *Journal of Speech, Language, and Hearing Research: JSLHR*, *41*, 458–466.

Reynolds, M. E., Isaacs-Duvall, C., Sheward, B., & Rotter, M. (2000). Examination of the effects of listening practice on synthesized speech comprehension. *Augmentative and Alternative Communication*, *16*, 250–259. doi:10.1080/07434610012331279104

Reynolds, M., & Jefferson, L. (1999). Natural and synthetic speech comprehension: Comparison of children from two age groups. *Augmentative and Alternative Communication*, *15*(3), 174–182. doi:10.1080/07434619912331278705

Rice, M., Hadley, P., & Alexander, A. (1993). Social bases towards children with speech and language impairments: A correlative causal model of language limitations. *Applied Psycholinguistics*, *14*, 445–471. doi:10.1017/S0142716400010699

Rigoll, G. (1987). The DECtalk system for German: A study of the modification of a text-to-speech converter for a foreign language. *Acoustics, Speech, and Signal Processing, IEEE International Conference on ICASSP '87, 12*, 1450-1453. Retrieved on March 14, 2009 from http://ieeexplore.ieee.org/stamp/stamp.jsp?arnumber=1169464&isnumber=26345

Ringeval, F., Chetouani, M., Sztahó, D., & Vicsi, K. (2008). *Automatic Prosodic Disorders Analysis for Impaired Communication Children.* Paper presented at the Workshop on Child, Computer and Interaction, Chania, Greece.

Robey, R. R. (1998). A meta-analysis of clinical outcomes in the treatment of aphasia. *Journal of Speech, Language, and Hearing Research: JSLHR*, *41*, 172–187.

Robillard, A. (1994). Communication problems in the intensive care unit. *Qualitative Sociology*, *17*, 383–395. doi:10.1007/BF02393337

Robinson, R. O. (1973). The frequency of other handicaps in children with cerebral palsy. *Developmental Medicine and Child Neurology*, *15*, 305–312.

Roddenberry, G. (Writer) & Allen, C. (Director). (1987). Encounter at Farpoint [Television series episode]. In G. Roddenberry (Executive Producer). *Star Trek: The Next Generation.* Los Angeles: Paramount Television.

Roddenberry, G. (Writer) & Butler, R. (Director). (1966). The Cage [Television series episode]. In G. Roddenberry (Producer), *Star Trek.* Culver City, CA: Desilu Studios.

Roddenberry, G. (Writer) & Hart, H. (Director). (1966). Mudd's Women [Television series episode]. In G. Roddenberry (Producer), *Star Trek*. Culver City, CA: Desilu Studios.

Rodman, R. D. (1999). *Computer Speech Technology*. Boston: Artech.

Rodríguez, W.-R., & Lleida, E. (2009). *Formant Estimation in Children's Speech and its Application for a Spanish Speech Therapy Tool*. Paper presented at the Workshop on Speech and Language Technologies in Education (SLaTE), Abbey Wroxall State, UK.

Rodríguez, W.-R., Saz, O., Lleida, E., Vaquero, C., & Escartín, A. (2008a). *COMUNICA - Tools for Speech and Language Therapy*. Paper presented at the Workshop on Child, Computer and Interaction, Chania, Greece.

Rodríguez, W.-R., Vaquero, C., Saz, O., & Lleida, E. (2008b). *Speech Technology Applied to Children with Speech Disorders*. Paper presented at the 4th Kuala Lumpur International Conference on Biomedical Engineering, Kuala Lumpur, Malaysia.

Rodríguez. V. (2008). *El uso de herramientas multimedia para la práctica de la pronunciación en clases de ELE con adolescentes*. Unpublished master dissertation, Antonio de Nebrija University, Spain.

Romski, M. A., & Sevcik, R. A. (1996). *Breaking the speech barrier: Language development through augmented means*. Baltimore: Paul H. Brookes Publishing.

Romski, M. A., & Sevcik, R. A. (2000). Children and adults who experience difficulty with speech. In D. Braithwaite & T. Thompson (Eds.), *Handbook of communication and people with disabilities: Research and application* (pp. 439-449). Hillsdale, NJ: Erlbaum.

Romski, M. A., Sevcik, R. A., Cheslock, M., & Barton, A. (2006). The System for Augmenting Language: AAC and emerging language intervention. In R. J. McCauley & M. Fey (Eds.), *Treatment of language disorders in children* (pp. 123-147). Baltimore: Paul H. Brookes Publishing Co.

Romski, M. A., Sevcik, R. A., Robinson, B., & Bakeman, R. (1994). Adult-directed communications of youth with intellectual disabilities using the system for augmenting language. *Journal of Speech and Hearing Research*, *37*, 617–628.

Rosenberg, S. (1982). The language of the mentally retarded: Development, processes, and intervention. In S. Rosenberg (Ed.), *Handbook of applied psycholinguistics: Major thrusts of research and theory* (pp.329-392). Hillsdale, NJ: Erlbaum.

Rosenberg, S., & Abbeduto, L. (1993). *Language & communication in mental retardation: Development, processes, and intervention*. Hillsdale, NJ: Erlbaum.

Rosenberg, W., & Donald, A. (1995). Evidence based medicine: An approach to clinical problem-solving. *BMJ (Clinical Research Ed.)*, *310*, 1122–1126.

Rosselli, F., Skelly, J. J., & Mackie, D. M. (1995). Processing rational and emotional messages: The cognitive and affective mediation of persuasion. *Journal of Experimental Social Psychology*, *31*, 163–190. doi:10.1006/jesp.1995.1008

Rostron, A., Ward, S., & Plant, R. (1996). Computerised augmentative communication devices for people with dysphasia: Design and evaluation. *European Journal of Disorders of Communication*, *31*, 11–30. doi:10.3109/13682829609033149

Rotholz, D., Berkowitz, S., & Burberry, J. (1989). Functionality of two modes of communication in the community by students with developmental disabilities: A comparison of signing and communication books. *The Journal of the Association for Persons with Severe Handicaps*, *14*, 227–233.

Rounsefell, S., Zucker, S. H., & Roberts, T. G. (1993). Effects of listener training on intelligibility of augmentative and alternative speech in the secondary classroom. *Education and Training in Mental Retardation*, *28*, 296–308.

Roux, J. C., & Visagie, A. S. (2007). Data-driven approach to rapid prototyping Xhosa speech synthesis. *SSW6-2007*, 143-147.

Rudman, L. A. (2004). Sources of implicit attitudes. *Current Directions in Psychological Science*, *13*, 79–82. doi:10.1111/j.0963-7214.2004.00279.x

Ruscello, D., Stutler, S., & Toth, D. (1983). Classroom teachers' attitudes towards children with articulatory disorders. *Perceptual and Motor Skills*, *57*, 527–530.

Sagisaka, Y. (1988). Speech synthesis by rule using an optimal selection of non-uniform synthesis units. *IEEE ICASSP1988*, 679-682.

Saz, O., Lleida, E., & Rodríguez, W.-R. (2009c). *Avoiding Speaker Variability in Pronunciation Verification of Children' Disordered Speech.* Paper presented at the Workshop on Child, Computer and Interaction, Cambridge, MA.

Saz, O., Rodriguez, V., Lleida, E., Rodríguez, W.-R., & Vaquero, C. (2009b). *An Experience with a Spanish Second Language Learning Tool in a Multilingual Environment.* Paper presented at the Workshop on Speech and Language Technologies in Education (SLaTE), Abbey Wroxall State, UK.

Saz, O., Rodríguez, W.-R., Lleida, E., & Vaquero, C. (2008). *A Novel Corpus of Children's Impaired Speech.* Paper presented at the Workshop on Child, Computer and Interaction, Chania, Greece.

Saz, O., Yin, S.-C., Lleida, E., Rose, R., Rodríguez, W.-R., & Vaquero, C. (2009a). Tools and Technologies for Computer-Aided Speech and Language Therapy. *Speech Communication*, *51*(10), 948–967. doi:10.1016/j.specom.2009.04.006

Schepis, M. M., & Reid, D. H. (1995). Effects of a voice output communication aid on interactions between support personnel and an individual with multiple disabilities. *Journal of Applied Behavior Analysis*, *28*, 73–77. doi:10.1901/jaba.1995.28-73

Schepis, M. M., Reid, D. H., & Behrman, M. M. (1996). Acquisition and functional use of voice output communication by persons with profound multiple disabilities. *Behavior Modification*, *20*, 451–468. doi:10.1177/01454455960204005

Schlosser, R. W. (2003). Roles of speech output in augmentative and alternative communication: Narrative review. *Augmentative and Alternative Communication*, *19*, 5–27. doi:10.1080/0743461032000056450

Schlosser, R. W. (2003). Roles of speech output in augmentative and alternative communication: Narrative review. *Augmentative and Alternative Communication*, *19*, 5–28. doi:10.1080/0743461032000056450

Schlosser, R. W., & Blischak, D. M. (2001). Is there a role for speech output in interventions for persons with autism? A review. *Focus on Autism and Other Developmental Disabilities*, *16*(3), 170–178. doi:10.1177/108835760101600305

Schlosser, R. W., & Raghavendra, P. (2003). Toward evidence-based practice in AAC. In R.W. Schlosser, H.H. Arvidson, & L.L. Lloyd, (Eds.), *The efficacy of augmentative and alternative communication: Toward evidence-based practice* (pp. 259-297). San Diego, CA: Academic Press.

Schlosser, R. W., & Raghavendra, P. (2004). Evidence-based practice in augmentative and alternative communication. *Augmentative and Alternative Communication*, *20*, 1–21. doi:10.1080/07434610310001621083

Schlosser, R. W., & Wendt, O. (2006). *The effects of AAC intervention on speech production in autism: A coding manual and form.* Unpublished manuscript, Northeastern University, Boston.

Schlosser, R. W., Belfiore, P. J., Nigam, R., Blischak, D., & Hetzroni, O. (1995). The effects of speech output technology in the learning of graphic symbols. *Journal of Applied Behavior Analysis*, *28*, 537–549. doi:10.1901/jaba.1995.28-537

Schlosser, R. W., Blischak, D. M., & Koul, R. J. (2003). Roles of speech output in AAC. In R. W. Schlosser (Ed.), *The efficacy of augmentative and alternative communication: toward evidenced-based practice*. (pp. 472 – 532). Boston: Academic Press.

Schlosser, R. W., Blischak, D. M., & Koul, R. K. (2003). Roles of speech output in AAC: An integrative review. In R.W. Schlosser, H.H. Arvidson, & L.L. Lloyd, (Eds.), *The efficacy of augmentative and alternative communication: Toward evidence-based practice* (pp. 471-531). San Diego, CA: Academic Press.

Schlosser, R. W., Lee, D. L., & Wendt, O. (2008). Application of the percentage of non-overlapping data in systematic reviews and meta-analyses: A systematic review of reporting characteristics. *Evidence-Based Communication Assessment and Intervention, 2*, 163–187. doi:10.1080/17489530802505412

Schlosser, R. W., Sigafoos, J., Luiselli, J. K., Angermeier, K., Harasymowyz, U., Schooley, K., & Belfiore, P. J. (2007). Effects of synthetic speech output on requesting and natural speech production in children with autism: A preliminary study. *Research in Autism Spectrum Disorders, 1*, 139–163. doi:10.1016/j.rasd.2006.10.001

Schlosser, R. W., Sigafoos, J., Luiselli, J. K., Angermeier, K., Harasymowyz, U., Schooley, K., & Belfiore, P. J. (2007). Effects of synthetic speech output on requesting and natural speech production in children with autism: A preliminary study. *Research in Autism Spectrum Disorders, 1*, 139–163. doi:10.1016/j.rasd.2006.10.001

Schlosser, R. W., Wendt, O., & Sigafoos, J. (2007). Not all systematic reviews are created equal: considerations for appraisal. *Evidence-Based Communication Assessment and Intervention, 1*, 138–150. doi:10.1080/17489530701560831

Schlosser, R., Belfiore, P., Nigam, R., Bilischak, D., & Hetzroni, O. (1995). The effects of speech output technology in the learning of graphic symbols. *Journal of Applied Behavior Analysis, 28*, 537–549. doi:10.1901/jaba.1995.28-537

Schlosser, R.W., & Wendt, O. (2008). Effects of augmentative and alternative communication intervention on speech production in children with autism: A systematic review. *American Journal of Speech-language Pathology: A Journal of Clinical practice, 17*, 212-230.

Schroeder, M. (2004).*Computer Speech: recognition, compression, synthesis.* Berlin: Springer.

Schwab, E. C., Nusbaum, H. C., & Pisoni, D. B. (1985). Some effects of training on the perception of synthetic speech. *Human Factors, 27*, 395–408.

Schwartz, J. L., Boë, L. J., & Abry, C. (2007). Linking the Dispersion-Focalization Theory (DFT) and the Maximum Utilization of the Available Distinctive Features (MUAF) principle in a Perception-for-Action-Control Theory (PACT). In M. J. Solé & P. Beddor & M. Ohala (Eds.), Experimental approaches to phonology (pp. 104-124): Oxford University Press.

Schwartz, J.-L., Boë, L.-J., Vallée, N., & Abry, C. (1997). The Dispersion -Focalization Theory of vowel systems. *Journal of Phonetics, 25*, 255–286. doi:10.1006/jpho.1997.0043

Schwartz, L. L. (1999). *Psychology and the media: A second look.* Washington, DC: American Psychological Society.

Schwartz, R., Klovstad, J., Makhoul, J., Klatt, D., & Zue, V. (1979). Diphone synthesis for phonetic vocoding. In *Proceedings of IEEE International Conference on Acoustics, Speech, and Signal Processing,* (pp. 891 – 894). New York: IEEE.

Scott, R. (Director). (1979). *Alien* [Motion picture]. United States: Brandywine Productions.

Scruggs, T. E., Mastropieri, M. A., & Castro, G. (1987). The quantitative synthesis of single subject research methodology: Methodology and validation. *Remedial and Special Education, 8*, 24–33. doi:10.1177/074193258700800206

Segers, E., & Verhoeven, L. (2005). Effects of lengthening the speech signal on auditory word discrimination in kindergartners with SLI. *Journal of Communication Disorders, 38*, 499–514. doi:10.1016/j.jcomdis.2005.04.003

Sevcik, R. A., & Romski, M. A. (2002). The role of language comprehension in establishing early augmented conversations. In J. Reichle, D. Beukelman, & J. Light (Eds.), *Exemplary practices for beginning communicators: Implications for AAC* (pp. 453-474). Baltimore: Paul H. Brookes Publishing Co., Inc.

Shane, H. (2009, April 3). Telephone Interview.

Shane, H., Higginbotham, D. J., Russell, S., & Caves, K. (2006). *Access to AAC: Present, Past, and Future.* Paper presented to the State of the Science Conference in AAC. March, Los Angeles.

Sigafoos, J., Arthur-Kelly, M., & Butterfield, N. (2006). *Enhancing everyday communication for children with disabilities*. Baltimore: Paul H. Brookes Publishing Co.

Sigafoos, J., Didden, R., & O'Reilly, M. (2003). Effects of speech output on maintenance of requesting and frequency of vocalizations in three children with developmental disabilities. *Augmentative and Alternative Communication, 19*, 37–47. doi:10.1080/0743461032000056487

Sigafoos, J., Didden, R., Schlosser, R. W., Green, V., O'Reilly, M., & Lancioni, G. (2008). A review of intervention studies on teaching AAC to individuals who are deaf and blind. *Journal of Developmental and Physical Disabilities, 20*, 71–99. doi:10.1007/s10882-007-9081-5

Sigafoos, J., Drasgow, E., Halle, J. W., O'Reilly, M., Seely-York, S., Edrisinha, C., & Andrews, A. (2004). Teaching VOCA use as a communicative repair strategy. *Journal of Autism and Developmental Disorders, 34*, 411–422. doi:10.1023/B:JADD.0000037417.04356.9c

Sigafoos, J., O'Reilly, M., & Green, V. A. (2007). Communication difficulties and the promotion of communication skills. In A. Carr, G. O'Reilly, P. Noonan Walsh, & J. McEvoy (Eds.), *The handbook of intellectual disability and clinical psychology practice* (pp. 606-642). London: Routledge.

Sigafoos, J., Woodyatt, G., Keen, D., Tait, K., Tucker, M., Roberts-Pennell, D., & Pittendreigh, N. (2000). Identifying potential communicative acts in children with developmental and physical disabilities. *Communication Disorders Quarterly, 21*, 77–86. doi:10.1177/152574010002100202

Sigelman, C. K., Adams, R. M., Meeks, S. R., & Purcell, M. A. (1986). Children's nonverbal responses to a physically disabled person. *Journal of Nonverbal Behavior, 10*, 173–186. doi:10.1007/BF00987614

Silverman, K., Beckman, M. E., Pitrelli, J., Ostendorf, M., Wightman, C., Price, P., et al. (1992). ToBI: a standard for labeling English prosody. *Proceedings of the Second International Conference on Spoken Language Processing*, 867-870.

Simmons-Mackie, N. N., & Damico, J. S. (2007). Access and social inclusion in aphasia: Interactional principles and applications. *Aphasiology, 21*, 81–97. doi:10.1080/02687030600798311

Sivertsen, E. (1961). Segment inventories for speech synthesis. *Language and Speech, 4*(1), 27–90.

Skillings, J. (2009, May 27). *Look out, Rover. Robots are man's new best friend*. Retrieved from http://news.cnet.com/Look-out%2C-Rover.-Robots-are-mans-new-best-friend/2009-11394_3-6249689.html?tag=mncol

Slowiaczek, L. M., & Nusbaum, H. C. (1985). Effects of speech rate and pitch contour on the perception of synthetic speech. *Human Factors, 27*, 701–712.

Smith, M. M. (2005). The dual challenges of aided communication and adolescence. *Augmentative and Alternative Communication, 21*(1), 76–79. doi:10.1080/10428190400006625

Smith, M. M. (2008). Looking back to look forward: Perspectives on AAC research. *Augmentative and Alternative Communication, 24*, 187–189.

Smith, M. M., & Connolly, I. (2008). Roles of aided communication: perspectives of adults who use AAC. *Disability and Rehabilitation. Assistive Technology, 3*, 260–273. doi:10.1080/17483100802338499

Smithsonian Institution. (2002a). *Haskins Laboratories*. Retrieved from http://americanhistory.si.edu/archives/speechsynthesis/ss_hask.htm

Smithsonian Institution. (2002b). *Kurzweil Company Products, Inc.* Retrieved from http://americanhistory.si.edu/archives/speechsynthesis/ss_kurz.htm

Snell, M. E., & Brown, F. (Eds.). (2006). *Instruction of students with severe disabilities* (6th ed.). Upper Saddle River, NJ: Pearson.

Snyder, M. L., Kleck, R. E., Strenta, A., & Mentzer, S. J. (1979). Avoidance of the handicapped: An attributional ambiguity analysis. *Journal of Personality and Social Psychology, 37*, 2297–2306. doi:10.1037/0022-3514.37.12.2297

Sobsey, D., & Reichle, J. (1989). Components of reinforcement for attention signal switch activation. *Mental Retardation & Learning Disability Bulletin, 17*, 46–59.

Soto, G., Belfiore, P. J., Schlosser, R. W., & Haynes, C. (1993). Teaching specific requests: A comparative analysis on skill acquisition and preference using two augmentative and alternative communication aids. *Education and Training in Mental Retardation, 28*, 169–178.

Spanias, A. S. (1994). Speech coding: A tutorial review. *Proceedings of the IEEE, 82*(10), 1541–1582. doi:10.1109/5.326413

Spiegel, B. B., Benjamin, B. J., & Spiegel, S. A. (1993). One method to increase spontaneous use of an assistive communication device: Case study. *Augmentative and Alternative Communication, 9*, 111–117. doi:10.1080/07434619312331276491

Spielberg, S. (Director). (1982). *E.T.: The Extra-Terrestrial.* United States: Universal Pictures.

Spielberg, S. (Director). (2001). *AI: Artificial Intelligence* [Motion picture]. United States: Warner Brothers.

Sproat, R., Möbius, B., Maeda, K., & Tzoukermann, E. (1998). Multilingual text analysis. In R. Sproat (Ed.), *Multilingual text-to-speech synthesis: The Bell Labs Approach.* (pp. 31–87). Dordrecht, The Netherlands: Kluwer Academic Publishers.

Stanton, A. (Director). (2008). *WALL-E* [Motion picture]. United States: Pixar Animation Studios.

Stern, S. E. (2008). Computer synthesized speech and perceptions of the social influence of disabled users. *Journal of Language and Social Psychology, 27*(3), 254–265. doi:10.1177/0261927X08318035

Stern, S. E., & Mullennix, J. W. (2004). Sex differences in persuadability of human and computer-synthesized speech: Meta-analysis of seven studies. *Psychological Reports, 94*, 1283–1292. doi:10.2466/PR0.94.3.1283-1292

Stern, S. E., Dumont, M., Mullennix, J. W., & Winters, M. L. (2007). Positive prejudice towards disabled persons using synthesized speech: Does the effect persist across contexts? *Journal of Language and Social Psychology, 26*, 363–380. doi:10.1177/0261927X07307008

Stern, S. E., Mullennix, J. W., & Wilson, S. J. (2002). Effects of perceived disability on persuasiveness of computer synthesized speech. *The Journal of Applied Psychology, 87*, 411–417. doi:10.1037/0021-9010.87.2.411

Stern, S. E., Mullennix, J. W., & Yaroslavsky, I. (2006). Persuasion and social perception of human vs. synthetic voice across person as source and computer as source conditions. *International Journal of Human-Computer Studies, 64*, 43–52. doi:10.1016/j.ijhcs.2005.07.002

Stern, S. E., Mullennix, J. W., Dyson, C., & Wilson, S. J. (1999). The persuasiveness of synthetic speech versus human speech. *Human Factors, 41*, 588–595. doi:10.1518/001872099779656680

Stevens, K. N., & Bickley, C. A. (1991). Constraints among parameters simplify control of Klatt formant synthesizer. *Journal of Phonetics, 19*, 161–174.

Stevens, K. N., & House, A. S. (1955). Development of a quantitative description of vowel articulation. *The Journal of the Acoustical Society of America, 27*(3), 484–493. doi:10.1121/1.1907943

Stone, D. L., & Colella, A. (1996). A framework for studying the effects of disability on work experiences. *Academy of Management Review, 21*, 352–401. doi:10.2307/258666

Street, R. L., & Giles, H. (1982). Speech accommodation theory: a social cognitive approach to language and speech. In M. Roloff, & C. R. Berger, (Eds.), *Social cognition and communication* (pp. 193–226). Beverly Hills, CA: Sage.

Strik, H., Neri, A., & Cucchiarini, C. (2008). *Speech Technology for Language Tutoring.* Paper presented at the LangTech 2008, Rome, Italy.

Styger, T., & Keller, E. (1994). Formant synthesis. In E. Keller (ed.), *Fundamentals of speech synthesis and speech recognition: Basic concepts, state of the art, and future challenges* (pp. 109-128). Chichester, UK: John Wiley.

Stylianou, Y. (2000). *On the Implementation of the Harmonic Plus Noise Model for Concatenative Speech Synthesis.* Paper presented at ICASSP 2000, Istanbul,

Turkey. Retrieved on March 14, 2009 from: http://www.research.att.com/projects/ tts/papers/2000–ICASSP/fastHNM.pdf

Stylianou, Y. (2001). Applying the harmonic plus noise model in concatenative speech synthesis. *IEEE Transactions on Speech and Audio Processing*, *9*(1), 21–29. doi:10.1109/89.890068

Summerfield, A., MacLeod, A., McGrath, M., & Brooke, M. (1989). Lips, teeth, and the benefits of lipreading. In A. W. Young & H. D. Ellis (Eds.), Handbook of research on face processing (pp. 223-233). Amsterdam: Elsevier Science Publishers.

Sundar, S. S., & Nass, C. (2000). Source orientation in human-computer interaction: Programmer, networker, or independent social actor? *Communication Research*, *27*, 683–703. doi:10.1177/009365000027006001

Suzuki, M. (2009, April 5). *Japan child robot mimicks infant learning.* Retrieved from http://www.physorg.com/news158151870.html

Sweidel, G. (1989). Stop, look and listen! When vocal and nonvocal adults communicate. *Disability & Society*, *4*, 165–175. doi:10.1080/02674648966780171

Sweidel, G. (1991/1992). Management strategies in the communication of speaking persons and persons with a speech disability. *Research on Language and Social Interaction*, *25*, 195–214.

Syrdal, A. K. (1995). Text-to-speech systems. In A.K. Syrdal, R. Bennet, & S. Greenspan (Eds.), *Applied speech technology* (pp. 99-126). Boca Raton, FL: CRC Press.

Tajfel, H. (1978). *Differentiation between groups: Studies in the social psychology of intergroup relations.* London: Academic Press.

Takeda, K., Abe, K., & Sagisaka, Y. (1992). On the basic scheme and algorithms in non-uniform unit speech synthesis. In G. Bailly, C. Benoît & T. R. Sawallis (Eds.), *Talking machines: Theories, models, and designs* (pp. 93-105). Amsterdam, The Netherlands: North-Holland Publishing Co.

Tamura, M., Masuko, T., Tokuda, K., & Kobayashi, T. (2001). Adaptation of pitch and spectrum for HMM-based speech synthesis using MLLR. In *Proceedings of ICASSP*, (pp.805–808).

Tang, H., Fu, Y., Tu, J., Hasegawa-Johnson, M., & Huang, T. S. (2008). Humanoid audio–visual avatar with emotive text-to-speech synthesis. *IEEE Transactions on Multimedia, 10*(6), 969–981. doi:10.1109/TMM.2008.2001355

Tang, H., Fu, Y., Tu, J., Huang, T. S., & Hasegawa-Johnson, M. (2008). EAVA: A 3D Emotive Audio-Visual Avatar. *IEEE Workshop on Applications of Computer Vision, 2008. WACV 2008,* (pp. 1-6).

Taylor, P., Black, A. W., & Caley, R. (1998). The architecture of the Festival speech synthesis system. In *Proceedings of the 3rd ESCA Workshop in Speech Synthesis* (pp. 147–151), Jenolan Caves, Australia.

Taylor, R. L., Sternberg, L., & Richards, S. B. (1995). *Exceptional children: Integrating research and teaching* (2nd ed.). San Diego: Singular.

TED Conferences, LLC. (Producer). (2008, April) Stephen Hawking asks big questions about the universe. *Talks.* Video posted to http://www.ted.com/talks/stephen_hawking_asks_big_questions_about_the_universe.html

Tedeshi, B. (2006, November 6). Do the Rights of the Disabled Extend to the Blind on the Web? *New York Times.* Retrieved from http://www.nytimes.com/2006/11/06/technology/06ecom.html?_r=1&scp=1&sq=Do%20the%20Rights%20of%20the%20Disabled%20Extend%20to%20the%20Blind%20on%20the%20Web?&st=cse

Tepperman, J., Silva, J., Kazemzadeh, A., You, H., Lee, S., Alwan, A., & Narayanan, S. (2006). *Pronunciation Verification of Children's Speech for Automatic Literacy Assessment.* Paper presented at the 9th International Conf. on Spoken Language Processing (ICSLP - Interspeech), Pittsburgh, PA.

Terkel, S. (2008). Looking for the human voice. *NPR Morning Edition*, Nov. 07, 2008. Retrieved Nov. 10, 2008 from http://www.npr.org/templates/story/story.php?storyId=96714084&ft=1&f=1021.

Thalheimer, W., & Cook, S. (2002, August). *How to calculate effect sizes from published research articles: A simplified methodology.* Retrieved on July 28, 2008, from http://work- learning.com/effect_sizes.htm

The Guardian. (2005). *Return of the time lord.* Retrieved September 14, 2009, from http://www.guardian.co.uk/science/2005/sep/27/scienceandnature.highereducationprofile

Toback, S. (2008). *Wonder why everything isn't speech controlled?* Retrieved from http://news.cnet.com/8301-13555_3-10023024-34.html?tag=mncol

Toda, T., & Shikano, K. (2005). NAM-to-Speech Conversion with Gaussian Mixture Models. Paper presented at the InterSpeech, Lisbon - Portugal.

Toda, T., & Tokuda, K. (2007). A speech parameter generation algorithm considering global variance for HMM-based speech synthesis. *IEICE Transactions on Information and Systems . E (Norwalk, Conn.), 90-D*(5), 816–824.

Toda, T., Black, A. W., & Tokuda, K. (2004). Mapping from articulatory movements to vocal tract spectrum with Gaussian mixture model for articulatory speech synthesis. Paper presented at the International Speech Synthesis Workshop, Pittsburgh, PA.

Toda, T., Black, A. W., & Tokuda, K. (2005). Spectral conversion based on maximum likelihood estimation considering global variance of converted parameter. Paper presented at the International Conference on Acoustics, Speech and Signal Processing (ICASSP), Philadelphia, PE.

Toda, T., Ohtani, Y., & Shikano, K. (2006). Eigenvoice conversion based on gaussian mixture model. Paper presented at the InterSpeech, Pittsburgh, PE.

Todman, J. (2000). Rate and quality of conversations using a text-storage AAC system: Single-case training study. *Augmentative and Alternative Communication, 16*, 164–179. doi:10.1080/07434610012331279024

Todman, J., & Rzepecka, H. (2003). Effect of pre-utterance pause length on perceptions of communicative competence in AAC-aided social conversations. *Augmentative and Alternative Communication, 19*, 222–234. doi:10.1080/07434610310001605810

Todman, J., Alm, N., Higginbotham, D. J., & File, P. (2008). Whole utterance approaches in AAC. *Augmentative and Alternative Communication, 24*, 235. doi:10.1080/08990220802388271

Tokuda, K., Yoshimura, T., Masuko, T., Kobayashi, T., & Kitamura, T. (2000). Speech parameter generation algorithms for HMM-based speech synthesis. Paper presented at the IEEE International Conference on Acoustics, Speech, and Signal Processing, Istanbul, Turkey.

Tokuda, K., Zen, H., Yamagishi, J., Masuko, T., Sako, S., Black, A., & Nose, T. (2008) *The HMM-based speech synthesis system (HTS) Version 2.1.* Retrieved June 27, 2008, from http://hts.sp.nitech.ac.jp/.

Tomasello, M. (1999). *The cultural origins of human cognition.* London: Harvard University Press.

Tóth, B., & Németh, G. (2008). Hidden-Markov-Model based speech synthesis in Hungarian. *Infocommunications Journal, 63*, 30-34. Retrieved on June 21, 2009: http://www.hiradastechnika.hu/data/upload/file/2008/2008_7/HT_0807_5TothNemeth.pdf

Tran, V.-A., Bailly, G., & Loevenbruck, H. (submitted). Improvement to a NAM-captured whisper-to-speech system. Speech Communication - special issue on Silent Speech Interfaces.

Tran, V.-A., Bailly, G., Loevenbruck, H., & Jutten, C. (2008). Improvement to a NAM captured whisper-to-speech system. Paper presented at the Interspeech, Brisbane, Australia.

Tran, V.-A., Bailly, G., Loevenbruck, H., & Toda, T. (2008). Predicting F0 and voicing from NAM-captured whispered speech. Paper presented at the Speech Prosody, Campinas - Brazil.

Tran, V.-A., Bailly, G., Loevenbruck, H., & Toda, T. (2009). Multimodal HMM-based NAM-to-speech conversion. Paper presented at the Interspeech, Brighton.

Tsurutami, C., Yamauchi, Y., Minematsu, N., Luo, D., Maruyama, K., & Hirose, K. (2006). *Development of a Program for Self Assessment of Japanese Pronunciation by English Learners.* Paper presented at the 9th International Conference on Spoken Language Processing (ICSLP - Interspeech), Pittsburgh, PA.

U. S. Department of Education. (2002). *Implementation of the Individuals with Disabilities Education Act: Twenty-first annual report to congress.* Washington, DC: Author.

Ulanoff, L. (2009, March 31). *Honda Asimo Responds to Thought Control--Horror Film Makers Rejoice.* Retrieved from http://www.gearlog.com/2009/03/honda_asimo_responds_to_though.php

Umanski, D., Kosters, W., Verbeek, F., & Schiller, N. (2008). *Integrating Computer Games in Speech Therapy for Children who Stutter.* Paper presented at the Workshop on Child, Computer and Interaction, Chania, Greece.

van de Sandt-Koenderman, M., Wiegers, J., & Hardy, P. (2005). A computerized communication aid for people with aphasia. *Disability and Rehabilitation, 27*, 529–533. doi:10.1080/09638280400018635

van Santen, J. P. H. (1992). Deriving text-to-speech durations from natural speech. In G. Bailly, C. Benoît & T. R. Sawallis (Eds.), *Talking machines: Theories, models, and designs* (pp. 275-285). Amsterdam, The Netherlands: North-Holland Publishing Co.

Vanderheiden, G. (2003). A journey through early augmentative communication and computer access. *Journal of Rehabilitation Research and Development, 39*, 39–53.

Vaquero, C., Saz, O., Lleida, E., & Rodríguez, W.-R. (2008). *E-Inclusion Technologies for the Speech Handicapped.* Paper presented at the International Conference on Acoustics, Speech and Signal Processing (ICASSP), Las Vegas, NV.

Vargas, P., von Hippel, W., & Petty, R. E. (2004). Using "partially structured" attitude measures to enhance the attitude-behavior relationship. *Personality and Social Psychology Bulletin, 30*, 197–211. doi:10.1177/0146167203259931

Venkatagiri, H. S. (1991). Effects of rate and pitch variations on the intelligibility of synthesized speech. *Augmentative and Alternative Communication, 7*(4), 284. doi:10.1080/07434619112331276023

Venkatagiri, H. S. (1994). Effect of sentence length and exposure on the intelligibility of synthesized speech. *Augmentative and Alternative Communication, 10*, 96–104. doi:10.1080/07434619412331276800

Venkatagiri, H. S. (1996). The quality of digitized and synthesized speech: What clinicians should know. *American Journal of Speech-Language Pathology, 5*, 31–42.

Venkatagiri, H. S. (2002). Speech recognition technology applications in communications disorders. *American Journal of Speech-Language Pathology, 11*(4), 323–332. doi:10.1044/1058-0360(2002/037)

Venkatagiri, H. S. (2003). Segmental intelligibility of four currently used text-to-speech synthesis methods. *The Journal of the Acoustical Society of America, 113*, 2094–2104. doi:10.1121/1.1558356

Venkatagiri, H. S. (2003). Segmental intelligibility of four currently used text-to-speech synthesis methods. *The Journal of the Acoustical Society of America, 113*(4), 2094–2104. doi:10.1121/1.1558356

Venkatagiri, H. S. (2004). Segmental intelligibility of three text-to-speech synthesis methods in reverberant environments. *Augmentative and Alternative Communication, 20*, 150–163. doi:10.1080/07434610410001699726

Venkatagiri, H., & Ramabadran, T. (1995). Digital speech synthesis: Tutorial. *Augmentative and Alternative Communication, 11*(1), 14–25. doi:10.1080/07434619512331277109

Verma, A., & Kumar, A. (2003). Modeling speaking rate for voice fonts. Paper presented at the Eurospeech, Geneva, Switzerland.

Vicsi, K., Roach, P., Öster, A., Kacic, P., Barczikay, P., & Sinka, I. (1999). *SPECO: A Multimedia Multilingual Teaching and Training System for Speech Handicapped Children.* Paper presented at the 6th European Conference on Speech Communication and Technology (Eurospeech-Interspeech), Budapest, Hungary.

von Tetzchner, S., & Grove, N. (2003). The development of alternative language forms. In S. von Tetzchner & N. Grove (Eds.), *Augmentative and Alternative Communication: Developmental Issues* (pp. 1–27). London: Whurr/Wiley.

von Tetzchner, S., & Jensen, M. H. (1996). Introduction. In S. von Tetzchner & M. Jensen (Eds.), *Augmentative and alternative communication: European perspectives* (pp. 1–18). London: Whurr/Wiley.

von Tetzchner, S., & Martinsen, H. (1996). Words and strategies: Communicating with young children who use aided language. In S. von Tetzchner & M. Jensen (Eds.), *Augmentative and alternative communication: European perspectives* (pp. 65–88). London: Whurr/Wiley.

von Tetzchner, S., & Martinsen, H. (2000). *Introduction to augmentative and alternative communication* (2nd ed.). London: Whurr/Wiley.

Vygotsky, L. (1962). *Thought and language.* Cambridge, MA: MIT Press.

Wacker, D. P., Wiggins, B., Fowler, M., & Berg, W. K. (1988). Training students with profound or multiple handicaps to make requests via microswitches. *Journal of Applied Behavior Analysis, 21*, 331–343. doi:10.1901/jaba.1988.21-331

Walden, B. E., Montgomery, A. A., Gibeily, G. J., Prosek, R. A., & Schwartz, D. M. (1978). Correlates of psychological dimensions in talker similarity. *Journal of Speech and Hearing Research, 21*(2), 265–275.

Wang, H., & Kawahara, T. (2008). *A Japanese CALL system based on Dynamic Question Generation and Error Prediction for ASR.* Paper presented at the 10th International Conference on Spoken Language Processing (ICSLP - Interspeech), Brisbane, Australia.

Wasson, C., Arvidson, H., & Lloyd, L. (1997). Low technology. In L. Lloyd, D. Fuller & H. Arvidson (Eds.), *Augmentative and alternative communication: A handbook of principles and practices* (pp. 127–136.). Boston: Allyn and Bacon.

Watts, O., Yamagishi, J., Berkling, K., & King, S. (2008). HMM-Based Synthesis of Child Speech. *1st Workshop on Child, Computer and Interaction (ICMI'08 post-conference workshop).*

Wegener, D. T., & Petty, R. E. (1997). The flexible correction model: The role of naive theories of bias in bias correction. In M. P. Zanna (Ed.) *Advances in experimental social psychology* (Vol 29, pp. 141-208). New York: Academic Press.

Weinrich, M., Boser, K. I., McCall, D., & Bishop, V. (2001). Training agrammatic subjects on passive sentences: Implications for syntactic deficit theories. *Brain and Language, 76*, 45–61. doi:10.1006/brln.2000.2421

Weinrich, M., Shelton, J. R., McCall, D., & Cox, D. M. (1997). Generalization from single sentence to multisentence production in severely aphasic patients. *Brain and Language, 58*, 327–352. doi:10.1006/brln.1997.1759

Weitzel, A. (2000). Overcoming loss of voice. In D. O. Braithwaite & T. L. Thompson, (Eds.), *Handbook of communication and people with disabilities: Research and application,* (pp. 451-466). Mahwah, NJ: Erlbaum.

Wells, J. C. (1982). *Accents of English: an introduction.* Cambridge, UK: Cambridge Univ. Press.

Whalen, D. H., Iskarous, K., Tiede, M. T., Ostry, D., Lehnert-LeHoullier, H., & Hailey, D. (2005). The Haskins optically-corrected ultrasound system (HOCUS). *Journal of Speech, Language, and Hearing Research: JSLHR, 48*, 543–553. doi:10.1044/1092-4388(2005/037)

Whalen, D. H., Kang, A. M., Magen, H. S., Fulbright, R. K., & Gore, J. C. (1999). Predicting midsagittal pharynx shape from tongue position during vowel production. *Journal of Speech, Language, and Hearing Research: JSLHR, 42*(3), 592–603.

Whiteford, W. A. (2000). *King Gimp.* VHS Tape, HBO.

Wicklegran, W. A. (1969). Context-sensitive coding associative memory and serial order in (speech) behavior. *Psychological Review, 76*, 1–15. doi:10.1037/h0026823

Wightman, C. W., Syrdal, A. K., Stemmer, G., Conkie, A. D., & Beutnagel, M. C. (2000). *Perceptually based automatic prosody labeling and prosodically enriched unit selection improve concatenative text-to-speech synthesis.* A paper presented at the ICSLP 2000 Conference, Beijing, China.

Wik, P., Hincks, R., & Hirschberg, J. (2009). *Responses to Ville: A virtual language teacher for Swedish.* Paper presented at Speech and Language Technology for Education Workshop, Wroxall Abbey Estate, UK.

Wilkins, D. (2006). *General Overview Linguistic and Pragmatic Considerations in the Design of Frametalker/Contact.* Unpublished manuscript. University at Buffalo, Department of Communicative Disorders and Sciences, Buffalo, NY.

Wilkins, D. P., & Higginbotham, D. J. (2005). The short story of Frametalker: An interactive AAC device. *Perspectives on Augmentative and Alternative Communication, 15*, 18–22.

Williams, M. B., Krezman, C., & McNaughton, D. (2008). "Reach for the stars": Five principles for the next 25 years of AAC. *Augmentative and Alternative Communication, 24*, 194–206. doi:10.1080/07434610802387851

Williams, S. M., Nix, D., & Fairweather, P. (2000). Using speech recognition technology to enhance literacy instruction for emerging readers. In B. Fishman & S. O'Connor-Divelbiss (Eds.), *Fourth international conference of the learning sciences.* (pp. 115-120). Mahwah, NJ: Erlbaum.

Willis, L., Koul, R., & Paschall, D. (2000). Discourse comprehension of synthetic speech by individuals with mental retardation. *Education and Training in Mental Retardation and Developmental Disabilities, 35*, 106–114.

Wilson, S. M., Saygin, A. P., Sereno, M. I., & Iacoboni, M. (2004). Listening to speech activates motor areas involved in speech production. *Nature Neuroscience, 7*, 701–702. doi:10.1038/nn1263

Witt, S., & Young, S.-J. (1997). *Computer-Assisted Pronunciation Teaching based on Automatic Speech Recognition.* Paper presented at the International Conference on Language Teaching, Language Technology, Groningen, The Netherlands.

Witten, I. H. (1982). *Principles of computer speech.* London: Academic Press.

Wolsko, C., Park, B., Judd, C. M., & Wittenbrink, B. (2000). Framing interethnic ideology: Effects of multicultural and colorblind perspectives of judgments of groups and individuals. *Journal of Personality and Social Psychology, 78*, 635–654. doi:10.1037/0022-3514.78.4.635

World Health Organization. (2001). *International classification of functioning, disability and health.* Geneva: World Health Organization.

Wortzel, A. (2001). *Camouflage Town homepage.* Retrieved from http://www.adriannewortzel.com/robotic/camouflagetown/index.html

Wortzel, A. (n.d.). *Homepage.* Retrieved July 1, 2009 from http://www.adriannewortzel.com/

Yamagishi, J., & Kobayashi, T. (2007). Average-voice-based speech synthesis using HSMM-based speaker adaptation and adaptive training. *IEICE Transactions on Information and Systems . E (Norwalk, Conn.), 90-D*(2), 533–543.

Yamagishi, J., Kobayashi, T., Nakano, Y., Ogata, K., & Isogai, J. (2009). Analysis of speaker adaptation algorithms for HMM-based speech synthesis and a constrained SMAPLR adaptation algorithm. *IEEE Transactions on Audio . Speech and Language Processing, 17*(1), 66–83. doi:10.1109/TASL.2008.2006647

Yamagishi, J., Nose, T., Zen, H., Ling, Z., Toda, T., & Tokuda, K. (2009). A robust speaker-adaptive HMM-based text-to-speech synthesis. *IEEE Transactions on Audio . Speech and Language Processing, 17*(6), 1208–1230. doi:10.1109/TASL.2009.2016394

Yamagishi, J., Zen, H., Toda, T., & Tokuda, K. (2007). Speaker-independent HMM-based speech synthesis system – HTS-2007 for the Blizzard challenge 2007. In *Proceedings of the Blizzard Challenge 2007* (paper 008), Bonn, Germany.

Yamagishi, J., Zen, H., Wu, Y.-J., Toda, T., & Tokuda, K. (2008). The HTS-2008 system: yet another evaluation of the speaker-adaptive HMM-based speech synthesis system in the 2008 Blizzard challenge. In *Proceedings of the Blizzard Challenge 2008*, Brisbane, Australia. Retrieved March 2, 2009, from http://festvox.org/blizzard/bc2008/hts_Blizzard2008.pdf.

Yang, M. (2004). Low bit rate speech coding . *IEEE Potential*, *23*(4), 32–36. doi:10.1109/MP.2004.1343228

Yarrington, D., Bunnell, H. T., & Ball, G. (1995). Robust automatic extraction of diphones with variable boundaries. *EUROSPEECH*, *95*, 1845–1848.

Yarrington, D., Pennington, C., Gray, J., & Bunnell, H. T. (2005). A system for creating personalized synthetic voices. In [Baltimore.]. *Proceedings of ASSETS*, *2005*, 196–197.

Yin, S.-C., Rose, R., Saz, O., & Lleida, E. (2009). *A Study of Pronunciation Verification in a Speech Therapy Application.* Paper presented at the International Conference on Acoustics, Speech and Signal Processing (ICASSP), Taipei, Taiwan.

Yorkston, K. M., Strand, E. A., & Kennedy, M. R. T. (1996). Comprehensibility of dysarthric speech: Implications for assessment and treatment planning. *American Journal of Speech-Language Pathology*, *5*, 55–66.

Yuker, H. E., & Block, J. R. (1986). *Research with the Attitude Toward Disabled Persons Scales (ATDP): 1960-1985.* Hempstead, NY: Center for the Study of Attitudes Toward Persons with Disabilities, Hofstra University.

Zangari, C., Lloyd, L., & Vicker, B. (1994). Augmentative and alternative communication: An historical perspective. *Augmentative and Alternative Communication*, *10*, 27–59. doi:10.1080/07434619412331276740

Zen, H., Nose, T., Yamagishi, J., Sako, S., & Tokuda, K. (2007a). The HMM-based speech synthesis system (HTS) version 2.0. In *Proceedings of the 6th International Speech Communication Association Speech Synthesis Workshop (SSW6)* (pp. 294–299), Bonn, Germany.

Zen, H., Toda, T., Nakamura, M., & Tokuda, K. (2007b). Details of the Nitech HMM-based speech synthesis system for the Blizzard challenge 2005. *IEICE Transactions on Information and Systems . E (Norwalk, Conn.)*, *90-D*(1), 325–333.

Zen, H., Tokuda, K., & Black, A. W. (2009). Statistical parametric speech synthesis. *Speech Communication*, *51*(11), 1039–1064. doi:10.1016/j.specom.2009.04.004

Zen, H., Tokuda, K., & Kitamura, T. (2007). Reformulating the HMM as a trajectory model by imposing explicit relationships between static and dynamic feature vector sequences. *Computer Speech & Language*, *21*(1), 153–173. doi:10.1016/j.csl.2006.01.002

Zen, H., Tokuda, K., Masuko, T., Kobayashi, T., & Kitamura, T. (2007c). A hidden semi-Markov model-based speech synthesis system. *IEICE Transactions on Information and Systems . E (Norwalk, Conn.)*, *90-D*(5), 825–834.

Zue, V. W., & Glass, J. R. (2000). Conversational Interfaces: Advances and Challenges. *Proceedings of the IEEE*, *88*(8), 1166–1180. doi:10.1109/5.880078

About the Contributors

John Mullennix is a Professor of Psychology at the University of Pittsburgh at Johnstown. He received a B.S. in Psychology from the University of Pittsburgh and a Ph.D. in Psychology from SUNY-Buffalo. His area of research encompasses speech perception, psycholinguistics, and speech technology. He has numerous scholarly publications in the areas of psychology and speech & hearing and has received federal research funding for his work on speech perception. Currently, he is working on research projects related to earwitness testimony and the attitudes toward users of computerized speech technology.

Steven Stern is a Professor of Psychology at the University of Pittsburgh at Johnstown. He received a B.A. in Psychology from Clark University and a Ph.D. in Psychology from Temple University. He is one of a small group of psychologists who study the social psychological implications of technology. He has published several articles on how technologies affect how people view themselves and with each other. As well as examining how people react toward assistive technologies, he is currently studying how cellular telephones alter interpersonal communication and peoples' relationships.

* * *

Pierre Badin is a senior CNRS Research Director at the Speech and Cognition Department, GIPSA-lab, Grenoble. Head of the 'Vocal Tract Acoustics" team from 1990 to 2002, associate director of the Grenoble ICP from 2003 to 2006, he is adjunct to the Department head since 2007. He has worked in the field of speech communication for more than 30 years. He gained international experience through extended research periods in Sweden, Japan and UK, and is involved in a number of national and international projects. He is associate editor for speech at *Acta Acustica*, and reviewer for many international journals. His current interest is speech production and articulatory modelling, with an emphasis on data acquisition, development of virtual talking heads for augmented speech, and speech inversion.

Gérard Bailly is a senior CNRS Research Director at the Speech and Cognition Department, GIPSA-lab, Grenoble. He is now the head of the department. He has worked in the field of speech communication for more than 25 years. He supervised 20 PhD Thesis and authored 32 journal papers and more than 200 book chapters and papers in major international conferences. He coedited "Talking Machines: Theories, Models and Designs" (Elsevier, 1992) and "Improvements in Speech Synthesis" (Wiley, 2002). He is associate editor for the Journal of Acoustics, Speech & Music Processing and reviewer for many international journals. He is a founder member of the ISCA SynSIG and SproSIG special-interest groups. His current interest is multimodal and situated interaction with conversational agents using speech, facial expressions, head movements and eye gaze.

Denis Beautemps is a CNRS Researcher at the Speech and Cognition Department, GIPSA-lab, Grenoble. He has worked in the field of speech communication for more than 10 years. He is now the head of the 'Talking Machine, Communicants agents, Face to Face interaction' team. His current interest is multimodal and supplemented speech, fusion of multi components as it has been the case in the Cued Speech modelling.

H. Timothy Bunnell received his Ph.D. in Experimental Psychology from The Pennsylvania State University in 1983. From 1983 until 1989 he was a Research Scientist at Gallaudet University studying speech enhancement and speech perception by deaf and hard of hearing individuals. Since 1989, Dr Bunnell has directed the Speech Research Laboratory at the duPont Hospital for Children and held research faculty appointments in the Departments of Linguistics and Computer and Information Sciences at the University of Delaware. Currently, Dr. Bunnell is the director of the Nemours Center for Pediatric Auditory and Speech Sciences. His research interests are in speech perception, speech synthesis, speech recognition and the application of speech technologies to the diagnosis and treatment of hearing and speech disorders in children and adults. With his colleague Irene Vogel, he is the Co-Editor of the journal *Language and Speech.*

Jeff Chaffee is a speech-language therapist with the Easter Seals Society of Mahoning, Trumbull, and Columbiana Counties in Youngstown, OH. He received his B.S. in speech-language pathology from Clarion University of Pennsylvania, and his M.S. in speech-language pathology from Indiana University of Pennsylvania. He has practiced in both in- and outpatient settings, working with children and adults, and recently was asked to lead expansion into a long-term acute care hospital for Easter Seals. This chapter is his first publication, and he dedicates it to his wife Kelli and son Sean. Currently, he is pursuing development of an "Augmentative Communication Specialist" position with Easter Seals and is preparing for trials with a new AAC client who may be a candidate for eye gaze technology.

Sarah Creer is a PhD student in the Clinical Applications of Speech Technology (CAST) group at the University of Sheffield, UK, working on personalizing synthetic voices for individuals with progressive speech loss. She received a BA (Hons) degree from the University of York, UK, and an MSc in Speech and Language Processing from the University of Edinburgh, UK. Before starting her PhD, she worked at the University of Reading, UK, on the compilation of the BASE (British Academic Spoken English) corpus.

Stuart Cunningham received a BEng in Software Engineering and PhD in Computer Science from the University of Sheffield. His PhD was concerned with modelling the recognition of filtered speech using missing data techniques, and continued these investigations as a Research Associate at the University of Sheffield. In 2002 he joined the Medical Physics and Clinical Engineering department at Barnsley Hospital to work on the development of speech recognition for people with severe speech impairment. Subsequently he assumed his current position as a lecturer in the Department of Human Communication Sciences at the University of Sheffield. His primary research interests are in clinical applications of speech technology, robust speech recognition, and the perception of speech in adverse conditions. He is currently a co-investigator on two projects funded by the National Institute for Health Research on the development of speech recognition for people with speech impairment.

James Dembowski is an assistant professor at Texas Tech University Health Sciences Center. He received his graduate education at the University of Texas at Dallas, and at the University of Wisconsin – Madison. He is a speech pathologist with a clinical background in augmentative communication, as well as in neurogenic speech-language disorders, stuttering, and voice disorders. His research interests focus on acoustic and articulatory phonetics in both normal and disordered speakers, and the physiology of voice production. His most recent research projects have focused on cross-linguistic acoustic patterns of consonant production in English and Japanese speakers. He is also interested in the application of laboratory technology to clinical practice, particularly the use of acoustic analysis. Currently, he is working on projects which attempt to apply acoustic analysis to the differential diagnosis of motor and language deficits in aphasic speakers.

Kathryn Drager, Ph.D., CCC-SLP, is an Associate Professor in the Department of Communication Sciences and Disorders at the Pennsylvania State University in Pennsylvania, USA. Her research interests include augmentative and alternative communication (AAC) and applications for young children, beginning communicators, and children with autism, listeners' comprehension of speech output, and assessment and intervention for individuals with severe disabilities with challenging behaviors. She is involved in a series of multidisciplinary collaborative research projects designed to enhance language development for beginning communicators who require AAC; enhance the communicative competence of people who require AAC; and improve the design of AAC technologies for individuals with significant speech and motor impairments. Dr. Drager serves as an Associate Editor for *Augmentative and Alternative Communication*. She teaches undergraduate and graduate courses in Augmentative and Alternative Communication, graduate courses in Swallowing Disorders, and undergraduate and graduate courses in Autism.

Frédéric Elisei is a CNRS Research Engineer at the Speech and Cognition Department, GIPSA-lab, Grenoble. He is responsible for the development and exploitation of the MICAL experimentation platform, designed to study multimodal face-to-face speech communication. He works on audiovisual speech i.e. modelling and synthesis of 3D talking heads, addressing several speakers and target languages. His current interest is multimodal and situated interaction with conversational agents, in particular giving agents adaptive skills such as varying speech styles (whisper, hyper-articulation...), displaying various facial expressions or adapting the language or the phonological repertoire to the human interlocutor.

Ashley Davis Fortier completed her B.S. in psychology from the University of Pittsburgh at Johnstown in 2005. Currently, she works in Maryland for the Medicaid Older Adult Waiver and Money Follows the Person Initiative.

Phil Green founded the Speech and Hearing group at the University of Sheffield in 1985. He has around 80 publications in topics ranging from Automatic Speech Recognition to Auditory Scene Analysis and Speech Perception and has coordinated a number of major research grants in these areas. Besides clinical applications of speech technology he is currently researching robust recognition techniques based on sound source separation.

Jeff Higginbotham, Ph.D is a Professor and Director of the Communication and Assistive Device Laboratory in the Department of Communicative Disorders and Sciences and State University of New

York at Buffalo. At UB, Dr. Higginbotham teaches courses in AAC and research design. A partner in the RERC on Communication Enhancement, Dr. Higginbotham's research focuses interactions in real-time and how AAC technologies can be designed to improve conversational performance. He has received federal research funding for his work in augmentative communication and assistive technology. Dr. Higginbotham also consults with industry on the design and development of augmentative communication devices.

Rajinder Koul earned his doctorate in speech-language pathology at the Purdue University. He is a speech-language pathologist, having received his undergraduate and master's degree in speech and hearing sciences in India. He is now professor and Chairperson in the Department in the Department of Speech, Language, and Hearing Sciences at the Texas Tech University Health Sciences Center-Lubbock. He also serves as the Associate dean (Research) for the School of Allied Health Sciences. Dr. Koul received 2001 Mary E. Switzer Distinguished Fellowship from the National Institute on Disability and Rehabilitation Research. In 2005, he was named a Fellow of the American Speech-Language –Hearing Association. Dr. Koul is the author of research publications and book chapters concerning augmentative and alternative communication (AAC) and developmental and acquired communication impairments. His research work has focused on understanding the factors that influence perception of synthetic speech in persons with developmental disabilities and on evaluating the efficacy of AAC intervention in persons with aphasia.

Giulio E. Lancioni received his Ph.D. in Child Development and Psychology from the University of Kansas. He is Professor at the Department of Psychology, University of Bari, Italy. Prior to this position, he spent many years at the Department of Psychology, University of Leiden, The Netherlands. His research interests include development and assessment of assistive technologies, training of social and occupational skills, and evaluation of strategies for examining preference and teaching choice in individuals with severe/profound and multiple disabilities. He has published widely in these areas and serves in the editorial board of several international journals concerned with these topics.

Pearl Langan works as a speech and language therapist with a specialist service for children and adolescents with mental health difficulties. She graduated with an honors BSc from Trinity College Dublin, where her dissertation focused on comparisons of aided communication systems from 'insider' and 'outsider' perspectives. She continues to maintain her interest in research in speech and language therapy, particularly as it relates to the development of language and communication skills.

Eduardo Lleida is a Professor of the Department of Electronical Engineering and Communications at the University of Zaragoza in Zaragoza, Spain. He received a B.Sc. and Ph.D. in Telecommunication Engineering from the Polytechnic University of Catalonia in Barcelona, Spain. His area of research covers all elements related to the acoustics, from noise and echo cancellation in automotive environments to acoustic modeling in advanced speech recognition or speaker verification systems. His research has led to many publications in international conferences and journals in the field of speech technologies.

Janice Murray is head of speech pathology and therapy at Manchester Metropolitan University, UK. Her first degree was in speech and language therapy and her Doctorate explored language development in children with cerebral palsy and limited speech intelligibility. She has developed a centre of excellence focusing on the research, education and service users needs in the field of augmentative and alternative communication (AAC). Her research interests include atypical language development, memory and its impact on aided language use, and personal histories of adults who use AAC. She has published in these areas. The educational and professional development of speech and language therapy students remains a keen focus of her work and she is particularly interested in the development of inter-professional learning opportunities for health and educational professionals.

Mark F. O'Reilly received his Ph.D. in Special Education from the University of Illinois at Urbana-Champaign in 1992. He is Professor of Special Education and the Mollie Villeret Davis Endowed Professor in Learning Disabilities at the University of Texas at Austin. His research focuses on the assessment and treatment of challenging behavior, communication and social skills interventions, and assistive technology with individuals with low incidence disabilities.

Christopher A. Pennington has over 20 years of research and software development experience in augmentative communication, computational linguistics and assistive technology. Formerly research staff at the University of Delaware, he is now a project coordinator and research developer at AgoraNet, Inc., a small company in Newark, Delaware that specializes in custom software and web development. Chris is currently coordinating the AgoraNet team that is commercializing the ModelTalker speech system software. He has also recently worked with projects investigating word prediction and customizing graphics for language representation.

Diana Petroi is a speech-language pathologist and a doctoral student in communication sciences and disorders at Texas Tech University Health Sciences Center. She is interested in neurologically based communication disorders.

Joe E. Reichle is a Professor in the Department of Speech-Language-Hearing Sciences and the Department of Educational Psychology at the University of Minnesota, USA. Currently he is Co-PI on a subcontract for an IES clinical trial examining the efficacy comprehensive curricula for preschoolers with ASD. Dr. Reichle has published over 55 articles in the area of augmentative and alternative communication and challenging behavior in rigorous refereed journals. He has been Associate Editor for the *Journal of Speech Language and Hearing Research* and *Augmentative and Alternative Communication.* His current research focuses on examining parameters of intervention intensity and procedural fidelity in translating experimental research into educational applications for preschoolers with autism spectrum disorders. Dr. Reichle directs the Autism Certificate Program at the University of Minnesota and is Co-PI of the Minnesota LEND interdisciplinary Leadership Training Grant in Neurodevelopmental Disorders. He is a Fellow of the American Speech Language and Hearing Association.

Victoria Rodriguez is a teaching member of Spanish as a foreign language in the Romance Language Department at the Vienna International School in Vienna, Austria. She has long term experience in teaching Spanish as a second language to secondary students in a multilingual environment. Her professional interest focuses in the development and testing of new pedagogical and multimedia tools to improve the oral skills of students learning one or more foreign languages.

W.-Ricardo Rodríguez is an assistant researcher at the University of Zaragoza in Zaragoza, Spain. He received a B.Sc. in Biomedical Engineering from the Corporación Universitaria de Ciencia y Desarrollo and the Universidad Distrital Francisco José de Caldas in Bogotá (Colombia) and a M.Sc. in Biomedical Engineering by the University of Zaragoza. His area of research gathers the study of acoustic and articulatory features in young children' speech for the development of speech therapy tools.

Debbie Rowe is a doctoral candidate in Rensselaer Polytechnic Institute's Communication and Rhetoric program. As both a Humanities, Arts, and Social Sciences Fellow and a Joanne Wagner Memorial Fellow at the university, she has pursued research in the application of text-to-speech technology to the field of composition, specifically to the practices of editing, and proofreading. She is currently wrapping up her dissertation research, documenting how experienced writers use reading aloud to themselves as a mode of revision, and what role text-to-speech technology can play during that process. As a former Information Technology manager in the non-profit sector, she applies her knowledge of technology, written composition, and communication in classrooms and volunteer venues in New York and South Korea.

Oscar Saz is an assistant researcher at the University of Zaragoza in Zaragoza, Spain. He received a B.Sc. and M.Sc. in Telecommunications Engineering from the University of Zaragoza. His area of research gathers the personalization of speech technology-based systems like Automatic Speech Recognition and speech assessment to speech variants like disordered or non-native speech. He is also interested in the application of this knowledge to the development of speech-based tools for the handicapped.

Ralf W. Schlosser received his Ph.D. in Special Education from Purdue University in 1994. He has held Research Director/Clinical positions at the Oklahoma Assistive Technology Center in Oklahoma City and Bloorview MacMillan Centre in Toronto. His current appointment is Professor in and Chair of the Department of Speech-Language Pathology and Audiology at Northeastern University in Boston, U.S.A. He also has a joint appointment in the School Psychology Program of the Department of Counseling and Applied Educational Psychology at Northeastern and serves as Director of Clinical Research at the Communication Enhancement Center of Children's Hospital Boston at Waltham. He teaches in the areas of research methods, evidence-based practice and augmentative and alternative communication (AAC). His research focuses on AAC intervention for children with developmental disabilities in general and autism in particular. He serves on several editorial boards and is co-editor-in-chief of *Evidence-based Communication Assessment and Intervention.*

Jeff Sigafoos received his Ph.D. in Educational Psychology from The University of Minnesota in 1990. He has held academic appointments at The University of Queensland, University of Sydney, and the University of Texas at Austin. His current appointment is Professor in the School of Educational Psychology and Pedagogy at Victoria University of Wellington, New Zealand. He teaches in the areas of educational psychology and developmental disabilities. His research focuses on communication intervention for individuals with developmental and physical disabilities. He has co-authored numerous intervention studies related to teaching individuals with developmental disabilities. He serves on several editorial boards and is co-editor-in-chief of *Evidence-based Communication Assessment and Intervention* and editor of *Developmental Neurorehabilitation.*

Martine Smith is Senior Lecturer in Speech Language Pathology in Trinity College Dublin. She has worked clinically as a speech and language therapist with children and adults with a range of communication difficulties, including severe speech and physical impairments. Her research interests and publications are primarily in the areas of language acquisition in exceptional circumstances, the impact of augmentative and alternative communication on language acquisition and social functioning across the lifespan, and links between spoken and written language. She is a Past President of the International Society for Augmentative and Alternative Communication (ISAAC) and has a particular interest in multidisciplinary research and intervention.

Elizabeth Steinhauser completed her B.S. in psychology from the University of Pittsburgh at Johnstown in 2006. In 2008, Elizabeth completed her M.S. in Industrial/Organizational Psychology from the Florida Institute of Technology. Currently, she is pursuing her doctorate degree in Industrial/ Organizational Psychology from Florida Institute of Technology and working as a contractor at the Defense Equal Opportunity Management Institute. Her current research interests include employment law and affective experiences in the workplace.

Dean Sutherland, Ph.D., is a Lecturer in the Health Science Centre at the University of Canterbury, Christchurch, New Zealand. He teaches AAC, child development, and early intervention. Dr. Sutherland received his PhD in speech-language therapy from the University of Canterbury in 2006. His research interests include AAC intervention for children and adults with complex communication needs and phonological development in young children with severe speech impairments. He is also interested in the role of families in early intervention for children who experience developmental disabilities. Dr. Sutherland is an executive board member of the New Zealand Speech-language Therapists Association.

Carlos Vaquero is a teaching assistant at the University of Zaragoza in Zaragoza, Spain. He received a B.Sc. and M.Sc. in Telecommunications Engineering from the University of Zaragoza in Zaragoza, Spain. His area of research has covered the development of speech therapy tools for the handicapped and now is oriented to the study of the acoustic part in speaker verification and speaker recognition systems.

Horabail Venkatagiri is an associate professor of Psychology and Communication Disorders at Iowa State University. His research interests include stuttering, speech technology, augmentative and alternative communication, and computer applications in Communication Disorders. He is an associate editor of the Journal of Augmentative and Alternative Communication. His research has been published the Journal of Augmentative and Alternative Communication, Journal of Fluency Disorders, Journal of Communication Disorders, American Journal of Speech-Language Pathology, Journal of Speech, Language, and Hearing Research, International Journal of Speech Technology, and the Journal of the Acoustical Society of America.

Stephen von Tetzchner is professor of developmental psychology at the Department of Psychology, University of Oslo, Norway. He has worked both academically and clinically with children having a range of disabilities, including children with motor impairment, intellectual impairment, deafness, blindness, Rett syndrome, Tourette syndrome, autism and Asperger syndrome. His research includes issues related to typical and atypical development in general, and communication and language development in particular, including the development of children who fail to acquire spoken language in the normal manner and may need intervention with an on-speech communication form. He has addressed communication and language from a developmental perspective, with a focus on understanding the transactional processes that govern typical and atypical development. He has published textbooks on developmental psychology, signed and spoken language development, augmentative and alternative communication, habilitation, challenging behavior and Asperser syndrome.

Junichi Yamagishi received the B.E. degree in computer science, M.E. and Ph.D. degrees in information processing from Tokyo Institute of Technology, Tokyo, Japan. He pioneered the use of speaker adaptation techniques in HMM-based speech synthesis in his doctoral dissertation 'Average-voice-based speech synthesis', which won the Tejima Doctoral Dissertation Award 2007. He held a research fellowship from the Japan Society for the Promotion of Science (JSPS) 2004-2007. He was an intern researcher at ATR spoken language communication Research Laboratories (ATR-SLC) 2003-2006. He was a visiting researcher at the Centre for Speech Technology Research (CSTR), University of Edinburgh, U.K., 2006-2007, where he is currently a senior research fellow, continuing research on speaker adaptation for HMM-based speech synthesis in an EC FP7 collaborative project: EMIME (www.emime.org). His research interests include speech synthesis, speech analysis and speech recognition. He is a member of IEEE, ISCA, IEICE, and ASJ.

Index

D

E

F

G

H

Q

R

S